Emergency Medicine

AN ILLUSTRATED COLOUR TEXT

For Elsevier
Commissioning Editor: Laurence Hunter
Development Editor: Lulu Stader
Project Manager: Emma Riley/Frances Affleck
Designer: Kirsteen Wright
Illustration Manager: Gillian Richards
Illustrator: Graeme Chambers

Emergency Medicine

AN ILLUSTRATED COLOUR TEXT

Edited by

Paul Atkinson BSc(Hons) MB BCh BAO MRCP FCEM
Consultant in Emergency Medicine, Addenbrooke's Hospital, Cambridge;
Associate Lecturer, University of Cambridge, UK

Richard Kendall BSc(Hons) MBBS FCEM
Consultant in Emergency Medicine, Addenbrooke's Hospital, Cambridge;
Associate Lecturer, University of Cambridge, UK

Lee Van Rensburg MBBCh FRCS(Orth)
Consultant in Trauma and Orthopaedics, Addenbrooke's Hospital,
Cambridge, UK

Section Editor

Duncan McAuley MBBChir MA FRCS(Ed) MRCP FCEM DipIMC
Consultant in Emergency Medicine, Addenbrooke's Hospital, Cambridge, UK

Foreword by

Jerome R. Hoffman MA MD
Professor of Medicine/Emergency Medicine, UCLA School of Medicine;
Attending Physician, UCLA Emergency Medicine Center;
Director, The Doctoring Program, UCLA School of Medicine, Los Angeles, USA

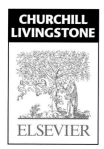

CHURCHILL LIVINGSTONE

ELSEVIER

EDINBURGH   LONDON   NEW YORK   OXFORD   PHILADELPHIA   ST LOUIS   SYDNEY   TORONTO   2010

CHURCHILL
LIVINGSTONE
ELSEVIER

First published 2010 © Elsevier Limited. All rights reserved.

ISBN 9780443069628
  Reprinted 2010

British Library Cataloguing in Publication Data
A catalogue record for this book is available from the British Library

Library of Congress Cataloging in Publication Data
A catalog record for this book is available from the Library of Congress

Notice
Knowledge and best practice in this field are constantly changing.
As new research and experience broaden our knowledge,
changes in practice, treatment and drug therapy may become
necessary or appropriate. Readers are advised to check the most
current information provided (i) on procedures featured or (ii)
by the manufacturer of each product to be administered, to
verify the recommended dose or formula, the method and
duration of administration, and contraindications. It is the
responsibility of the practitioner, relying on their own experience
and knowledge of the patient, to make diagnoses, to determine
dosages and the best treatment for each individual patient, and
to take all appropriate safety precautions. To the fullest extent of
the law, neither the Publisher nor the Editors assume any
liability for any injury and/or damage to persons or property
arising out of or related to any use of the material contained in
this book.

The Publisher

The
publisher's
policy is to use
**paper manufactured
from sustainable forests**

Printed in China

Foreword

In medicine's version of geologic time, Emergency Medicine is still an infant. That's true even in North America, where although well established as both a clinical and academic discipline, it remains one of the very youngest specialties. For a generation of practitioners, however, it has been around for most of our career – and thus it is exciting for me to watch as it develops and matures in many parts of the world. The publication of a new text in EM always represents a further step in that process – particularly when it represents the work of a group as talented and committed as the editors of 'Emergency Medicine – An Illustrated Colour Text' – whom I was fortunate enough to get to know, and work with, during my year-long sabbatical at Cambridge University.

To some of us, EM is both the most exciting and the most challenging of specialties. To understand why I believe this – and why I think those of you to whom this book is directed, early on in your medical career, may come to agree with me – we need to explore a little where EM came from, and how its derivation was different from that of other medical specialties.

When the first neurologists decided to concentrate on diseases of the nervous system, it was surely because there was a particular *body of knowledge* that was becoming more and more complex, and demanded the full attention of those who wished to become expert. The same was true for cardiologists, or gynaecologists, or radiation oncologists, etc. But that *wasn't* the case for EM. Don't misunderstand – this is not because EM doesn't have a special body of knowledge – as even a glance at this book will demonstrate. Expertise in resuscitation, and diagnostic decision-making, and trauma care, and pre-hospital systems, and medical toxicology are a few of the areas that immediately jump to mind. EM *shares* some aspect of these with other specialties, but the same is generally true of every specialty.

Surgical specialties tend to be a little different. Training in neurosurgery is a great deal longer than training in neurology, and in cardiac surgery a lot longer than in cardiology. This is *not* because their body of knowledge is larger – if anything, the opposite is likely to be true. It's because surgical training is about acquiring *skills* (rather than simply *knowledge*). The same is fundamentally true, I believe, about EM – it is a set of *skills* that makes one a specialist in EM (as we will address shortly). Even so, EM didn't arise because a group of us decided to concentrate on the special skills it requires; EM was born because patients demanded it. The discovery of penicillin made it clear that *acute treatment* of infectious disease was possible, and important; wartime advances in surgery did the same for trauma (spawning the UK notion of 'casualty' and 'accident and emergency'). Patients soon understood that *many* symptoms would benefit from acute attention, and that they didn't need to suffer while waiting for a delayed visit to a doctor. This was true not only for a host of life threatening conditions – acute MI, hyperkalaemia, overdose, dehydration in an infant, or 3rd-degree heart block, etc but also for less serious, but nevertheless *treatable* conditions; there was no reason to suffer without medical attention from a ureteric stone, or a moderate asthma attack, or even a headache or sore throat. This patient-centered realization had added force in a society like the US, which both had a faltering primary care safety net at the time that EM began to develop, and a population less likely to share the capacity for patience and forbearance famous on the other side of the Atlantic.

So EM arose, de facto, from patient demand. But as more and more, and sicker and sicker, patients began to show up, it became eminently clear that ministering to their needs was no simple matter, and couldn't be left in the hands of those without training, or appropriate skills. Patients created the need for EDs; EDs created the need for the *specialty* of EM.

While procedural skills have a role in EM (and sometimes seem its most exciting aspect, to beginners), it is quintessentially a diagnostic specialty that is relatively unique in that *undifferentiated* disease presentation is a core feature. That's why the book you're holding is organized around *symptoms* and *findings* – unlike standard textbooks in almost every other medical specialty, which are organized around *disease entities*. Imagine if patients came to the ED with a complaint of 'I'm having a pulmonary embolism' or 'I need care for my acute heart failure' or 'it's an exacerbation of COPD,' or 'this time it's pneumonia' – instead of 'I can't breathe' which could be any one, or two, or *all* of the above, among many other things; that would make EM a whole lot easier … and a whole lot less interesting!

The *skills* needed by an EM specialist also involve appropriate decision-making in the face of a number of rather extraordinary stresses. An emergency physician (EP) not only has to establish priorities rapidly in any given patient, he has to do the same *among* a large group of patients, where in a busy ED several may have an obvious need for emergency intervention, but the same is *possible* in many others, even if far less apparent. The EP also doesn't have the luxury of taking a history, and doing an exam, and reviewing the records, and ordering labs, etc, in the orderly fashion we learn about in medical school; she has to *act* entirely out of order, based on brief interactions, and rapid assessment, without time to gather much of the information that could be helpful. As if that weren't complicated enough, she's got to do this with a patient she's never met before, and who may be not be at his best – frightened, or in pain, or demanding, or altered, or intoxicated, or all of the above. The patient's never met you before either, so there's a level of trust that has to be earned. And you may not be at your very best (every shift), either. And finally, choices have to be made, and acted upon, while other (potentially unstable) patients wait.

In the midst of such turmoil, perhaps the most important trait of an expert EP is the ability to remain calm. Not because you don't find it *exciting* but because staying levelheaded is absolutely essential if you want to make good decisions. EM is not for everyone; if you're not comfortable with uncertainty, or capable of calm amidst controlled chaos, you will never be a good fit for EM. But being born with the right temperament – while necessary – is not sufficient; this is also a *skill* that takes time and experience to develop. (Don't be discouraged; if you thrive on trying to spin several plates at once, *and* you are helped to learn, in a safe environment where patients will not be harmed ... *and* are patient with yourself ... it will happen.)

If it is ironic that personal serenity is an essential element of expert emergency care, it will seem equally so that another key skill is the ability to use *time* in your favor ... to *do nothing* – 'don't just do something, stand there!' This isn't the case for every ED patient, of course, but for a great many of them it is essential to understand that you indeed have time and to allow that time to provide the answer to key questions ('Is this early appendicitis?' or 'Can I send this patient home without a CT scan, as long as there is good follow-up?' or 'Will pain relief be adequate as the only treatment in this case?' etc).

Many people are attracted to EM because of the very sick patients – the so-called 'true emergencies.' But only a small minority of our patients are acutely unstable, and in fact it is the *other* patients who can be the most challenging. It's relatively easy to take care of a crashing patient with a stab wound to the abdomen; it can be very hard to pick the epidural abscess needle out of the low back pain haystack. Furthermore, sending a patient away from medical care – which we do with the large majority of 'minor' ED patients – can be the toughest decision one ever has to make in medicine.

Which is why another skill you will need to learn is the EM *approach* to differential diagnosis. This is addressed in the Introduction to Emergency Medicine chapter.

A specialist in EM is someone who's learned these skills well, as they relate to the entire broad set of problems seen in a typical ED. This may seem daunting at first – but we develop expertise in anything through a combination of *training* and *experience*. I expect my residents in EM to be as skilled as anyone in medicine at dealing with the emergency airway – because over time they have lots of training, and lots of experience, with just that issue. Same for head trauma (minor as well as severe), and the diagnosis of abdominal pain, and undifferentiated 'dizziness,' and ... all the things we do (and learn, and teach) every day. (They can't be great at *everything* – which is why in EM we can't take out the inflamed appendix we just diagnosed, or fix a blocked V-P shunt, or take care of chronic renal disease, or ...)

This book cannot substitute for the training, or the experience, that are essential to developing the skills of a specialist; no book can, of course. Still, no amount of training and experience is enough, without being based on a framework of knowledge. It is precisely such a framework that every good text should endeavour to provide. Knowing everything in this book (if that were even possible) wouldn't make you a specialist in EM ... but becoming familiar with what it has to teach you can help you think about and organize the experiences you have in the ED – and that is certainly a worthwhile place to start!

Jerome R Hoffman
Los Angeles
2010

Preface

Emergency Medicine: An Illustrated Colour Text is a readily accessible, up-to-date resource that we hope those beginning on their journey into the exciting new specialty of emergency medicine will find useful. Medical students and newly-graduated doctors will have knowledge and experience of the core specialties that look after patients. They may not, however, have an approach to, or experience of, the undifferentiated patient who approaches the nurse, paramedic or doctor with a problem. Yes, a problem; not a diagnosis or a disease. This book aims to take a look at medicine from the front door of the hospital and as such we have tried to make this book as symptom-based as possible.

The first section introduces the purpose of emergency medicine and outlines the way to approach an emergency patient. This is followed by a section on resuscitation – the core skill of the emergency practitioner. We then look at the principal investigations commonly used in the emergency department. The remainder of the book is divided into sections representing problems and disease categorized both by type of injury or illness and by regions of the body. In common with other titles in the series, each of these sections is subdivided into single or double page spreads looking at particular presenting problems. Each topic has a box highlighting key points and also,

where relevant, points specific to children. There is a separate paediatric section outlining common and important paediatric emergencies. Finally we look at violence and social problems, all too common but often overlooked topics.

We hope that this text will help to introduce this exciting specialty to a new generation of medical students and junior doctors and enable them to be better equipped at dealing with all manner of emergency presentations.

PA, RK, LVR, DM

The only true wisdom is in knowing you know nothing
Socrates

Acknowledgements

We are grateful to all of our friends, colleagues and family members who have helped and encouraged us during the writing and preparation of this book. In particular we would like to thank those in the Emergency Department and Medical Photography Department at Addenbrooke's Hospital for their patience and cooperation during the taking and re-taking of the many photographs (Fig. 1, p. 2; Fig. 1, p. 4; Fig. 4, p. 5; Fig. 1, p. 6; Fig. 2, p. 9; Fig. 1, p. 35; Fig. 1, p. 36; Figs 2 and 3, p. 36; Fig. 3, p. 38; Figs 1 and 2, p. 40; Fig. 1, p. 42; Fig. 3, p. 43; Fig. 2b, p. 50; Fig. 1, p. 52; Figs 3 and 4, p. 55; Fig. 4, p. 85; Fig. 1, p. 110; Fig. 2, p. 161; Fig. 1, p. 168).

Photos in the 'Plant and animal toxins' section (pp. 112–113) are by Elke Rohn (Fig. 1), Stefanie Leuker (Fig. 2), José Antonio de Assis (Fig. 3), Andrew Lee (Fig. 4) and Jeffrey Collingwood (Fig. 5). Photos in the 'Electrical and water induced injury' section (pp. 116–117) are by James Stratton (Fig. 1) and Benjamin Earwicker (Fig. 3).

We are grateful for permission from Elsevier to reproduce figures and tables from other titles in the 'Illustrated Colour Text' series as follows: Fig. 2 (p. 3), Figs 1 and 2 (p. 16&17), Fig. 2 (p. 31), Fig. 2 (p. 33), Fig. 4 (p. 39), Fig. 3 (p. 127) from M Avidan et al (2003) *Perioperative Care, Anaesthesia, Pain Management and Intensive Care*; Fig. 2 (p. 19), Fig. 1 (p. 64), Fig. 2 (p. 67), Fig. 2 (p. 142), Fig. 2 (p. 165) from D E Newby and N Grubb (2005) *Cardiology*; Figs 2, 3 and 4 (p. 57), Figs 3, 4 and 5 (p. 151&152), Fig. 1 (p. 154) from R S Dhillon and C A East (2006) *Ear, Nose and Throat and Head and Neck Surgery*, 3rd edn; Fig. 1 (p. 73), Figs 1 and 3 (p. 94&95), Table 1 (p. 100), Fig. 1 (p. 102), Table 1 (p. 102) from G Fuller and M Manford (2005) *Neurology*, 2nd edn; Fig. 2 (p. 78), Figs 3 and 4 (p. 133), Fig. 1 (p. 142) from P D Welsby (2002) *Clinical History Taking and Examination*, 2nd edn; Fig. 3 (p. 79), Fig. 2 (p. 80) from G P Butcher (2003) *Gastroenterology*; Fig. 3 (p. 81), Fig. 3 (p. 83), Figs 1 and 2 (p. 88&89) from P Renton (2004) *Medical Imaging*; Fig. 2 (p. 85), Figs 1, 2, 3 and 4 (p. 90&91), Fig. 1 (p. 124), Figs 1, 2, 3 and 4 (p. 126&127) from N Bullock et al (2008) *Urology*; Fig. 1 (p. 118), Figs 3 and 4 (p. 119), Fig. 1 (p. 122) from R McRae and A W G Kinninmonth (1997) *Orthopaedics and Trauma*; Fig 1 (p. 130) and Figs 1 and 2 (p. 132) from D J Gawkrodger (2008) *Dermatology*, 4th edn; Fig. 2 (p. 137), Figs 2, 3 and 4 (p. 142&143), Figs 1 and 3 (p. 144&145) from M Batterbury and B Bowling (2005) *Ophthalmology*, 2nd edn; Fig. 1 (p. 139) from M R Howard and P J Hamilton (2008) *Haematology*, 3rd edn; Figs 1 and 2 (p. 146&147) from J Pitkin et al (2003) *Obstetrics and Gynaecology*.

Fig. 2 (p. 11) is reproduced courtesy of GlideScope®. Fig. 2 (p. 13), Fig. 2 (p. 131) and Fig. 1 (p. 166) are reproduced courtesy of the Resuscitation Council UK. Fig. 2 (p. 62) is reproduced from W Köstler, P C Strohm and N P Südkamp (2004) Acute compartment syndrome of the limb. *Injury* 35(12): 1221–1227 (Fig. 2), with permission from Elsevier. Fig. 2 (p. 111) is reproduced courtesy of the Health Protection Agency (June 2008) and Fig. 2 (p. 155) is reproduced with kind permission of the Meningitis Society.

We could not have completed this text without the patience of our families, especially our wives – thank you Julie, Katie, Gemma and Sharon-Anne.

Cover Image: GlideScope® Video Laryngoscope, with kind permission of Verathon Ltd.

PA, RK, LVR, DM

Contributing authors

Oshaani Abeyakoon BSc(Hons) MBBS
Clinical Fellow in Emergency Medicine,
  Addenbrooke's Hospital, Cambridge,
  UK

Vazeer Ahmed BM MRCP FCEM
Consultant in Emergency Medicine,
  Addenbrooke's Hospital, Cambridge,
  UK

Paul Atkinson BSc(Hons)
MB BCh BAO MRCP FCEM
Consultant in Emergency Medicine,
  Addenbrooke's Hospital, Cambridge,
  UK

Jonathan Baird BSc(Hons) MBChB
MRCS(Ed) MCEM
Specialty Registrar in Emergency
  Medicine, Addenbrooke's Hospital,
  Cambridge, UK

Berto Bauza-Rodriguez MD MRCS
Specialist Registrar in Emergency
  Medicine, Addenbrooke's Hospital,
  Cambridge, UK

Adrian Boyle BM MRCP FCEM
MPhil MD
Consultant in Emergency Medicine,
  Addenbrooke's Hospital, Cambridge,
  UK

Catherine Hayhurst BMBCh
MA(Cantab) MRCP DTM&H
Specialist Registrar in Emergency
  Medicine, Addenbrooke's Hospital,
  Cambridge, UK

Peter Heinz State Exam Med MD
MRCP(UK) MRCPCH
Consultant in Acute Paediatrics and
  Paediatric Emergency Medicine,
  Addenbrooke's Hospital, Cambridge,
  UK

Jerome R. Hoffman MA MD
Professor of Emergency Medicine and
  Internal Medicine, University of
  California, Los Angeles, USA

Mike Iacovou MBBS MRCS
Specialist Registrar in Emergency
  Medicine, Addenbrooke's Hospital,
  Cambridge, UK

Wayne Kark MBBS MCEM
Specialty Registrar in Emergency
  Medicine, Addenbrooke's Hospital,
  Cambridge, UK

Richard Kendall BSc(Hons) MBBS
FCEM
Consultant in Emergency Medicine,
  Addenbrooke's Hospital, Cambridge,
  UK

David Lewis MBBS FRCS FCEM
Consultant in Emergency
  Medicine, Ipswich Hospital,
  London, UK

Simon Lewis BSc(Hons) MBBS
MCEM DIMC RCSEd
Specialist Registrar in Emergency
  Medicine, Addenbrooke's Hospital,
  Cambridge, UK

Duncan McAuley MBBChir MA
FRCS(Ed) MRCP FCEM DipIMC
Consultant in Emergency Medicine,
  Addenbrooke's Hospital, Cambridge,
  UK

Sharon-Anne McAuley MB BCh
BAO MSc MRCP MRCPCH
Specialist Registrar in Paediatrics,
  Addenbrooke's Hospital, Cambridge,
  UK

Sarah MacFarlane MB BCh BAO
MRCS(Ed)
Clinical Fellow in Emergency Medicine,
  Addenbrooke's Hospital, Cambridge,
  UK

Russell E. McLaughlin MB BCh
BAO FRCSI FCEM MMedSci
Clinical Director in Emergency
  Medicine, Royal Victoria Hospital,
  Belfast Trust, Belfast, UK

Chris Maimaris MBChB FRCS FCEM
Consultant in Emergency Medicine,
  Addenbrooke's Hospital, Cambridge,
  UK

Rhys Roberts MBBChir BA(Hons)
MA MRCP PhD
Research Fellow in Neurology,
  Addenbrooke's Hospital, Cambridge,
  UK

Susan Robinson BM FRCP FRCS(Ed)
FCEM
Consultant in Emergency Medicine,
  Addenbrooke's Hospital, Cambridge,
  UK

Steffen Schickerling MRCS(A&E)
DRCOG DCH DTM&H(Liverpool)
Specialist Registrar in Emergency
  Medicine, Addenbrooke's Hospital,
  Cambridge, UK

Daniel Stanciu DM MRCS(Ed)
Specialist Registrar in Emergency
  Medicine, Addenbrooke's Hospital,
  Cambridge, UK

John Sutherland MBChB
FRCS(A&E) FCEM
Consultant in Emergency Medicine,
  Redland Hospital, Queensland,
  Australia

Catriona Thompson BM
MRCS(Eng) FCEM
Consultant in Emergency Medicine,
  Peterborough District Hospital,
  UK

Lee Van Rensburg MBBCh
FRCS(Orth)
Consultant in Trauma and
  Orthopaedics, Addenbrooke's
  Hospital, Cambridge, UK

Dhakshinamoorthy Vijayasankar
MBBS, MRCS(A&E) FCEM
Consultant in Emergency Medicine,
  Peterborough District Hospital, UK

Contents

Introduction to emergency medicine

The fact that your patient gets well does not prove that your diagnosis was correct

Samuel J. Meltzer

Introduction to emergency medicine

Overview and history

Emergency medicine, one of the youngest specialties, has grown to become a challenging and increasingly popular career choice. It is the specialty defined by its patients rather than by any physician-derived classification system. It challenges the traditional medical model of maximizing knowledge of ever decreasing areas of the disease spectrum and in doing so challenges its practitioners to safely and expertly provide care for the broadest possible spectrum of disease.

Emergency care is an essential part of any healthcare system and as such must be available 24 hours per day. The number of patients presenting to emergency departments (Fig. 1) in the developed world has been increasing significantly over recent years and departments have had to develop strategies to deal with overcrowding, difficulties with admitting patients into hospital beds and changes in workforce such as decreased doctors' hours of work.

Although emergency medicine has been practised for decades, if not centuries, it has taken until the later third of the twentieth century for the specialty to establish itself independently. The Casualty Surgeons Association was formed in London in 1967. In 1972 the UK Department of Health funded thirty consultant posts creating a new specialty, *accident and emergency medicine*. In 1979, emergency medicine became the twenty-third recognized medical specialty in the USA, and was recognized as a medical specialty in Australia in 1993 and in New Zealand in 1995. In 2004, the name *emergency medicine* became official in the UK.

Emergency medicine:

'To evaluate, manage, treat and prevent unexpected illness and injury.' Society of Academic Emergency Medicine

The challenges faced in the emergency care system include:

- availability at any time for any complaint
- unfamiliarity of patients
- a wide spectrum of presentations
  - simple to complex problems
  - neonates to the very elderly
  - patients and relatives
- a need to be able to act on limited information and lack of patient records
- expertise in trauma management
- time pressures and unpredictable numbers of patients
- differentiating trivia from subtle symptoms of serious disease.

The approach to the emergency patient

All these challenges, not least the lack of prior knowledge of the patient, mean that each patient's problem requires careful attention, thoughtful enquiry and honest informed opinion.

When dealing with the patient who is actually or potentially critically ill or injured, an approach that differs from the traditional model is required. To take a full history, perform a full examination, and order and review appropriate tests in a patient who may require immediate intervention and treatment, may threaten their very survival. Irrespective of the nature of the clinical emergency, maintenance of adequate oxygenation and ventilation, adequate blood pressure and adequate blood flow to vital organs are important guiding principles. The approach adopted by the various life-support courses is the one used instinctively by emergency teams (Fig. 2) for all patients:

- The primary survey (ABCDE)
  - Airway (with cervical spine control in trauma)
- Breathing and oxygenation
- Circulation (with haemorrhage control)
- Disability (neurology)
- Exposure and environment
- Resuscitation and treatment of life threats
- Secondary survey – history and examination
- Emergency treatment and investigations
- Disposition and definitive care.

This approach ensures that the most immediately life-threatening problems are recognized and treated in the order of their likely impact.

Treat first what kills first.

The ability to be able to treat recognized problems, even without a diagnosis, is key to the practice of emergency medicine. The mark of an emergency physician is the ability to manage the airway (intubate, provide a surgical airway), to manage the breathing of a patient (perform emergency respiratory interventions: ventilation, chest decompression) and to be able to provide cardiovascular support (such as Advanced Life Support).

The 'Emergency Medicine (EM) approach' to differential diagnosis

This is often phrased in terms of 'worst first' – in the emergency department, acute coronary syndrome (ACS) is at the top of the differential of chest pain, and common things like costochondritis almost nowhere to be

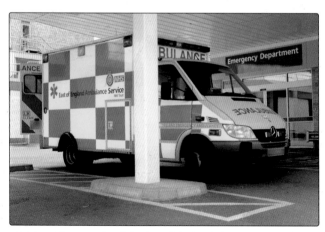

Fig. 1 **The emergency department** – front door of the hospital.

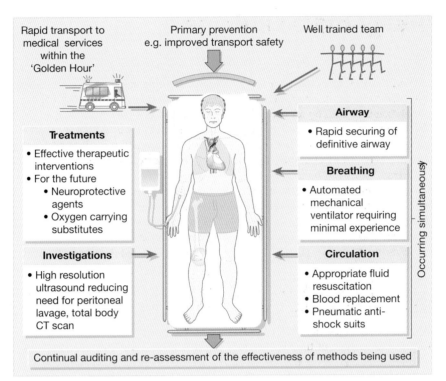

Fig. 2 **Modern resuscitation.**

found. But that's not nearly all of it; we also emphasize disease that is at least reasonably *likely* (which is why Boerhaave's Syndrome is rarely part of that same list). In addition, it has to be *treatable* (so end-stage metastatic disease is only peripherally a topic in EM). And finally (and perhaps most important) it has to matter that you diagnose and treat it *today*, rather than tomorrow (which is why a brain tumor is not high on the differential of headache ... but bleeding into a tumor, with acute rise in ICP, most certainly is.)

All of these considerations lead the expert emergency physician to use a diagnostic approach that centers around *red flags* – the cardinal signs and symptoms – in back pain, or skin rash, or 'dizzy,' or any patient presentation imaginable – that make us look further, right now. Only when such red flags are eliminated can you consider discharging a patient ... away from medical care.

Tests in emergency medicine

A test is useful only if interpreted in the appropriate clinical setting, and used to address a specific question. Aim to undertake the test that will provide the best answer to your clinical question, rather than the test that is easiest to arrange.

Tests tend to fall into two broad categories: those used for screening and those used for diagnosis. Screening tests are designed to identify the possibility that disease *might be* present and to prompt further evaluation in those who screen positive. Diagnostic tests provide the user with some certainty that a disease *is* present.

Sensitivity and specificity

Sensitivity of a test is a measurement of how well a test identifies all with a particular condition. A sensitivity of 100% means that the test recognizes all sick people. The specificity is the proportion of individuals without the condition who are correctly identified by the test as not having it. A specificity of 100% means that the test recognizes all well people. (SpIN and SnOUT – SPecificity rules IN and SeNsitivity rules OUT.)

Positive and negative predictive values

Sensitivity and specificity are characteristics of how accurate a test is. A patient is more likely to want an answer to the questions 'If my test result is positive, what is the likelihood that I have the disease?' or 'If my result is negative, what is the likelihood I don't have the disease?' These values are the positive and negative predictive value (PPV/NPV) of the test.

Unlike sensitivity and specificity, the PPV and NPV will change depending on how common the disease is in the population. For rare diseases, the PPV will always be low, even when a test is near perfect in terms of sensitivity and specificity.

Likelihood ratios (LR)

The positive likelihood ratio (LR^+) and negative likelihood ratio (LR^-) for a test combine the sensitivity and specificity results into single measures that tell us how useful a positive or negative test result is in clinical practice.

Pre- and post-test probabilities

To apply likelihood ratios, it is important to have an estimate of the probability that a condition is present before the test is done (pre-test probability). For example:

- If a patient is seen who is unconscious, what is the probability that he has a severe head injury?
- If a young man is seen at midnight and he smells of alcohol what is the probability that he has a severe head injury?
- If a young man is seen at midnight, he smells of alcohol, and has blood pouring out of his ear, what is the probability that he has a severe head injury?

Once an estimate has been made, the use of a screening or diagnostic test with a known likelihood ratio can then provide a post-test probability, aiding formulation of a safe treatment plan. As the pre-test probability rises, to be able to rule out disease, the LR^- needs to be low (e.g. a normal CT scan of the head).

> ### Key points
> - Treat life-threatening problems first.
> - Treatment can proceed initially without an exact diagnosis.
> - Use appropriate tests, always have a pre-test probability for the disease/finding.
> - Be cautious with high risk groups (elderly, very young).
> - Focus the examination on the key systems involved, being aware that a broad screening examination of other systems may be required.
> - Review all available documents (paramedic, nursing, previous notes).
> - Think of abuse and violence.
> - Document everything clearly.
> - Practise within your abilities and ask for help when needed.

Learning in emergency medicine

The emergency department is an invaluable learning environment. It is essential to develop strategies for learning rather than to depend passively on scheduled teaching sessions. Nowhere else in the hospital setting will a medical student or doctor gain exposure to such a wide variety of patients, in terms of age, symptoms and signs, severity, procedures and underlying diagnoses. The key concept that should be embraced is that learning is the responsibility of the individual.

Learning objectives

Try to set learning objectives, ideally as part of a formal appraisal with a mentor. When setting objectives the question should be asked as to whether it is knowledge, skill or attitude development that is being sought. These are learned in different ways:

Knowledge

This is probably the most testable form of learning and, at its most crude, represents the retention and regurgitation of facts. Doctors who have a good knowledge base will do well in multiple choice question (MCQ) examinations but this is often a poor measure of their actual clinical ability. We accumulate knowledge actively by reading or casually by experience.

Skills

These can be broken down into psychomotor skills (doing) and deductive skills (reasoning). Psychomotor skills, such as suturing or scanning, are learned by repetition (Fig. 1). Deductive skills, such as x-ray interpretation, are a higher order of thinking; a synthesis of knowledge and experience. Skills can be tested in a number of ways including Objective Structured Clinical Examinations (OSCEs) and Directly Observed Procedural Skills (DOPSs).

Attitude

Similar to deductive skills, attitude cannot easily be learned from a book or taught on a course. Attitude is developed by reflection and feedback from positive role models. Attitude is tested in a number of ways including formal testing at interview or informally by casual observation of workplace interaction.

As part of the learning strategy one must endeavour to appreciate the different approaches required to achieve certain objectives. To pass an MCQ a considerable amount of reading is required. To learn how to place a chest drain is more difficult as it requires knowledge, supervision, skill and enough clinical exposure to allow the opportunity to arise.

Pitfalls

There are a number of common pitfalls that may occur despite the best intentions of a well-motivated learner. These pitfalls may represent a clinical risk as well as an education loss.

Pitfall: Failure to actively pursue knowledge-gaps in clinical situations; for example being too busy to follow up clinical outcomes.

Solution: When encountering a knowledge-gap in a clinical situation ask a senior colleague or look it up at the time. Keep a record of difficult cases and follow them up to confirm/refute your initial clinical impression.

Pitfall: Reliance on self-contained knowledge in stressful situations. We naturally struggle to recall essential knowledge in very stressful situations.

Solution: Some knowledge is best kept outside of your head, on posters, PDAs or department handbooks. This strategy is known as 'cognitive load reduction'.

Pitfall: Lack of constructive feedback. Traditionally the feedback loop in emergency medicine was long and non-constructive, informing a doctor of their error three weeks previously. Timely and constructive feedback is essential for skills eminence and good patient care.

Solution: Seek regular feedback from your colleagues not just at appraisal time (Fig. 2).

Pitfall: Passive learning. This is where doctors expect to be given knowledge and skills during protected teaching sessions without the need to contribute. This is demoralizing for teacher and learner.

Solution: Use your teaching programme as a syllabus to your background reading and come prepared to teaching sessions. This leads to a much more rewarding teaching session for both parties.

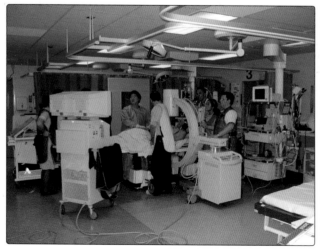
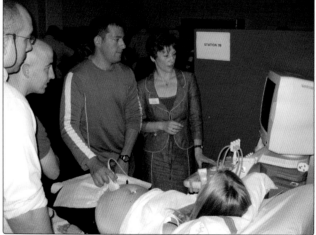

Fig. 1 **'Hands on' learning for a practical skill.**

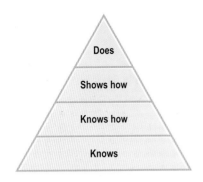

Miller's triangle

Fig. 2 **A framework for assessing clinical competence.**

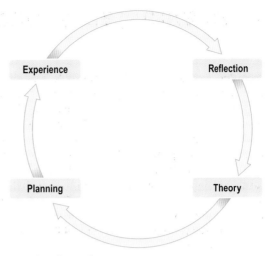

Fig. 3 **The experiential learning cycle.**

Experiential learning

Much of the learning that occurs in the emergency department is experiential learning; learning based on experience. This can be improved by adopting a process, often described as a cyclical process, linking experience with reflection and planning (Fig. 3).

Simulation

Simulation is becoming an increasingly useful teaching method in emergency medicine. Medical simulation has evolved from simulation training in the airline industry. Human factors have been implicated in contributing to numerous air crashes and near misses. These events involve a complex series of various human factors such as communication failure, poor leadership and unfamiliarity with equipment or procedures. The airline industry developed the use of simulation training where aircrew were placed in a simulated 'crisis' and their management analysed. The real value of simulation training lies in the teaching of skills such as team working, communication and leadership. Medical emergencies are inherently stressful situations and poor performance can occur despite excellent knowledge. Simulation aims to address this by training individuals utilizing a sophisticated simulator mannequin and carefully designed

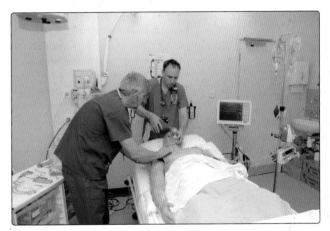

Fig. 4 **Learning in a simulation suite.**

patient environment. The mannequin has numerous variable features such as reactive pupils, palpable pulses and breath sounds (Fig. 4). It is operated from a control room which has a two-way mirror and closed circuit television, enabling the whole simulated area to be viewed. Common emergencies can be simulated such as anaphylaxis, acute life-threatening asthma or gastrointestinal bleeding. On completion of a scenario, a debriefing with video clips is undertaken to demonstrate particular behaviour with good practice being highlighted and encouraged.

Key points

- The emergency department is an invaluable learning environment.
- Try to set learning objectives.
- Plan for and reflect on learning experiences.
- Supervised practice on simulators or mannequins provides a safe learning environment for emergency management and procedures.

Good clinical care and communication skills

Working in the emergency department commonly involves working under pressure. It requires a breadth of knowledge and the ability to deal with the unexpected. This can only be achieved as a team where individual members communicate well with patients and with one another.

Prioritizing

Emergency medical staff should quickly learn to deal with the immediate:

- Sick patients need an A (airway), B (breathing), C (circulation) approach.
- Patients in pain need analgesia at their initial assessment.
- Unwell patients will need to be reviewed at appropriate intervals.

The emergency department consultation

Conditions that the emergency physician may deal with every day are not everyday occurrences for the patient (Fig. 1). Patients may come with problems that shock, surprise or annoy, but a doctor should remain non-judgemental, giving good care to everyone.

Some of the skills required for a good consultation are listed below. Many of these techniques have been shown to save time and improve diagnostic accuracy as well as improving patient satisfaction.

- Listening without interrupting.
- Using open questions.
- Screening: 'Is there anything else you have noticed?'
- Summarizing what the patient has told you.
- Signposting: 'I need to ask you about your risk factors for heart disease.'

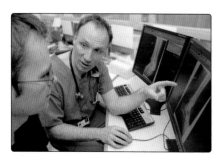

Fig. 1 **Communicating clearly with a patient.**

- Giving information in small 'chunks' and 'checking' the patient understands.
- Discussing options and agreeing a plan with the patient where possible.
- Safety netting: 'Come back if x or y happens.'

Breaking bad news

Bad news is unfortunately common in the emergency department. Preparing when, where and how to give bad news will help.

- Take another member of staff to give support.
- Introduce yourself and make sure you know who you are talking to.
- Give a warning shot that you are going to break bad news.
- Use simple everyday language without euphemisms.
- Do not be embarrassed when people are upset, be sympathetic.
- Wait to see if they need more information or just more time to take the news in.

Note keeping

Good, concise, legible notes are vital in the emergency department. Each entry should be dated, timed and the staff member's name should be printed. Notes are used by many staff members at the time as well as being a legal record.

Communication and teamwork within the emergency department

A patient's experience of the emergency department hinges on good teamwork and communication, with many adverse events and complaints being due to poor communication. Referrals to other specialties require politeness and precise information to allow the specialist to assess the urgency of the referral. Communication with nurses should be clear and timely so that they can do their job well.

Teamwork in cardiac arrests and major trauma

Teamwork is essential in the resuscitation room but can be difficult as teams may never have worked together before. The leader (usually a senior emergency department doctor) should be obviously in charge but will often stand back to get an overview. Team members can help by identifying themselves as they arrive and whilst fulfilling their roles should be prepared to do any task they are assigned, however trivial. If relatives are in the room watching the resuscitation, a team member should be assigned to stay with them and explain events to them.

'Housekeeping'. Work in the emergency department can be busy and stressful. Staff must look after their own and others' needs to enable them to work effectively and safely. This can be as simple as taking breaks so as to eat and drink regularly. More complex is how to recover from a frustrating or upsetting encounter with a patient or colleague and start the next consultation afresh. This may require time to talk with colleagues, a break or just a change of scene, switching from one area of the department to another.

Paediatric considerations

- Talk to children as well as their parents; explain things honestly and simply.
- Treat pain early. Reducing pain reduces fear.
- Take parents concerns seriously; they know their child better than you do.
- Always consider non-accidental injury.

Key points

- Many adverse events and complaints are due to failures in communication.
- Take time and care to communicate effectively.
- Look after yourself and your colleagues.

Resuscitation and initial management

No doctor is better than three

German proverb

Pre-hospital care and major incidents

Pre-hospital care

Background

Hospitals have existed in one form or another for over two thousand years. They function as centres where clinical expertise and specialist resources are focused in order to efficiently care for patients. Care provided to the ill and injured has always started outside hospitals in the pre-hospital phase.

Pre-hospital care has been heavily shaped by warfare. An early example of pre-hospital care was the introduction of the first 'flying ambulance' (*ambulance volante*) by Baron Larrey to retrieve the injured from the Napoleonic battlefields. The modern care of the acutely ill or injured in the pre-hospital phase is a specialist endeavour requiring specific skills and knowledge (Fig. 1).

Systems

There is no best way of delivering an emergency medical service, and so pre-hospital systems vary widely throughout the world. All share the aim of providing treatment to those in need of urgent medical care, with the goal of either satisfactorily treating the illness, or arranging for timely removal of the patient to a point of definitive care. This is most likely to be the emergency department. Pre-hospital care providers respond to incidents as diverse as a fall out of bed, to a myocardial infarction, to a family trapped inside their car after a collision, to a major incident involving many people.

In most countries, the Emergency Medical Service/System (EMS) is summoned by members of the public via an emergency telephone number (such as 999, 911 and 112). This puts them in contact with the control centre for the EMS, which then dispatches a suitable resource to deal with the situation. This resource usually consists of a transport platform (rapid response vehicle, motorcycle, ambulance, helicopter, fixed wing plane) and one or more equipped, trained medical professionals. The transport system varies according to the terrain, the distances and costs involved. The medical professional may be part of a dedicated ambulance organization, or be a police, fire or volunteer responder with medical skills.

Care and skills

Pre-hospital care is provided by professionals with differing skill levels and includes first aiders, paramedics and advanced pre-hospital critical care physicians. Pre-hospital care practitioners can deal with the complete spectrum of emergencies and are trained to assess and stabilize, deliver appropriate meaningful interventions, and either discharge or transport to further care. This is all undertaken in a different environment for each patient, and the challenges this presents should never be underestimated. To cope with these environments, additional training and equipment is required.

Major incidents

A major incident in health terms may be defined as a significant event where the number, severity or type of live casualties exceeds the normal resources available. A major incident for one emergency service may not be so for another emergency service. For example, a plane crash with no survivors may be a major incident for the police and fire services, but not for health services. Similarly, an outbreak of SARS may overwhelm the health services, but not impact the fire service. From the perspective of the hospital emergency department, a major incident can be either internal (within the hospital) or external (in the community).

Classification

Incidents can be classified into:

- Simple or compound – compound incidents damage the infrastructure aiming to deal with the incident such as communications, transport links or the hospital itself.
- Compensated or uncompensated – when all possible resources available as part of the major incident response are allocated to the incident, can it be managed?
- Man-made (war, terrorist attack, mass gathering, plane crash) or natural (earthquake, tidal wave, volcano).

Most major incidents are man-made, simple and compensated, and also uncommon, for example a train crash.

Planning

The key to dealing with rare events or incidents that overwhelm is in the planning. All organizations that could potentially be involved in a major incident should have robust and coordinated plans in place that are regularly rehearsed (Fig. 2). These major incident plans will have to take into account topics such as:

- Staffing – getting appropriate extra personnel to assist either from within the organization, or through

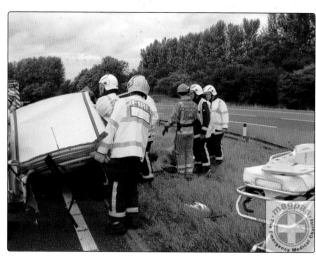

Fig. 1 **The emergency services, including a pre-hospital care team, treating a casualty at the roadside.**

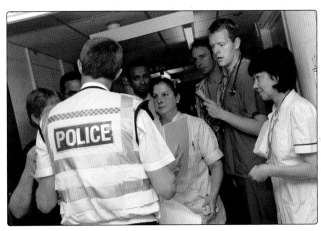

Fig. 2 **Communication between the police and members of the hospital major incident management team.**

mutual aid from other similar civilian or military organizations.

- Equipment – what supplies will be needed to deal with a large number of patients? Where will these supplies be stored and how will they get to where they are needed?
- Training – staff will need to have a plan to work to that gives clear roles and instructions. In the UK, the Major Incident Medical Management and Support Course (MIMMS) teaches a systematic approach to scene and casualty management.
- Special incidents – dealing with chemical, biological, radiological or terrorist incidents (see 'Hazardous material and CBRN incidents' chapter).
- Organization – there is great potential for chaos at such an incident, and structures have been developed to provide organization.

In the UK, a Gold – Silver – Bronze command structure (also termed Strategic – Tactical – Operational) is used by emergency services to establish a hierarchical framework for the command and control of major incidents and disasters. This system does not explicitly signify hierarchy of rank, since the roles are not rank-specific, but the chain of command will often be the same as the order of rank. Although the Gold – Silver – Bronze command structure was designed for disasters, it has been successfully utilized for all manner of pre-planned operations.

Gold Command

The Gold Commander is in overall control of their organization's resources at the incident. They will not be on site, but at a distant control room, Gold Command, where they will formulate the strategy for dealing with the incident with Gold Commanders from various organizations.

Silver Command

The Silver Commander is the senior member of the organization at the scene, in charge of all their resources. They decide how to utilize these resources to achieve the strategic aims of the Gold Commander. At the scene of the incident, they will closely coordinate with other organizations' Silver Commanders, usually situated in purpose-built command vehicles, at a Joint Emergency Services Control Centre (JESCC).

Bronze Command

A Bronze Commander directly controls the organization's resources at the incident and will be found with their staff working on scene. If an incident is widespread geographically, different Bronzes may assume responsibility for different areas. If complex, differing Bronzes can command differing tasks or responsibilities at an incident.

Triage

With an overwhelming number of casualties, they must be prioritized in order of need in order to direct resources. Triage is a dynamic, structured method of sorting based upon basic physiology and ABCs. Labels can be attached to patients showing the triage category, and stay with the patient from scene to hospital.

Key points

Pre-hospital care

- As a specialty, pre-hospital care is inextricably linked to emergency medicine.
- Emergency medical systems should provide seamless and appropriate care from the moment the patient is injured, taken ill, or seeks help.
- The many different demands for emergency or 'unscheduled' health care can only be met by new and innovative working patterns and practices.

Major incidents

- A major incident is any emergency situation that requires the implementation of special arrangements by one or more of the emergency services, the health services, or the local authority.
- It is important to recognize and declare a major incident early to optimize coordination of the response.
- Always use a standard structured approach when dealing with a major incident.

Airway management and ventilation

Control of the airway is arguably the single most important intervention during the resuscitation and management of a seriously ill or injured patient. Airway, being the 'A' of the ABC approach, comes first because each subsequent stage depends upon the patency of the airway. Delivery of oxygenated blood to vital organs can be achieved only after adequate ventilation of the lungs. The only circumstance in which another procedure might take precedence over airway management is when defibrillation is required for a shockable rhythm and the patient is in cardiac arrest.

Airway management in the resuscitation setting is based upon these principles:

1. assessment of the airway
2. airway opening manoeuvres
3. simple airway management and adjuncts
4. advanced airway management.

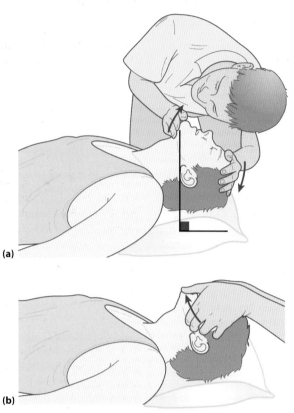

(a)

(b)

Fig. 1 **Assessing the airway using the Look, Listen and Feel technique**; opening the airway using the head tilt, chin lift **(a)** and jaw thrust **(b)**.

Assessment of the airway

This assessment focuses on whether the airway is open and whether breathing is present and adequate. Assessment is made by **Looking** for thoracic and abdominal movement, for objects in the mouth, for tongue swelling and for anterior neck trauma or swelling; **Listening** for normal airflow through the mouth and nose, and for abnormal sounds suggesting airway obstruction; and **Feeling** for air movement at the mouth, for crepitus, or airway shift from the midline.

Airway opening manoeuvres

In the unconscious patient, airway obstruction may be caused by the tongue or palate blocking the oropharynx. After carefully removing any obstructive objects from the mouth, open the airway using the head tilt, chin lift technique. This method is contraindicated in injured patients, where cervical spine injury is a possibility, and jaw thrust is preferred (Fig. 1). An appropriate flow of oxygen should be initiated via either a non-rebreathing mask or bag-valve-mask apparatus.

If the patient is choking, effective coughing should be encouraged. Ineffective coughs can be assisted by back blows and abdominal thrusts (Heimlich manoeuvre), whereas in the unconscious patient, cardiopulmonary resuscitation (CPR) is started.

Simple airway management and adjuncts

Patients who vomit or have excess secretions in the airway require suctioning. If no equipment is available, a vomiting unconscious patient should be turned onto their side (recovery position) to avoid aspiration.

Simple airway adjuncts such as the nasopharyngeal airway (NPA) and the oropharyngeal airway (OPA) assist in maintaining a patent airway, but do not provide a 'definitive' airway, as the potential for aspiration still exists. Care should be taken when inserting an NPA in any patient with head or facial injuries, as there is a risk of advancing the airway through a base of skull fracture.

Advanced airway management

In the emergency setting, the goal is always to obtain a definitive airway, i.e. either endotracheal intubation, or establishment of a surgical airway.

Endotracheal intubation

Endotracheal (ET) intubation is the placement of a (cuffed) tube into the trachea. In emergency practice, the most common route is orotracheal intubation. Common indications for emergency endotracheal intubation are:

- coma – for airway protection or controlled ventilation
- respiratory support
- during CPR.

Endotracheal intubation is most often performed by direct laryngoscopy, with a laryngoscope being used to obtain a view of the glottis. The ET tube is then inserted under direct vision.

In the deeply unconscious patient, or in a respiratory arrest or peri-arrest setting, the patient may be intubated expediently and without induction drugs. In the patient who is self-ventilating, the most usual form of intubation is under general anaesthesia using the technique of RSI – rapid sequence induction (or intubation).

Rapid sequence induction (intubation)

Intubation is accomplished by sedating and paralysing the patient, while applying cricoid pressure to prevent aspiration (Table 1). Always optimize the approach and plan for a 'first pass' intubation.

Laryngeal mask airway (LMA)

This device consists of a wide bore tube with a distal cuff designed to fit around the laryngeal opening. It may also be useful for the unconscious patient when the clinician has been unable to intubate.

The difficult airway

A patient may have an airway that is difficult to intubate. Extra equipment and highly skilled airway clinicians should be immediately available for such patients. Equipment such as the gum elastic bougie or a video laryngoscope (Fig. 2) will aid intubation in this group of patients.

Should intubation fail, emergency alternatives include reverting to ventilation with a bag-valve-mask, LMA or proceeding to a surgical airway such as a cricothyroidotomy. Needle cricothyroidotomy may be undertaken to oxygenate the patient while preparing for a definitive surgical airway. It is essential to continue to oxygenate the patient through whatever means. Patients die from hypoxia not from an inability to intubate.

Ventilation

Non-intubated patients can be ventilated using a bag-valve-mask with supplemental oxygen. Intubated patients should be attached to a ventilator, unless the patient is in cardiac arrest when manual (bag-valve) ventilation is preferable.

Non-invasive ventilation (NIV) and continuous positive airway pressure (CPAP) are discussed in the 'Breathlessness' chapter.

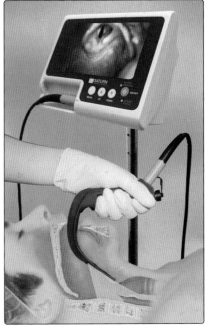

Fig. 2 **View of vocal cords using a video laryngoscope.**

Paediatric considerations

- Hypoxaemia occurs more quickly in infants.
- The airway is narrower and tidal volumes are less.
- The neutral head position is optimal for opening the airway.
- Children come in different sizes, and as such airway size is less predictable. It is important to have at least three different sized ET tubes (a half size above and below the estimated diameter). Uncuffed ET tubes may be used for children up to 10 years of age.
- For infants use size 3 to 4 ET tubes.
- For children aged 1 to 10 the appropriate uncuffed ET tube size may be determined by the following formula (age in years):

  ET tube size = 4 + (age/4)
  e.g. For an 8-year-old: 4 + (8/4) = size 6

Key points

- Airway assessment is the first priority in the seriously ill patient.
- Simple manoeuvres and basic adjuncts will open most airways.
- Adequate ventilation and oxygenation is the first priority.
- Always consider the need for a definitive airway.

Table 1 **Optimizing 'first pass' success for rapid sequence intubation (The 10 'P's)**
1. Preparation
2. Predict a difficult intubation
If the oral route is impossible then do not begin an RSI – consider other options (e.g. senior anaesthetic help/ surgical airway)
Have an alternative oral intubation device (e.g. GlideScope) ready
3. Patient position – head elevation will improve the glottic view
4. Pre-oxygenation – if the patient is hypoxic then ventilate gently with bag-valve-mask
5. Premedication
Consider atropine in children or an opiate for neuroprotection
6. Paralysis and sedation
Etomidate, ketamine, propofol or thiopental as sedatives for induction
Suxamethonium or rocuronium for paralysis
7. Cricoid pressure
8. Pass the tube
Identify the epiglottis first – then the posterior structures of the laryngeal opening – then the cords
Use external laryngeal manipulation to optimize your view of the glottis
Use a straight-to-cuff shaped tube (bougie or stylet)
9. Prevent hypoxia – move to rescue ventilation (LMA, bag-valve-mask) rather than allow hypoxia through prolonged intubation attempts
10. Confirm position
Direct vision, auscultate, end-tidal CO_2

Cardiac arrest

Cardiac arrest is absent or inadequate contraction of the heart that causes complete circulatory failure with no palpable pulses in major arteries, loss of consciousness and shallow breathing progressing to apnoea.

Sudden cardiac arrest is a leading cause of death in the western world. The most common underlying cause is a ventricular arrhythmia resulting from cardiac ischaemia. In the remaining out-of-hospital arrests, non-cardiac aetiologies such as lung disease and cerebrovascular disease are common, as well as trauma, asphyxia, drug overdose and drowning.

Irreversible brain damage occurs after 5 minutes in an arrest, and recovery of normal neurological function is rare in patients who have been untreated for more than 10 minutes. The term 'cardiopulmonary resuscitation (CPR)' is used to describe a combination of rescue breaths (mouth to mouth or using a bag-valve-mask) and external chest compressions. CPR can generate up to 30% of baseline cardiac output but it is restoration of a perfusing rhythm that is required for survival. Survival is optimized when there is early recognition of warning signs with an early call to the emergency medical services (EMS) or cardiac arrest team (CAT), early initiation of CPR, early defibrillation and advanced life support measures, and effective post-resuscitation care. These steps are known as the 'chain of survival'.

All emergency personnel attending a cardiac arrest need a unified approach to the patient. The familiar Airway, Breathing, Circulation (ABC) approach is used.

Basic Life Support (BLS)

The initial response to a cardiac arrest is initiation of BLS. This includes checking the victim, shouting for help, opening the airway and checking for breathing (see 'Airway management and ventilation' chapter), alerting emergency services/cardiac arrest team, and initiating CPR at a compression-to-breath ratio of 30:2 in adults and 15:2 in infants and children. In a collapsed child or adult, with a pulse and suspected foreign body airway obstruction, perform abdominal thrusts (Heimlich). In infants, alternate between series of five back blows and five chest thrusts.

Lay rescuers do not need to assess for pulse or signs of circulation for an unresponsive victim and can perform chest compressions without providing rescue breathing (Fig. 1).

Advanced Life Support (ALS)

The priority for an adult in cardiac arrest is identification of a shockable rhythm (VF/VT) and early defibrillation. The only time when defibrillation is delayed is in an unwitnessed out-of-hospital arrest when a short period of CPR is performed first.

The ALS algorithm (Fig. 2) provides a uniform approach to the management of adult cardiac arrest by emergency personnel.

Management depends upon whether the underlying cardiac rhythm is shockable: VF/pulseless VT; or non-shockable: asystole or pulseless electrical activity (PEA).

Adrenaline (epinephrine) 1 mg is given intravenously every 3–5 minutes. Amiodarone 300 mg is given after three unsuccessful shocks. The airway and intravenous access should be secured during the phases of CPR. With all arrests, potentially treatable causes should be sought and treated. These are listed as the 'Hs and Ts':

- Hypoxia
- Hypovolaemia
- Hyperkalaemia, hypokalaemia, hypocalcaemia, H$^+$ ions (acidaemia), hypoglycaemia and other metabolic disorders
- Hypothermia
- Tension pneumothorax
- Tamponade (cardiac)
- Toxic substances (poisoning)
- Thromboembolism (pulmonary embolus/coronary thrombosis).

Atropine 3 mg is given in asystole or slow PEA where the heart rate is less than 60 bpm. Calcium chloride (10 mL of 10%) is indicated during resuscitation from PEA if this is thought to be caused by hyperkalaemia, hypocalcaemia, or an overdose of calcium-channel-blocking drugs or magnesium. The use of sodium bicarbonate is not routinely recommended.

If a rhythm change is noted during the rhythm check, move to the appropriate side of the algorithm. If a pulse is detected, move to the post-resuscitation care phase.

Ethical issues

Advance directives

In some countries, legally binding directives have been introduced which allow patients to express their wish that CPR and life support measures should not be initiated in the event of a cardiac arrest. Where there is any doubt regarding the wishes of a patient, resuscitation should be initiated.

Do not attempt CPR (DNACPR) orders

Many patients, such as those with terminal malignancy, will not benefit from CPR in the event of a cardiac arrest. This should be discussed with the patient and close family members where appropriate, and a DNACPR order may be signed for the patient.

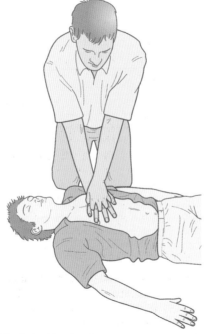

Fig. 1 **Position for chest compressions during BLS for an adult patient.**

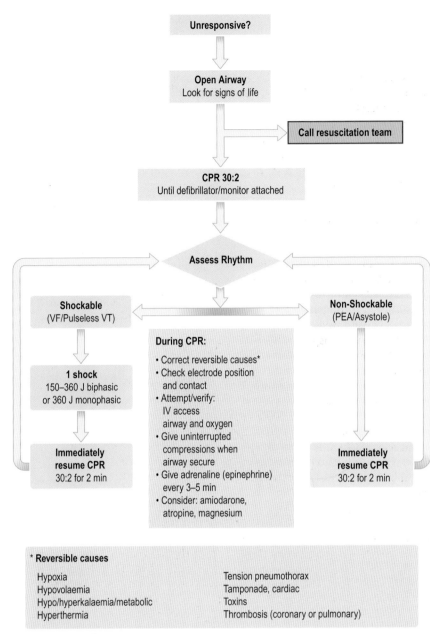

Fig. 2 **Adult Advanced Life Support algorithm.**

Post-resuscitation care

Return of spontaneous circulation should initiate the process of intensive post-resuscitation care. The underlying cause for the arrest should be sought, while stabilizing the patient. Standard investigations should be performed:

- 12-lead ECG
- arterial blood gas (and other laboratory blood tests)
- chest x-ray
- central venous access and monitoring.

The patient should have a primary and secondary survey completed using the ABCDE system. Seizure control, prevention of hyperthermia and blood glucose control are other important considerations. A period of induced hypothermia may benefit certain subgroups of patients, especially those who remain unconscious post arrest. Transfer to an appropriate high level unit should be arranged.

The latest versions of the UK resuscitation guidelines can be accessed at www.resus.org.uk.

Paediatric considerations

Most children have healthy hearts and therefore cardiac arrest in a child usually represents the endpoint of failure of another major system. Respiratory disease, sepsis and trauma contribute significantly to unexpected paediatric deaths.

The principles of management of a paediatric arrest concentrate on oxygenation and ventilation, and treating the underlying cause. Rhythm recognition and defibrillation, although important, are not commonly critical to outcome.

Major differences in the advance life support algorithm for children include:

- Commence basic life support and CPR prior to attaching monitor leads.
- Use a 15:2 ratio of chest compressions to breaths.
- Consider immediate intra-osseous access if no intravenous access available.
- Doses of drugs and energy levels should be calculated using actual or estimated weight of the child.

Stopping CPR

Many resuscitation attempts fail to obtain a return of spontaneous circulation (ROSC). At some point, CPR will have to be stopped. As a rule, while VF/VT is present, resuscitation should continue. Asystole for 20 minutes, despite Advanced Life Support measures, is generally accepted as an indication to stop CPR. Ensure that all likely reversible causes have been addressed adequately before stopping resuscitative attempts.

Relatives

A patient in cardiac arrest is often accompanied by a close relative or friend. Care should also be provided for them, and they should be offered the opportunity to stay during the resuscitation attempt.

Bedside echocardiography

Focused ultrasound can identify causes such as pericardial tamponade, or suspected pulmonary embolus, and assess ventricular motion. Ventricular akinesis is a very poor prognostic sign.

End-tidal CO₂ (ETCO₂)

Another prognostic indicator in cardiac arrest is end-tidal CO_2. A low $ETCO_2$ may be able to predict irreversible death in patients with pulseless electrical activity undergoing advanced cardiac life support.

Key points
- Early recognition/prevent cardiac arrest.
- Early CPR.
- Early defibrillation.
- Post-resuscitation care.

Arrhythmias and defibrillation

Arrhythmias

The normal adult heart beats in a regular, coordinated fashion at a rate of 60 to 100 beats per minute (bpm). Slower rates (sinus bradycardia) can occur in healthy young people, particularly athletes and during sleep. Faster rates (sinus tachycardia) occur with exercise, illness, or emotion through sympathetic neural and circulating catecholamine drive.

Arrhythmias are disturbances of the normal electrical rhythm of the heart. While most are benign, some can cause haemodynamic compromise and even cardiac arrest. As a pragmatic approach, arrhythmias can be classified as fast or slow, regular or irregular, and as narrow or broad complex. They can also be classified by site of origin (e.g. supraventricular or ventricular) and by duration (paroxysmal, persistent or permanent). Common causes are listed in Table 1.

Tachyarrhythmias

These are disturbances of the heart's rhythm resulting in a heart rate of over 100 bpm. The commonest causes of tachyarrhythmias are increased automaticity (that is increased spontaneous myocyte depolarization), and re-entry (the circular propagation

of an impulse around two interconnected pathways with different conduction characteristics and refractory periods). Assessment should always start with an ABC approach and a pulse check before carefully studying the ECG trace (see page 28).

Regular narrow complex tachycardia

Look carefully for P waves and determine if the patient has a sinus tachycardia secondary to underlying systemic pathology.

Supraventricular tachycardia (SVT) most commonly presents as a narrow complex tachycardia. It is caused by either automatic activity of the atria or re-entry circuits. Atrioventricular re-entrant tachycardia (AVRT) occurs when there is an accessory pathway between the atria and ventricles as for example in Wolff–Parkinson–White (WPW) syndrome. In sinus rhythm the characteristic ECG features of WPW syndrome are an up-sloping delta wave and a short PR interval. Some individuals have two pathways in their AV node (a slow and fast pathway). They may develop an AV nodal re-entrant tachycardia (AVNRT).

Atrial tachycardia occurs when there is re-entry within the atria or from an automatic atrial focus. The P waves often appear abnormal. In atrial flutter with 2:1 block the ventricular rate is 150 bpm (Fig. 1a).

Initial treatment

Regular narrow complex tachycardia may respond to vagal manoeuvres and is responsive to AV nodal blocking agents such as adenosine, beta-blockers and calcium channel blockers (verapamil). Adenosine should be given into a proximal vein as a flushed bolus. If there are signs of cardiovascular compromise, synchronized DC cardioversion may be considered. Recurrence is common on medical therapy, so refer for catheter ablation.

Irregular narrow complex tachycardia

Atrial fibrillation (AF) occurs when individual atrial muscle fibres contract independently (Fig. 1b). The AV node conducts irregularly and the ventricles therefore contract irregularly. The ECG

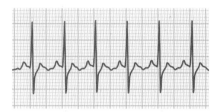

(a)

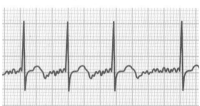

(b)

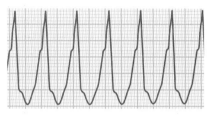

(c)

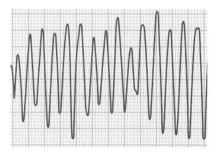

(d)

Fig. 1 **Rhythm strips** showing **(a)** a regular narrow complex tachycardia (atrial flutter), **(b)** an irregular narrow complex tachycardia (AF), **(c)** a broad complex tachycardia (VT), and **(d)** ventricular fibrillation (VF).

shows no P waves and irregular QRS complexes.

In these patients the risk of thromboembolism is approximately 5% per year but may be as high as 20% in high risk groups.

Management involves either rhythm control with an attempt at cardioversion (either electrical or pharmacological), or pharmacological rate control together with anticoagulation or antiplatelet therapy.

Traditionally digoxin has been used for atrial fibrillation but is ineffective at prevention and conversion, and may be profibrillatory as it decreases the atrial refractory period. Rate control may be attained with calcium channel

Table 1 **Causes and clinical features of arrhythmias**
Causes of arrhythmias
Cardiac
▪ Myocardial infarction
▪ Coronary artery disease
▪ Aberrant conduction pathway
▪ Mitral valve disease
▪ Cardiomyopathy
▪ Pericarditis
▪ Myocarditis
Non-cardiac
▪ Alcohol
▪ Pneumonia
▪ Drugs (beta-agonist, digoxin, tricyclics)
▪ Metabolic imbalance (K^+, Mg^{2+}, Ca^{2+}, hypoxia, hypercapnia)
▪ Caffeine
Clinical features
▪ Some arrhythmias are asymptomatic and incidental, e.g. AF
▪ Palpitation
▪ Chest pain
▪ Dyspnoea
▪ Syncope/Presyncope
▪ Hypotension
▪ Pulmonary oedema

blockers or beta-blockers in patients with normal LV function. Digoxin and amiodarone can be effective for rate control in patients with LV dysfunction and decompensated congestive heart failure to slow ventricular response.

Regular broad complex tachycardia

Ventricular tachycardia (VT) is a broad complex tachycardia defined as three or more successive ventricular beats at a rate above 120 bpm (Fig. 1c). The rhythm can be self-terminating or can be sustained. It can degenerate to ventricular fibrillation (VF). The ECG has broad QRS complexes and no P waves.

Other causes of regular broad complex tachycardia include supraventricular tachycardia (SVT) with bundle branch block, atrial flutter with bundle branch block and atrial flutter or SVT with pre-excitation (e.g. WPW syndrome).

The distinction between VT and an SVT with aberrant conduction can be difficult. *If in doubt always assume it is VT; in an emergency both can be treated with synchronized DC cardioversion.*

Irregular broad complex tachycardia

This group includes atrial fibrillation (AF), atrial flutter or multifocal tachycardia with bundle branch block, pre-excited AF (e.g. WPW syndrome) and torsades de pointes.

In atrial fibrillation with WPW, AV nodal blocking agents may paradoxically increase conduction through the accessory pathway and precipitate VF. Therefore in an irregular broad complex tachycardia, **avoid** AV nodal blockers (adenosine, verapamil), and consider amiodarone, or synchronized DC cardioversion if symptomatic with hypotension.

Torsades de pointes is a variant of VT which is associated with a long QT interval. It can precipitate ventricular fibrillation. The ECG shows broad complex tachycardia and variation in the QRS axis giving a sine wave appearance.

Ventricular fibrillation (VF) is a disorganized electrical activity of the heart (Fig. 1d). A heart in VF cannot sustain a perfusing cardiac output.

Emergency treatment

Patients with VF or pulseless VT require immediate diagnosis and defibrillation. Unstable patients with VT require DC cardioversion. In the cardiovascular stable patients with VT, management with IV antiarrhythmic drugs such as amiodarone may be appropriate. Magnesium can be used in torsades de pointes.

Bradyarrhythmias

Bradyarrhythmias result from decreased intrinsic pacemaker function or a block in conduction, principally within the AV node or the His–Purkinje system. For clinical purposes, bradycardia can be defined as a heart rate <50 bpm, though correlation with the clinical picture is essential. Sinus bradycardia is a slow sinus rhythm and can be caused by increased vagal stimulation or drugs.

AV nodal and His–Purkinje disease

First degree heart block is defined as prolongation of the PR interval (>0.2 s, >5 small squares). It rarely causes symptoms, but may impair diastolic ventricular filling.

There are two types of second degree heart block:

- Mobitz type 1 (Wenckebach) where there is a progressive increase in the PR interval with intermittent complete AV block when a P wave is not conducted (Fig. 2a). This is usually a benign rhythm.
- Mobitz type 2 where the PR interval is constant but there is intermittent failure to conduct the P waves, with either a 2:1 or 3:1 block being common. There is an increased risk of developing complete heart block.

In third degree (complete) heart block there is complete AV dissociation, and the ECG trace shows no correlation between P waves and QRS complex (Fig. 2b).

Patients with a symptomatic bradycardia should be assessed using an ABC approach. Atropine is the first-line drug treatment. Adrenaline (epinephrine) or isoprenaline, or external pacing may be required if the patient is hypotensive and unresponsive to atropine. These are all holding measures until a temporary pacing wire can be inserted.

Mobitz type 2 and third degree blocks are often symptomatic and require admission for monitoring and possible pacing.

Defibrillation

Cardiac output ceases almost immediately, and cerebral hypoxic injury starts within 3 minutes of the onset of ventricular fibrillation/pulseless ventricular tachycardia (VF/pulseless VT). Successful defibrillation must be achieved urgently if neurological recovery is to be achieved (see 'Cardiac arrest' chapter). Most hospitals now have biphasic defibrillators, and automated external defibrillators (AEDs) are available in many public places.

Online resources

Current guidelines are available at www.resus.org.uk.

> **Key points**
>
> - Always check the clinical state of the patient before treating the arrhythmia: pulse check.
> - Always use a synchronized shock when a pulse is present.

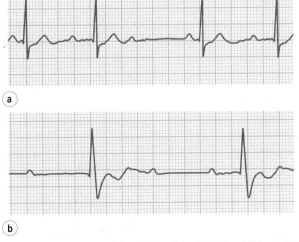

Fig. 2 **Rhythm strip** showing **(a)** second degree (Wenckebach) block and **(b)** complete heart block.

Shock

Shock is a state of inadequate perfusion and oxygenation of vital organs and tissues. This results in cellular hypoxia and cell death, if allowed to persist.

Classification

Tissue and organ perfusion is dependent upon a functioning circulatory system. This requires a functioning pump (heart) and delivery system (blood vessels) as well as an adequate volume of perfusing fluid (blood).

Shock can be classified according to failure of these systems (Fig. 1):

1. Hypovolaemic
   (a) acute blood loss – intraperitoneal bleeding, ruptured aortic aneurysm, gastrointestinal (GI) bleed, fractures, open wounds
   (b) fluid loss – burns, GI losses (vomiting or diarrhoea)
2. Cardiogenic – primary pump failure
   (a) myocardial infarction
   (b) arrhythmia
   (c) valve problems.
3. Obstructive – obstruction to outflow or venous return
   (a) cardiac tamponade
   (b) tension pneumothorax
   (c) massive pulmonary embolism.
4. Distributive – leaky or dilated blood vessels
   (a) sepsis
   (b) anaphylaxis
   (c) neurogenic shock.

Haemorrhage is the most common cause of shock in the injured patient.

Clinical features

The diagnosis of shock can be very difficult, as there may be very few obvious clinical signs, especially in the early stages. Shock may be recognized by:

- **Tachycardia (>100 bpm)** – the body responds to poor tissue perfusion by increasing sympathetic drive, resulting in increased heart rate. This is often the earliest sign of hypovolaemic shock, but may not be seen in elderly patients, or those taking beta-blockers.
- **Tachypnoea.**
- **Hypotension (systolic blood pressure <90 mmHg)** – hypotension may be a late sign, as the body is able to compensate for a significant loss of effective circulating volume. These compensatory mechanisms are particularly effective in young and fit patients. Postural hypotension may be an earlier sign.
- **Peripheral perfusion** – skin may appear cool, clammy and pale with a prolonged capillary refill time in hypovolaemic shock. Septic or anaphylactic shock results in peripheral vasodilatation and warm peripheries.
- **Oliguria** – decreased renal perfusion in shock leads to reduced urine output. Normal urine output should be 0.5 mL/kg/hour for adults and 1–2 mL/kg/hour for children.
- **Altered consciousness** – shocked patients may initially be agitated. As shock progresses, confusion, lethargy and a reduction in conscious level may be seen.
- **Metabolic (lactic) acidosis** – inadequate tissue perfusion leads to anaerobic metabolism in affected tissues. This results in the production of lactic acid and a metabolic acidosis.

Shock is a physiological state, rather than a diagnosis in its own right. Differentiate between the different types of shock and identify an underlying cause since this will direct further treatment.

Acute blood loss
It is essential that any potential sources of blood loss are identified. Occasionally, this may be obvious as in the case of open wounds, but consider the possibility of occult bleeding (GI bleed, leaking abdominal aortic aneurysm, damage to solid organs, pelvic fracture).

Cardiac failure
Signs of cardiac failure may be seen with a raised jugular venous pressure (JVP), peripheral oedema and a gallop rhythm. ECG changes may demonstrate an underlying pathology.

Cardiac tamponade
The classic triad of hypotension, muffled heart sounds, and raised JVP may be seen (Beck's triad). Pulsus paradoxus (pulse weaker on inspiration) and Kussmaul's sign (JVP rises on inspiration) may be present.

Tension pneumothorax
Acute respiratory distress with absent breath sounds plus hyperresonance on the affected side, distended neck veins and tracheal deviation.

Pulmonary embolism
Chest pain and dyspnoea may be associated with hypoxia and signs of right heart strain.

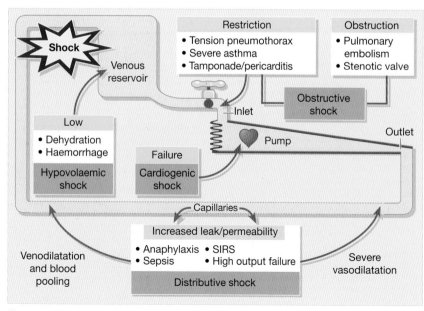

Fig. 1 **Mechanisms of shock.** SIRS, systemic inflammatory response syndrome.

Sepsis

There may be an obvious source of infection associated with pyrexia and rigors. These changes may not be obvious in elderly or immunocompromised patients.

Anaphylaxis

Generalized inflammatory response leads to systemic vasodilatation and increased vascular permeability. This results in hypotension with warm peripheries initially. This is often associated with a cutaneous manifestation such as urticaria, erythema or swelling of the face. There may be pruritus and bronchospasm.

Monitoring and investigations

Investigation is directed towards identifying the degree of shock and discriminating between the various causes of shock.

- Monitor vital signs.
- Perform FBC, coagulation screen, urea and electrolytes, LFTs, glucose, cross-match blood for transfusion.
- Consider blood cultures.
- Arterial blood gas including lactate.
- 12-lead ECG and cardiac monitoring.
- Chest x-ray.
- Urinary catheter – monitor urine output.
- Consider central line for CVP measurement and jugular venous gas measurement.
- Consider bedside ultrasound (abdominal and cardiac evaluation with sonography in shock – ACES).

Other tailored investigations may be required to confirm clinical suspicion of underlying disease (cardiac tamponade, pulmonary embolism).

Management

The aim is to restore tissue perfusion with adequately oxygenated blood. Priorities are:

- ensure adequate ventilation (airway and breathing) and oxygenation
- restore adequate circulating volume
- identify and treat cause of shock
- treat complications (coagulopathy, renal failure, other organ dysfunction).

As with all critically ill patients, the ABC approach directs immediate management (see 'Introduction to emergency medicine' chapter).

Fluid therapy allows expansion of the circulating volume, and can be achieved by giving a colloid, a crystalloid, or blood (Fig. 2). Large volumes may be required to replace losses as fluid may be redistributed to the interstitial and intracellular spaces. Boluses of 1 to 2 litres of crystalloid in adults, or 10 to 20 mL/kg in children, may need to be repeated to replace losses.

Treat the cause

Haemorrhagic shock
Continuing blood loss must be stopped. In the case of open wounds, this may be by applying a pressure dressing. Urgent surgery may be required. Continuing losses from fractures may be minimized by splinting.

STOP THE BLEEDING!

Consider hypotensive resuscitation (ensure a mean pressure adequate to perfuse cerebral and renal vessels) for aortic dissection or leaking aortic aneurysm or incompressible internal haemorrhage. This is generally appropriate only if the patient has a normal conscious level and is talking. It is a temporary measure whilst definitive treatment, such as surgery, is organized.

Cardiogenic shock
Cardiac failure may not respond to fluid therapy. Care must be taken to avoid volume overload since this will lead to further deterioration in cardiac function.

- Arrhythmias should be treated urgently (see 'Arrhythmias and defibrillation', chapter).
- Measures to assess the fluid volume status should be instituted early (central venous pressure measurement).
- Inotropic support may be required to maintain cardiac output.
- Cardiac ultrasound may be used to assess cardiac function and differentiate cardiogenic from other forms of shock.

Monitoring response to treatment

Response to treatment may be monitored by watching for changes in peripheral perfusion and monitoring vital signs.

Invasive monitoring allows continuous measurement of vital signs and assessment of the need for further treatment. This may include:

- CVP monitoring – measures filling pressure of right side of heart
- arterial line – continuous measure of blood pressure.

> **Key points**
> - Shock is underperfusion **not** hypotension.
> - Ensure oxygenation, adequate volume restoration and early treatment of the underlying cause.

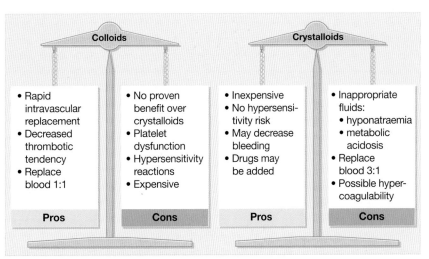

Colloids		Crystalloids	

• Rapid intravascular replacement
• Decreased thrombotic tendency
• Replace blood 1:1
	• No proven benefit over crystalloids
	• Platelet dysfunction
	• Hypersensitivity reactions
	• Expensive
		• Inexpensive
		• No hypersensitivity risk
		• May decrease bleeding
		• Drugs may be added
			• Inappropriate fluids:
			  • hyponatraemia
			  • metabolic acidosis
			• Replace blood 3:1
			• Possible hypercoagulability

Pros	**Cons**	**Pros**	**Cons**

Fig. 2 **Fluid resuscitation: which fluid?**

Acid–base and fluid balance

Acid–base balance

Junior doctors and students are often intimidated by acid–base physiology. Understanding of the principles and having a system for interpretation are key factors in the management of critically ill patients. In emergency medicine the most commonly encountered abnormalities of acid–base balance are respiratory acidosis, metabolic acidosis, and mixed metabolic and respiratory acidosis (Fig. 1).

Physiology

About 16 000 mmol of CO_2 is generated daily. If CO_2 is not eliminated via the lungs an excess of H^+ results, leading to acidosis (respiratory acidosis):

$$CO_2 + H_2O = H_2CO_3 = H^+ + HCO_3^-$$

The kidneys eliminate acid in a variety of ways such as combining hydrogen ions with ammonia and phosphate which is then excreted in the urine. The kidneys also regulate the amount of bicarbonate absorbed back into the blood.

If renal failure occurs metabolic acidosis will ensue.

If tissue perfusion is poor (e.g. shock) decreased oxygen delivery results in increased anaerobic metabolism, lactate production and a metabolic acidosis.

Blood gas definitions

The pH is a negative logarithmic representation of the H^+ concentration.

Normal arterial pH is between 7.35 and 7.45.
Acidosis, a process which leads to acidaemia: pH <7.35.
Alkalosis, a process which leads to alkalaemia: pH >7.45.
Base excess/deficit. The more negative the base excess the more severe the acidosis. Base excess is a measure of the metabolic component of acid–base disturbance. Normal values range from −2 to +2.
Standard bicarbonate. Normal standard HCO_3^- is 22–26 mmol/L.

The anion gap, the difference between the major plasma cations and anions. The normal anion gap is between 8 and 16 mmol/L.

$$\text{Anion gap} = ([Na^+] + [K^+]) - ([Cl^-] + [HCO_3^-])$$

Carbon dioxide. $PaCO_2$ is between 4.5 kPa and 6.0 kPa.
Oxygen. Normal range for arterial blood is 10.0–13.3 kPa.

Compensation

This is the process by which the lungs or kidneys tend to return arterial pH towards normal. Compensation never quite returns the pH to completely normal. For example, in type II respiratory failure the kidneys can compensate for the elevated CO_2 by increasing absorption of bicarbonate. In so doing the effect of elevated CO_2 on the pH is minimized. This response to elevated CO_2 takes days to develop and therefore only occurs with chronic CO_2 elevation.

In metabolic acidosis the lungs increase CO_2 elimination by increasing alveolar ventilation. This response is much more rapid, occurring over minutes. Increased alveolar ventilation reduces CO_2 until exhaustion supervenes.

Interpretation of the arterial blood gas

1. What is the PaO_2? Note the inspired oxygen concentration (FiO_2).
2. Is the pH normal, low or high?
3. What is the primary acid–base disturbance? Compensatory mechanisms tend to return pH towards normal but do not reverse the primary disturbance (Table 1).
4. Check the base excess; the more negative, the greater the metabolic acidosis.
5. Check the standard bicarbonate; this provides similar information to the base excess.
6. Check the lactate. In metabolic acidosis elevated lactate suggests poor tissue perfusion.

Common acid–base disturbances in emergency medicine

Acute respiratory acidosis

Increased $PaCO_2$ with normal HCO_3^- resulting from alveolar hypoventilation.

Common causes include life-threatening asthma, acute exacerbations of chronic obstructive pulmonary disease (COPD), severe pneumonia, severe pulmonary oedema,

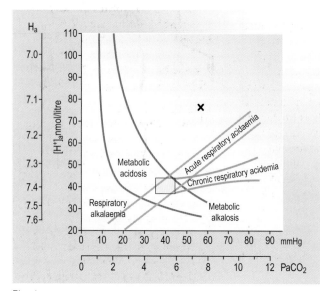

Fig. 1 **Arterial blood gas interpretation:** the point marked 'x' represents a mixed metabolic and respiratory acidosis.

Table 1 **The four main acid–base disturbances**				
Acid–base disturbance	pH	Primary disturbance	Compensation	Example
Respiratory acidosis	Low pH	Increased $PaCO_2$	Increased HCO_3^- takes 2 days	COPD, respiratory tract obstruction
Respiratory alkalosis	High pH	Reduced $PaCO_2$	Decreased HCO_3^- with chronicity	Hyperventilation
Metabolic acidosis	Low pH	Reduced HCO_3^-	Reduced $PaCO_2$	Diabetic ketoacidosis
Metabolic alkalosis	High pH	Increased HCO_3^-	Increased $PaCO_2$	Protracted vomiting

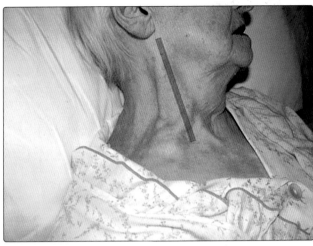

Fig. 2 **Estimation of the jugular venous pressure (JVP).** Look for pulsations of the internal jugular vein. Distension of external neck veins is not a reliable marker of right atrial pressure.

airway obstruction, opiate overdose and patient exhaustion with declining respiratory effort.

In chronic respiratory acidosis, renal compensation takes at least 72 hours to develop, e.g. COPD. Acute on chronic respiratory acidosis occurs frequently in exacerbations of COPD.

Metabolic acidosis
Metabolic acidosis can be subdivided into:

- metabolic acidosis with increased anion gap, i.e. increased acid load or an inability to excrete acid
- metabolic acidosis with normal anion gap, i.e. loss of bicarbonate.

Metabolic acidosis with increased anion gap
Causes can be remembered using the mnemonic: SIMPLE DR.

S: salicylates and solvents
I: iron and isoniazid
M: methanol
P: paraldehyde
L: lactic acidosis
E: ethylene glycol
D: diabetic ketoacidosis
R: renal failure.

Metabolic acidosis with normal anion gap
Causes include diarrhoea in children, pancreatic fistulae, ureter-sigmoidostomy, Addison's disease, acetazolamide and excessive saline administration.

Respiratory alkalosis
This is caused by alveolar hyperventilation.

Metabolic alkalosis
Protracted vomiting can result in loss of gastric hydrochloric acid. Conn's syndrome and chronic steroid therapy can also cause metabolic alkalosis.

Mixed acid–base disorders
Combined respiratory and metabolic acidosis occurs commonly in the setting of cardiogenic shock with pulmonary oedema, sepsis with pneumonia or acute respiratory distress syndrome (ARDS), severe anaphylaxis and severe trauma with chest injuries. Severe metabolic acidosis with initial respiratory compensation followed by patient exhaustion and decline in respiratory rate is often seen.

Fluid balance

Assessment of fluid balance (dehydration or fluid overload) relies heavily upon interpretation of physical signs such as dry or moist mucous membranes, skin turgor or oedema, estimation of the jugular venous pressure (JVP; Fig. 2) and measurement of urine output. Interpretation of these physical signs is fraught with difficulty and confounded by co-morbidities such as cardiac, renal and hepatic disease. Interpretation of clinical examination can be aided by measuring the central venous pressure (CVP), estimating CVP or right atrial pressure using bedside ultrasound, and observing the response to a fluid challenge.

The history may indicate whether a patient is likely to be fluid depleted or replete.

Daily fluid requirements vary widely and are influenced by underlying disease state. Fluid resuscitation aims to replace intravascular losses and should be tailored to the type of loss. Crystalloid solutions such as 'normal' saline, Hartmann's or Ringer's lactate solution are commonly used as the initial replacement fluids. With blood loss, it may be necessary to initiate replacement of red blood cells in conjunction with careful volume replacement. Typical volumes for resuscitation boluses are 1 to 2 litres in adults, or 10 to 20 mL per kg body weight in children.

Baseline daily (24 hours) fluid requirement for an adult is approximately 2500 mL; whereas in children it should be calculated by body weight: 100 mL/kg for the first 10 kg, 50 mL/kg for the second 10 kg, and 25 mL/kg for the remaining body weight.

The main electrolytes of interest in emergency medicine are potassium and sodium, and to a lesser extent magnesium and calcium. These are discussed further in the 'Biochemical and endocrine emergencies' chapter.

Key points

- Systematically review blood gas readings within the clinical context.
- Venous gases accurately reflect acid–base status.
- Arterial gases should be used in respiratory disease.
- Fluid replacement should be guided by a careful assessment of intravascular and extravascular fluid status.

Coma

Coma is a profound reduction in the level of consciousness. The level of consciousness is assessed using the Glasgow Coma Scale (GCS). This is a score that is derived using three components: eye opening, response to voice and motor response (Table 1). A patient with a GCS score of 8 or less is considered to be in coma.

Management is divided into two phases; an initial resuscitation phase using an ABCDE approach, and a second phase where a definitive diagnosis is made. Early assessment and management of the airway is key in the comatose patient as protective airway reflexes and muscle tone may be lost (see 'Airway management and ventilation' chapter). It is also essential to check the blood glucose in the initial phase. The differential diagnosis for a patient in coma is very wide (Table 2). During the initial resuscitative phase, certain clues to the underlying aetiology may become apparent. Look for pinpoint pupils or needle tracks suggestive of intravenous drug abuse and possible heroin overdose. Are there unequal pupils? Is there any evidence of head injury? Is there divergent gaze or abnormal body posturing suggestive of intracranial pathology such as an intracranial haemorrhage? Is the patient cold with a low core temperature, suggesting hypothermia as a cause for the coma?

Is the patient hypotensive, suggesting a lack of cerebral perfusion as a cause for the coma?

Once the patient has been adequately initially assessed and resuscitated, concentrate on determining the underlying aetiology for their depressed level of consciousness. It is important to gather as much information as possible at this stage.

Sources of information include friends and family, paramedics, and the patient's general practitioner. Ask if there were any empty packets of tablets or bottles of alcohol found near the patient suggesting poisoning as a possible cause. Were any paraphernalia of intravenous drug use evident? Was the patient's recent mental state normal, or had they been depressed, again suggesting poisoning as a possible cause? Where were they found? Was there any heating appliance nearby, or had they been working with a machine emitting fumes in a closed area suggesting possible carbon monoxide poisoning? Was the event very sudden, preceded by headache or vomiting, suggestive of intracranial haemorrhage, especially subarachnoid haemorrhage? What medications are they taking? Are they on warfarin, suggesting possible intracranial haemorrhage? Are they diabetic, suggesting possible

hypoglycaemia as a cause? Was there any history of head injury, suggestive of intracranial haemorrhage? Are they epileptic, suggesting a possible post-ictal state?

When satisfied that as much information as is possible has been gathered, examine the patient in a systematic manner.

Important bedside investigations include:

- Blood glucose measurement (include in the initial resuscitative phase).
- Electrocardiogram.
- Bedside blood testing. Point of care blood gas analysers give a wealth of information including electrolyte levels, acid–base details, haemoglobin, glucose, carboxy-haemoglobin levels as well as information about the respiratory function. They work equally as well with a heparinized venous sample (Fig. 1). This may rapidly identify a metabolic cause for the depressed level of consciousness such as hyponatraemia or carbon monoxide poisoning (Fig. 2).
- Urine toxicology screen. Bedside ELISA tests show recent ingestion of a range of substances including opiates, cocaine, cannabis, ecstasy and tricyclic antidepressants.
- Urinalysis and pregnancy test.
- Chest x-ray.

Other useful tests include laboratory blood tests and a CT scan of the head. A CT head scan is mandatory in any patient where the diagnosis is not immediately clear or where the level of consciousness does not improve with treatment.

Table 1 Glasgow Coma Scale: record the patient's best response in each category

Eye opening

Spontaneous	4
To voice	3
To pain	2
No response	1

Verbal response

Orientated	5
Confused, disorientated	4
Inappropriate words	3
Incomprehensible sounds	2
No response	1

Motor response

Obeys commands	6
Localizes pain	5
Withdraws to pain (flexion)	4
Abnormal flexion posturing	3
Extension posturing	2
No response	1

Table 2 Differential diagnosis of coma

Vascular causes	Intracranial haemorrhage, subarachnoid haemorrhage, brainstem infarction
Infectious causes	Meningitis, encephalitis, other (malaria, typhoid)
Toxic causes	Poisoning, drugs – opiates, sedatives (benzodiazepines, 5-HT₃ antagonists, tricyclic antidepressants)
	Poisoning, other – alcohol, carbon monoxide
Metabolic causes	Hyponatraemia, hypernatraemia, hypercalcaemia, hypoxia, hypercapnia, uraemia, hepatic encephalopathy, Wernicke's encephalopathy (thiamine deficiency)
Traumatic causes	Extradural haematoma, subdural haematoma, cerebral contusions/haematomas, diffuse axonal injury
Endocrine causes	Hypoglycaemia (antidiabetics, acute liver failure, alcohol, Addison's disease), hyperglycaemia (diabetic ketoacidosis, non-ketotic coma), myxoedema/thyroid storm, Addisonion crisis
Other causes	Hypothermia, hypotension

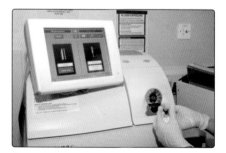

Fig. 1 **Point of care blood testing (POCT)**, traditionally called 'blood gas analyser'. The new generation analysers give a wealth of information from a heparinized venous sample.

Blood type	Venous			
FIO₂	0.21			
Temperature	37.0 °C			
pH	7.209 (-)	[	7.350 -	7.450]
H⁺	61.9 nmol/L			
PCO₂	6.80 kPa (+)	[	4.67 -	6.00]
PO₂	2.47 kPa (--)	[	10.67 -	13.33]
cHCO₃	19.9 mmol/L			
BE	-8.2 mmol/L			
pH'	7.209			
H''	61.9 nmol/L			
PCO₂'	6.80 kPa			
PO₂'	2.47 kPa			
Na⁺	140.0 mmol/L	[	135.0 -	148.0]
K⁺	4.63 mmol/L (+)	[	3.50 -	4.50]
Ca²⁺	1.083 mmol/L (-)	[	1.120 -	1.320]
Urea	7.3 mmol/L	[	2.5 -	6.4]
Glu	11.5 mmol/L (++)	[	3.3 -	6.1]
Lac	13.4 mmol/L (++)	[	0.4 -	2.2]
Bili	Out of range (-)	[	51 -	850]
Hct	44.0 %	[	35.0 -	50.0]
Hct(c)	39.8 %			
tHb	13.3 g/dL	[	11.5 -	17.4]
O₂Hb	28.0 % (--)	[	95.0 -	99.0]
COHb	23.4 % (++)	[	0.5 -	2.5]
MetHb	0.9 %	[	0.4 -	1.5]
HHb	47.7 % (++)	[	1.0 -	5.0]
SO₂	37.0 %	[	75.0 -	99.0]

Fig. 2 **Printout of a venous POCT sample** from a patient found at home with a GCS score of 7; note the carboxyhaemaglobin (COHb) level of 23.4%. The diagnosis was of carbon monoxide poisoning due to a faulty gas heater.

Common causes for coma

Hypoglycaemia

It is important to identify low blood sugar levels as soon as possible. It is essential to check a bedside glucose and correct any hypoglycaemia immediately in any patient with a reduced level of consciousness. Generally hypoglycaemia occurs in insulin-dependent diabetics who omit a meal and may have an intercurrent illness such as gastroenteritis. Occasionally patients on oral hypoglycaemics can become hypoglycaemic but this is never the case with metformin alone. Metformin acts by increasing the sensitivity of cells to insulin. If a patient on metformin is hypoglycaemic there will be an alternative cause. Treatment of hypoglycaemia is with dextrose, either 50 mL of 50%, which can be irritant to veins, or 500 mL of 10%, which is less irritant. Consider other possible causes for hypoglycaemia such as alcohol, fulminant liver failure, Addison's disease, cerebral malaria, insulin overdose (as deliberate self-harm; serum C-peptide will not be raised) and very rarely, insulinoma (serum C-peptide will be raised).

Intracranial haemorrhage

This is a very common and often catastrophic cause of coma. Massive subarachnoid haemorrhage may occur without any preceding symptoms; suspect when a previously well patient presents with sudden collapse and coma. Potential signs on examination

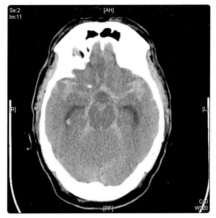

Fig. 3 **CT of the head showing subarachnoid haemorrhage**. CT of the head looking for blood is performed without contrast. Fresh blood appears white on CT and is visible on this CT around the basal cisterns.

include unequal pupils and an abnormal gaze; on fundoscopy there may be subhyaloid haemorrhage (retinal haemorrhage around the optic disc). If there is very extensive haemorrhage there may be abnormal posturing such as extension of the limbs. The diagnosis is made on unenhanced CT head scan (Fig. 3). Nimodipine helps to reduce vasospasm and prevent secondary brain injury. Further management depends upon the cause of the haemorrhage; commonly this is from an intracranial aneurysm. The aneurysm is identified with angiography. Traditionally this has been with digital subtraction angiography but increasingly CT or MR angiography is being utilized. Treatment of the aneurysm involves either surgical clipping or an interventional procedure such as coiling.

Intracerebral haemorrhage may present either as a stroke with focal signs, or as a sudden loss of consciousness and coma. Urgent head CT and coagulation screen testing are indicated. Anticoagulation should be urgently reversed in the presence of intracranial haemorrhage; discuss with a neurosurgeon as surgical intervention may be life-saving.

Key points

- Coma is a GCS score of 8 or less.
- Initial structured approach is ABCDE, then proceed to information gathering and systematic examination.
- Always check the blood glucose.
- CT head scan is mandatory if no definite cause is identified.

Plain radiographs

Although advanced imaging techniques are used with increasing frequency in the emergency department, plain x-rays still make up the bulk of imaging in this setting. Deciding who needs imaging and what form of imaging can be difficult. Rates of x-ray requesting vary between individual doctors, hospitals and countries. Clinical prediction rules have been devised to aid the decision-making process. These are based on multivariate analyses undertaken to identify a number of parameters that predict which patients require imaging. These rules have been validated prospectively and have a high sensitivity (but never 100%). Examples include the Ottawa ankle rules, Ottawa knee rules (see 'Lower limb and pelvic trauma' chapter) and the NEXUS cervical spine rules (see 'Head and spinal trauma' chapter).

Each medical specialty tends to have its own approach to looking at a particular x-ray. For example, with a chest x-ray a cardiologist will note the cardiothoracic ratio and contour of the aorta, a general surgeon will look for free air under the diaphragm, an orthopaedic surgeon will look for bony injury such as a clavicle fracture. In the emergency department it is important to have a systematic approach to ensure that nothing is missed. Do not get distracted by the obvious abnormality: go systematically and meticulously through the whole radiograph and identify all the abnormalities (Figs 1 and 2).

The ten commandments of emergency department radiology[1]:

1. Treat the patient, not the radiograph.
2. Take a history and examine the patient before requesting a radiograph wherever possible.
3. Request a radiograph only when necessary. Unnecessary x-rays include coccyx, nose, skull (in someone who needs a CT), ribs (chest x-ray indicated only to look at lung parenchyma and to exclude a haemo or pneumothorax).
4. Never look at a radiograph without seeing the patient, and never see the patient without looking at the radiograph.
5. Look at every radiograph, the whole radiograph, and the radiograph as a whole (ABCs approach).
6. Re-examine the patient if there is any incongruity between the radiograph and the expected findings.
7. The rule of twos:
   (a) Two views at right angles (orthogonal) – a fracture may be visible in only one view.
   (b) Two joints – include the joint above and below to exclude a dislocation or subluxation (e.g. Monteggia fracture) (Fig. 2).
   (c) Two sides – in children partially ossified epiphyses make radiograph interpretation difficult. It may be useful to compare the injured side to normal. Atlases of normal variants are available.
   (d) Two occasions – repeat radiographs 10–14 days after injury may reveal a fracture, for example scaphoid and stress fractures.
   (e) Two radiographs – certain fractures or injuries are difficult to spot, for example carpal injuries.
8. Take radiographs before and after procedures. After reduction of fractures and dislocations, after removal of foreign bodies.
9. If a radiograph does not look quite right there is probably something wrong.
10. Ensure you are protected by fail safe mechanisms – most emergency departments will have a reporting system in place for missed radiological abnormalities (including missed lung malignancies, missed fractures).

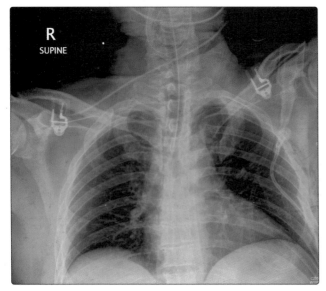

ABCs approach

A – Adequacy/alignment: slightly rotated to the left, no name visible.

B – Bones: multiple rib fractures left lower thorax.

C – Cartilage and joints: NOTE distraction between T9 and T10 increased disc space.

S – Soft tissues: ET tube well placed, Nasogastric tube coiled in back of throat.

Lung parenchyma, no opacification, vascular markings to the edge (BUT percutaneous tube thoracostomy in place and surgical emphysema on left).

Heart and mediastinum slightly enlarged, but underinflated and supine film.

Diaphragm, crisp outline, no free air, costophrenic angles clear.

Fig. 1 **Chest x-ray and ABCs approach;** particularly note distraction between T9 and T10 at the bottom of the radiograph suggesting unstable spinal injury. This injury would be easily missed unless a meticulous systematic approach is adopted.

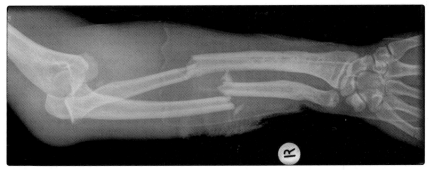

Fig. 2 **Radiograph of right forearm** with obvious fractures of radius and ulna midshaft; note dislocation of radial head, also note fracture neck of fifth metacarpal at edge of film. Don't get distracted by the obvious injury.

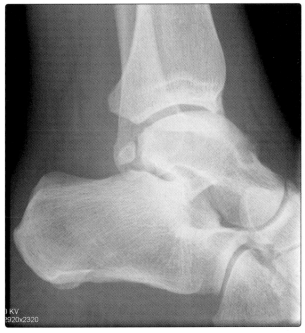

Fig. 3 **Radiograph of the ankle** showing os trigonum at the posterior aspect of the talus, a normal variant misdiagnosed as a fracture.

Approach to radiographs

One approach to interpreting radiographs that is easy to remember is based on 'ABCs' (Fig. 1):

- A – Adequacy, Alignment
- B – Bones
- C – Cartilage and joints
- S – Soft tissues.

Adequacy: check the name and date on each radiograph, ensure all of the areas of interest can be seen – for example in trauma ensure that a cervical spine x-ray series includes C7 and T1.

Alignment: of the patient to the radiograph (rotation).

Bones: follow the cortical outline looking for breaks or steps in the continuity. Observe the trabecular pattern of the medullary cavity for abnormalities.

Cartilage and joints: inspect all the joint spaces and articular surfaces and note abnormal calcification.

Soft tissues: soft tissue swelling may indicate an underlying skeletal injury. Examine soft tissue organs, lung parenchyma, bowel gas pattern (Fig. 1).

Normal variants are common and may lead to diagnostic confusion. The most common normal variants include accessory ossicles around the foot and ankle (Fig. 3).

Reference

1. Touquet R, Driscoll P, Nicholson D. Teaching in accident and emergency medicine: 10 commandments of accident and emergency radiology. *BMJ* 1995;310:642–655.

Key points

- Perform the most appropriate radiographic investigation first.
- Never accept suboptimal images, always ensure that adequate views have been taken.
- Adopt a careful structured approach for interpretation.

Emergency ultrasound

The use of ultrasound at the bedside to answer focused clinical questions is a relatively recent development in the field of emergency medicine. It is safe, rapid and non-invasive and can be performed by a wide range of specialists including non-radiologists, and is ideal in the setting of acute illness or the unstable patient. It does not replace the accurate diagnostic report provided by formal radiological modalities such as CT scanning and radiology departmental ultrasound.

Emergency ultrasound is used as an extension of the clinical examination to rule in or rule out key diagnoses in specific clinical settings. Examples of the clinical questions to be answered include:

- Does this hypotensive patient have an abdominal aortic aneurysm?
- In this trauma patient, is there free intraperitoneal fluid?
- In a patient in cardiac arrest is there pericardial tamponade?

Emergency bedside ultrasound can also be used to facilitate invasive procedures, including:

- placement of central venous catheters
- the draining of pleural effusions and ascites
- localization of subcutaneous foreign bodies.

The key question that any physician wishing to use emergency ultrasound should ask themselves is: will a bedside ultrasound scan change or assist the immediate management of the patient in the emergency department?

Bedside ultrasound can also be used to assess the haemodynamic status of a shocked patient; simple measures such as the amount by which the inferior vena cava collapses on inspiration (IVC collapse index), or an ultrasound estimation of the JVP in the patient who is able to sit at 45°, can provide an estimate of venous filling.

Background

Ultrasound technology allows the production of images by processing high frequency sound waves transmitted and received by a probe. The frequencies used for medical ultrasound range from 2 to 15 MHz, with lower frequencies used for abdominal and cardiac scanning and high frequencies used for superficial and detailed ultrasound. The modes of ultrasound used in emergency scanning include B mode (or 2D ultrasound), M mode used in cardiac ultrasound, and Doppler imaging when assessing flow. Some simple principles that help interpretation of ultrasound images are:

1. Different tissue types reflect or transmit ultrasonic waves in a variable manner leading to different appearances in the ultrasound picture. Bone or calcified structures, such as gallstones, are highly reflective and appear white with a black acoustic shadow behind them. Fluid transmits ultrasonic waves and appears black. Soft tissue structures and organs reflect some sound and transmit the remainder, therefore, appearing grey.
2. Air is the enemy! To prevent air distorting the picture, gel must be applied between the probe and the skin. Gentle pressure will also help to dislodge any air in the field.
3. Probe selection: A curved low frequency probe is used for abdominal scanning and often thoracic scanning. A high frequency linear probe is used for soft tissue scanning and vascular scanning. A phased ray probe is used for cardiac scanning.
4. High frequency settings provide a detailed picture but with less penetration, low frequency settings provide better penetration but with less detail.
5. Structures should be viewed in at least two planes, traditionally longitudinal and transverse.

Specific uses

Focused assessment with sonography in trauma (FAST)

The objective of the FAST scan is the detection of free intraperitoneal fluid or pericardial fluid in the trauma patient (Fig. 1). The scan involves four views: the right upper quadrant (hepatorenal angle/Morrison's pouch); the left upper quadrant (splenorenal angle); the pelvic view; and the

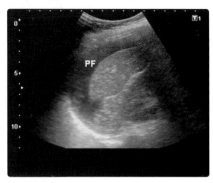

Fig. 1 **FAST scan showing free peritoneal fluid (PF).** This suggests intraperitoneal haemorrhage in the setting of trauma.

subxiphoid/pericardial view. The limitations of this study need to be understood, yet when used appropriately, it plays an invaluable role in the assessment of the multiply injured patient.

Focused aortic scanning

Emergency bedside scanning of the aorta again asks a binary question: is there an abdominal aortic aneurysm (AAA)? The scan does not determine whether this aneurysm is leaking, rather just that there is an aneurysm present. In the hands of appropriately trained emergency physicians or surgeons, ultrasound identification of AAA is both highly specific and sensitive. The overwhelming benefit of this test is the detection of unsuspected AAA in the shocked patient or patient with abdominal pain.

Focused cardiac scanning

Bedside cardiac ultrasound evaluation in the emergency department is limited to a global assessment of contractility and to the detection of pericardial effusions/tamponade. This is performed on patients who are in an arrest or in a shocked condition. The utility of this scan is to highlight the need for intervention such as pericardiocentesis, and also assist with decisions such as the appropriateness of ongoing resuscitation attempts (Fig. 2).

Detection of pleural disease

Bedside ultrasound can be used to differentiate between pleural effusions

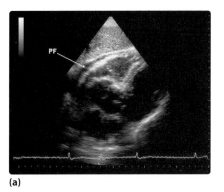

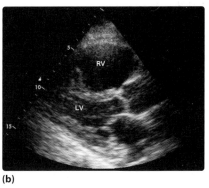

(a)   **(b)**

Fig. 2 **Focused cardiac ultrasound images** of **(a)** pericardial fluid (PF) on a subcostal view and **(b)** dilated right ventricle (RV) on a parasternal long axis view in a patient with pulmonary embolism.

Other bedside applications

Some emergency physicians use bedside ultrasound to help identify gallstones, cholecystitis, hydronephrosis, subcutaneous foreign bodies and also intrauterine pregnancy (in the evaluation of patients with possible ectopic pregnancy).

Shock ultrasound

Abdominal and cardiac evaluation by sonography in shock (ACES) is a combination of individual applications in the undifferentiated hypotensive patient (Fig. 3). It can provide a useful pointer to possible underlying aetiologies. This includes focused scans of the aorta, FAST (for free peritoneal and pleural fluid, pericardial tamponade and general cardiac wall motion) and an IVC collapse index. Again, this type of screen is an extension of the clinical examination and does not provide a formal report. With experience, focused ultrasound can be invaluable in the assessment of hypotensive or breathless patients. Identification of right ventricular dilatation may indicate possible pulmonary embolism, whereas a dilated hypocontractile left ventricle may indicate dilated cardiomyopathy.

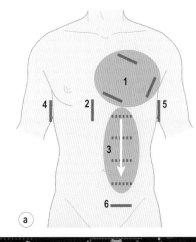

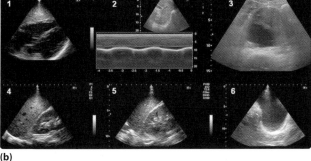

(b)

Fig. 3 **(a) The six windows for the ACES scan** and **(b) images of the views obtained.** (1, Cardiac. 2, IVC diameter and inspiratory collapse. 3, Aorta. 4, Right upper quadrant. 5, Left upper quadrant. 6, Pelvis.)

and consolidation, which may not be apparent on a plain chest x-ray. It can also be used to mark a safe point for aspiration. Ultrasound can also be utilized in the detection of pneumothorax. Normally, when both pleural surfaces are apposed, a sliding echogenic line, with comet tails, can be seen. This is lost with pneumothorax.

Procedural ultrasound

There is mounting evidence that ultrasound improves the safety and accuracy of interventional procedures, for example, placement of central venous catheters and aspiration of fluid collections such as pleural effusions and ascites. It is important to emphasize the need for the normal aseptic precautions to be taken in this setting.

Web resources

www.emergencyultrasound.org.uk
www.collemergencymed.ac.uk/CEM >
   Training and Examinations >
   Ultrasound training
www.acep.org > practice resources >
   ultrasound

Key points

■ Focused emergency ultrasound is an extension of the bedside clinical assessment.

■ Scans are performed to answer direct questions.

■ Bedside ultrasound is particularly useful in critically ill patients.

■ Appropriate training and assessment is essential.

CT and MRI

Computed axial tomography (CT scan) and magnetic resonance imaging (MRI) are very useful imaging modalities in the emergency department. They are being increasingly used as first line investigations. The use of intravenous (IV) contrast and manipulation of the data allows for three-dimensional (3-D) reconstruction of images and creation of angiograms (Figs 1 and 2).

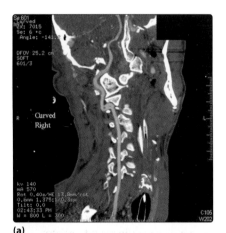

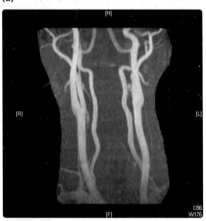

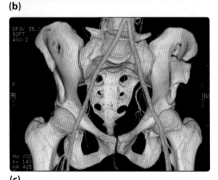

(a)

(b)

(c)

Fig. 1 **(a) CT angiogram, reconstruction of vertebral artery; (b) MRI angiogram of great vessels of the neck; and (c) three-dimensional CT angiogram of pelvis;** note comminuted iliac blade fracture of the left iliac crest.

Computed tomography

The first CT scanners developed in the early 1970s required the source/detector array to spin around 360 degrees. It would then reverse while the table advanced and the sequence repeated. This process took time and limited its use. Spiral or helical CTs were introduced in the 1980s and utilized the technology of the power slip ring, which enables the scanner to rotate continuously. This allows faster scanning and continuous acquisition of data allowing for 3-D reconstruction. Multislice technology began in the 1990s initially with two rings. It is now becoming standard to have 64-slice helical CT scanners. With 64-slice scanner technology it is possible to image the heart and great vessels in detail. Modern 256-slice scanners can image the heart in one beat, making it possible to scan patients with arrhythmias and reducing the radiation involved.

The use of CT for emergency department patients is increasing, as the diagnostic benefits become more apparent, and scanners more readily available. The early use of CT scanning in certain conditions such as abdominal pain and headache can help identify important pathology rapidly. Examples of some indications for emergency CT scanning are shown in Table 1.

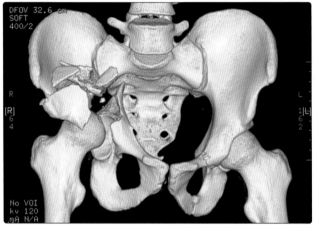

Fig. 2 **A 3-D CT reconstruction of the pelvis** showing an acetabular fracture of the right hip, with concomitant superior and inferior pubic rami fractures on the left.

Table 1 **Indications for emergency computed tomography (CT)**
CT head
■ Head trauma (see 'Head and spinal trauma' chapter)
■ Possible subarachnoid haemorrhage
■ Suspected CVA (stroke)
■ Decreased level of consciousness with no obvious cause (Fig. 3)
■ Patients with a ventriculoperitoneal (VP) shunt and headaches, vomiting and decreased level of consciousness, amnesia or confusion
CT spine
■ Suspected spinal fracture
■ Incomplete cervical spine plain x-rays
CT chest
■ Chest trauma
■ Pulmonary embolism (CT pulmonary angiogram, CTPA)
■ Suspected aortic dissection
CT abdomen
■ Abdominal trauma
■ Acute surgical abdomen, acute appendicitis (Fig. 4)
■ Abdominal aortic aneurysm (possible endovascular management)
CT musculoskeletal
■ Pelvic and acetabular fractures
■ Complex periarticular fractures (pilon ankle fracture, tibial plateau fracture)
■ Suspected fractured neck of femur (normal plain radiograph, persistent pain)
■ Scaphoid fracture (normal radiograph)

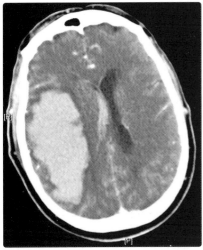

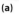
(a)

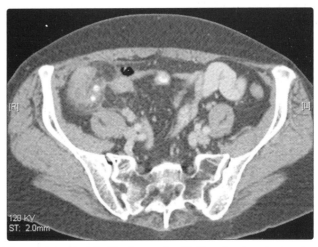

Fig. 4 **CT abdomen done for right iliac fossa pain with IV and oral contrast;** note appendicoliths in right iliac fossa.

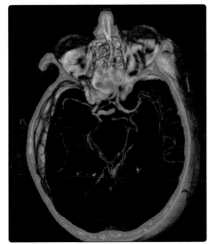
(b)

Fig. 3 **(a) CT brain** showing large right-sided frontoparietal haematoma with intraventricular blood **(b)** CT angiogram reconstruction showing haematoma and cerebral vascular anatomy, no obvious aneurysm.

Magnetic resonance imaging

Magnetic resonance imaging has been available since the early 1980s. It is excellent for imaging soft tissues and requires no radiation. The patient is placed inside a strong magnetic field, aligning all the hydrogen protons (water); a radiofrequency pulse specific to hydrogen is then passed through the body deflecting the hydrogen protons. The radio wave transmitter is then turned off allowing the hydrogen protons to re-align and release their excess stored energy. This signal is then converted into an image by a computer. MRI is very versatile, yet still has several disadvantages mostly related to the closed design and time taken to acquire the images.

Claustrophobia is a common problem, obese patients may not fit in the scanner, and access to acutely ill patients is limited. MRI scanning in young children often requires sedation and occasionally a general anaesthetic. MRI remains expensive to purchase, maintain and operate. Open MRI

scanners are becoming increasingly available, overcoming some of the limitations above.

An MRI is contraindicated in patients with:

- cardiac pacemaker, implanted cardiac defibrillator
- cerebral aneurysm clips
- carotid artery vascular clamp
- neurostimulator
- implanted drug infusion device
- bone growth/fusion stimulator
- cochlear, otologic or ear implant.

Key points

- Consider performing a CT or MRI early if the information required will not be available from plain x-rays.

- Do not consider CT or MRI to be 'special' tests – they are cost-effective as initial tests in many conditions, e.g. CT head through pelvis in major trauma; MRI in suspected spinal cord lesions.

- Avoid routine use of CT where there is no clinical need.

The electrocardiogram

Background

The electrocardiogram (ECG/EKG) is arguably the most important bedside test available to the emergency physician. With a simple system and careful consideration the ECG can reveal many aspects of the patient's condition from myocardial ischaemia to electrolyte disturbances, from pulmonary disease to hypothermia.

The ECG is obtained by measuring electrical potential between various points of the body. Each lead records the electrical signals of the heart by detecting tiny changes in electrical potential from the myocardium on the body surface from a particular combination of recording electrodes which are placed at specific points on the patient's body.

The electrical cardiac cycle is represented on the ECG trace as a sequence of deflections which are labelled P to T (or U). The x-axis represents time (at a paper speed of 25 mm/s, one small block of ECG paper (1 mm) translates into 0.04 seconds) while the y-axis indicates the direction of the overall depolarization vector. When a depolarization moves toward a positive electrode, it creates a positive deflection on the ECG in the corresponding lead, likewise creating a negative deflection when moving away from the lead (Fig. 1).

The chest leads and leads aVL, aVR and aVF are unipolar leads where the direction is from the 'centre' of the heart radially outward. The limb leads I, II and III are bipolar, giving a vector in the direction of a line between the two electrodes. For example, in lead I, the direction is from left to right. The 12 standard leads therefore map out the areas of the surface of the heart (Table 1, below; and Fig. 1, page 70).

The P wave represents atrial depolarization. This is followed by the PR interval before ventricular depolarization, represented by the QRS complex. The T wave represents ventricular repolarization.

A systematic approach to ECG interpretation

A stepwise approach is important even for those experienced at reading ECGs. The following approach should help detect all major abnormal findings.

1. What is the rate?

The ventricular rate can be calculated by dividing the average number of large (5 mm) squares between two R waves into 300. A normal resting heart rate is between 60 and 100.

Table 1 **ECG leads**	
Septum	V_1, V_2
Anterior	V_2–V_5
Lateral	I, aVL, V_5, V_6
Inferior	II, III, aVF
Posterior	V_8, V_9 (15-lead ECG)
Right ventricle	V_3R, V_4R (15-lead ECG)

2. What is the rhythm?

Is it regular or irregular? Are P waves present and related to each QRS complex? Absent P waves and an irregular rhythm are seen in atrial fibrillation.

3. Are the P waves normal?

If they are different, this may suggest the presence of ectopic atrial pacemakers or multifocal atrial tachycardia. The presence of inverted P waves in leads where this is abnormal (any lead except aVR) may suggest retrograde conduction of P waves from near the AV junction. Tall (>2.5 mm) P waves may indicate right atrial overload ('P pulmonale'). Broad, notched P waves in the limb leads or broad biphasic P waves in V_1 indicate left atrial overload ('P mitrale').

4. What is the PR interval?

The PR interval extends from the start of the P wave to the start of the QRS complex. The normal value is 120 to 200 milliseconds (3 to 5 small squares). There are three 'degrees' of AV nodal block (see the 'Arrhythmias and defibrillation' chapter). The PR segment may be depressed in pericarditis and is shortened in WPW syndrome.

5. What is the QRS axis?

The normal QRS axis (mean vector of depolarization) lies roughly along a line from sinoatrial node to apex. The normal range is from 15 to 105 degrees. It can be calculated by summating the vectors in leads I, II and III. Leads I and aVF will have positive QRS deflections with a normal axis.

6. Are the QRS complexes normal?

A narrow QRS complex (<120 ms) indicates a supraventricular origin whereas the QRS complex may be widened (>120 ms) for several reasons. These include a ventricular origin of the QRS complex (such as ventricular ectopics or ventricular tachycardia), a supraventricular rhythm that is conducted aberrantly, bundle branch blocks (Table 2), intraventricular conduction disturbance, and electrolyte disturbances.

The presence of Q waves may indicate a previous infarct.

Increased amplitude of the QRS deflections, with the sum of the S in

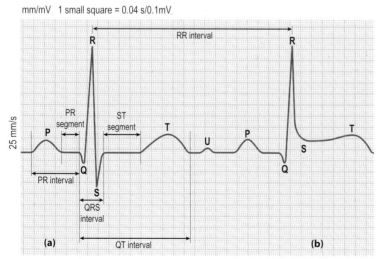

Fig. 1 **(a) A normal ECG complex** and **(b) a complex showing ST segment elevation.**

Table 2 **Bundle branch blocks (BBB):** small deflections are indicated using lower case, and larger deflections UPPER CASE	
Typical right BBB (see Fig. 2)	Wide QRS duration; rSR or rsR (tall R') in lead V_1 and wide terminal S wave in V_5 and V_6
Typical left BBB (see Fig. 2)	Wide QRS duration; no right BBB can be present; predominantly negative QRS complex in lead V_1; and upright QRS in V_6
Left BBB and acute myocardial infarction	Three independent ECG findings are highly specific for acute myocardial infarction in LBBB, but not found in all cases. These Sgarbossa criteria are: ST segment elevation of 1 mm or more that is concordant with (in the same direction as) the QRS complex ST segment depression of 1 mm or more in lead V_1, V_2 or V_3 ST segment elevation of 5 mm or more that was discordant with (in the opposite direction from) the QRS complex

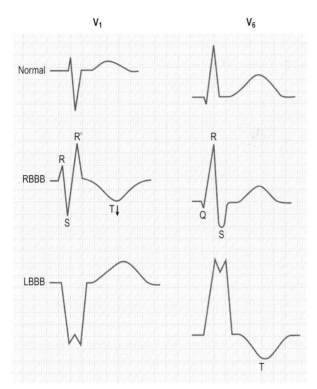

Fig. 2 **Bundle branch block patterns.** The QRS complex is widened (>120 ms).

V_1 and the R in V_5 or V_6 over 35 mm may indicate left ventricular hypertrophy. Predominant R waves in V_1 may be due to one of the following causes:

- posterior myocardial infarction
- right ventricular hypertrophy
- right bundle branch block
- WPW syndrome
- incorrect lead placement.

7. Are the ST segments normal, depressed or elevated?
In the normal ECG, the ST segment should be isoelectric (compare with the TP segment). Elevation or depression of the ST segment (see Fig. 1 in 'Acute coronary syndromes' chapter) above or below this level indicates a repolarization abnormality. Causes include cardiac ischaemia, ventricular hypertrophy, tachycardia,

pericarditis, drug effects or ventricular aneurysm. Dynamic changes are much more suggestive of cardiac ischaemia. A prominent J wave is seen in hypothermia (see 'Heat and cold emergencies' chapter).

8. Are the T waves normal?
T wave flattening or inversion occurs in ischaemia or ventricular hypertrophy. Tall or peaked T waves may indicate ischaemia or hyperkalaemia.

9. What is the QT interval?
This is the time from onset of QRS to end of T wave. It changes with heart rate and is corrected for by calculating the corrected QT interval (QTc = QT interval/√(RR interval)). A normal QT interval should be less than half the RR interval. The QTc should be less than 0.42 seconds. A value over 0.50 seconds may be seen in poisoning from a variety of drugs (tricyclic antidepressants, erythromycin, sotalol and amiodarone), congenital QT syndromes, and hypocalcaemia.

10. Are there abnormal U waves?
The U wave is not always seen. It is small and follows the T wave. Prominent U waves are seen in hypokalaemia, hypercalcaemia, thyrotoxicosis, and with digoxin.

11. Are any changes new, when compared to old or previous ECGs?
Comparison helps to determine if changes (such as left bundle branch block or T wave inversion) are old or new.

Key points
- Always adopt a systematic approach to ECG interpretation.
- Compare with previous ECGs wherever possible.

Haematology, biochemistry and other emergency blood investigations

Ordering investigations in the emergency department (ED)

Tests must be interpreted in the context of the clinical presentation. There are a number of factors that may influence the interpretation of these tests:

Timing

Some blood tests look at the specific level of a substance after a particular event and must be taken at a particular time.

- Paracetamol levels should be measured at least 4 hours after ingestion.
- Markers of myocardial damage peak at varying times, e.g. troponin I levels peak at least 12 hours after the myocardial injury was sustained.

Sensitivity and specificity

Will the test performed give an easily interpretable answer that can be used to aid diagnosis? For example, a D-dimer may not be sensitive or specific enough on its own when asking whether the patient has a pulmonary embolus.

Trends

Many patients have chronic disease, in addition to their acute illness. The ability to look at previous blood results over a period of time will assist with interpreting any abnormalities.

Values

Results are rarely reported as 'positive' or 'negative', but as a value that must be interpreted.

Point of care testing (POCT)

Increasing use is being made of technology to make testing blood easier and quicker. The blood glucose monitor was one of the first true bedside monitoring devices. Nowadays there are sophisticated analysers that can accurately give immediate results at the patient's bedside for haemoglobin, sodium, potassium, urea, lactate and glucose in addition to the traditional blood gas parameters.

Common investigations

Haematology

Haematological investigations include the full (or complete) blood count (FBC), clotting studies, erythrocyte sedimentation rate (ESR), products of fibrin degradation and blood product requests. A typical FBC will give results for the following:

Haemoglobin. The concentration of haemoglobin is given and should be compared to normal values for men, women, children or pregnant women (Table 1). A **low** level of haemoglobin may indicate a chronic process such as anaemia, or a more acute blood loss. Since haemoglobin is a measure of concentration, it depends upon the amount of solution present as well. A sudden loss of blood will cause an equal loss of solution and haemoglobin, and the concentration remaining will be the same as before the blood loss and so in acute blood loss the haemoglobin may be initially normal. To assist, look at the *haematocrit (or packed cell volume)* as a measure of cells per volume of blood. A high haemoglobin level (polycythaemia) is more unusual, and is associated with an increased risk of venous thrombosis.

White cell count (WCC). A raised WCC may indicate an acute infection but is also non-specifically raised in many other conditions such as following trauma or after a seizure. Very high WCCs often represent a malignant process such as leukaemia. A very low WCC usually represents immunosuppresion, either drug (chemotherapy) or disease (severe infection) induced. A normal WCC does not exclude the presence of infection.

Platelets. Low levels will increase the risk of bleeding and the patient may present with bruising. Transfusions are rarely needed until levels drop to a very low level ($<20 \times 10^9$/L) or if the patient is actively bleeding ($<50 \times 10^9$/L).

The erythrocyte sedimentation rate (ESR) is an indication of inflammation that is raised in many conditions. It may be helpful when considering endocarditis or temporal arteritis, but its main use lies outside the ED in monitoring chronic inflammatory conditions.

D-dimer is a product of fibrin degradation and is raised in many conditions such as liver disease, inflammatory conditions, pregnancy, trauma and malignancy. It is mainly used in the investigation of venothromboembolic disease. As it is a non-specific test, it can only be interpreted in these cases in conjunction with a clinical scoring system (see 'Thromboembolic disease' chapter).

Other. Haematology may also analyse samples for clotting screen (useful in those taking anticoagulants or with liver disease), malarial parasites and load, and blood group for administration of blood products such as packed cells and fresh frozen plasma.

Biochemistry

Biochemistry departments will perform a range of tests, some of which are relevant to managing patients in the ED.

Electrolytes. Sodium and potassium, maintained in homeostasis by the kidney, are integral to many physiological systems (see 'Biochemical and endocrine emergencies' chapter).

Urea and creatinine. Nitrogenous waste is excreted through the kidneys and measured as blood urea (or blood urea nitrogen, BUN). If excretion changes, urea levels will change and therefore it may be used as an indirect measure of renal function. It is also useful in the ED when considering upper GI bleeding. Blood in the GI tract, once digested, will increase the nitrogenous waste and therefore the

Table 1 **Normal values of haemoglobin in different groups**	
	Haemoglobin levels (g/dL)
Women	12.1–15.1
Men	13.8–17.2
Children	11–16
Pregnant women	11–12

urea level. As urea is a vital part of the countercurrent system in the kidney for water reabsorption, it is often used as a marker of hydration, with a raised level of urea indicating dehydration.

Creatinine is also used as a measure of renal function in a similar way to urea. It provides a better long-term indicator of renal function.

Creatine Kinase (CK). This is a marker for muscle damage such as rhabdomyolysis.

Liver function test (LFT). The LFT usually measures bilirubin, ALT or AST (measures of hepatic cellular function and damage), ALP (a measure of biliary duct damage), and albumin. (See the 'Jaundice and hepatic disorders' chapter for more detail.)

Amylase and lipase. A significantly raised amylase or lipase level in an ED patient can be used in the appropriate clinical context to confirm the diagnosis of acute pancreatitis. Other abdominal pathologies, such as a perforated viscus, can cause an increased serum amylase.

C-reactive protein (CRP). As a measure of both the presence and severity of infection, CRP, produced by the liver, is raised moderately in viral and often markedly in bacterial infections.

Cardiac markers. There are several markers of myocardial damage that can be easily measured (Fig. 1). Their use is further discussed in the 'Acute coronary syndromes' chapter.

Other biochemistry. Specific other tests may be requested depending on the clinical question being asked. Checking the serum calcium level may be of value in the constipated lung cancer patient. Magnesium levels may be of use in a patient presenting with a cardiac arrhythmia.

Drug levels. Levels of some therapeutic drugs can be measured in the blood, the most common being digoxin, lithium, anti-epileptics, and aminophylline. This may be useful in the ED in patients who present with the effects of over- or under-

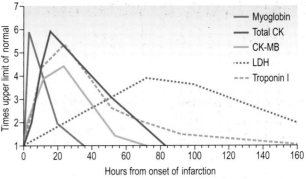

Fig. 1 **Changes in levels of cardiac markers after myocardial damage.** CK, creatine kinase; CK-MB, cardiac isomer of creatine kinase; LDH, lactate dehydrogenase.

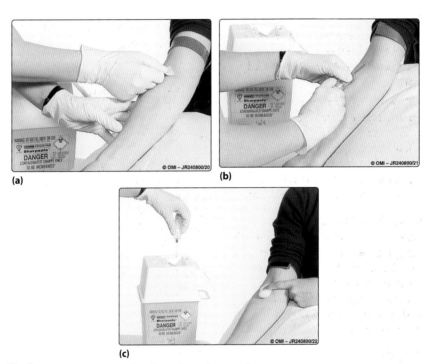

Fig. 2 **Taking a blood sample using universal precautions.**

medication. Levels of paracetamol and salicylate are commonly measured in overdose patients.

Arterial blood gases. These are discussed in detail on page 18.

Microbiology

Infections account for a large proportion of the medical caseload of an ED. Before commencing treatment, it is best practice to obtain samples to attempt to isolate the organism, especially in the sickest patients

(Fig. 2). Blood cultures taken aseptically, although not giving a result in the ED, can be critical in guiding management of the septic patient but should not delay emergency treatment.

Key points

- Blood tests should be used to answer specific questions.
- Always consider the clinical probability of disease when interpreting a result.
- Treat the patient – not the test results.

Pain management and procedural sedation

An essential component of modern emergency practice is to manage a patient's pain and anxiety to facilitate appropriate medical care in a safe, effective and humane fashion.

The first step in pain management is to avoid unnecessary painful procedures. If possible, utilize techniques such as steristrips and skin adhesives rather than suturing. Consider whether a patient requires a cannula or an arterial blood gas – invasive procedures should not be performed because they are 'routine'.

All invasive procedures cause pain unless steps are taken to prevent it. There is almost always preparation time, allowing systematic analgesia or local anaesthesia.

Pain management

Pain is commonly under-recognized and under-treated, especially in children. There is often difficulty in assessing the severity of pain, as the patient may not appear distressed or may have difficulty describing/admitting to pain.

Recognition and alleviation of pain should be a priority and this process should start at triage, be monitored during the patient's time in the emergency department and finish with ensuring adequate analgesia at, and if appropriate, beyond discharge.

When treating pain, especially in children, pay attention to the other distressing factors such as fear of an unfamiliar environment and people, parental distress, people in uniforms and fear of injury severity.

Pain assessment

The pain ladder contains objective and subjective descriptions with a numerical scale. For children some scales are based solely on faces (Fig. 1).

The experience of the member of staff assessing the patient will help in estimating the severity of the pain. Visual clues such as crying or loss of movement of a limb, which can be measured by behavioural scoring systems such as the CHEOPS score, are particularly useful in non-verbal children.

How to treat pain

In children, psychological strategies such as involving parents, cuddles, child-friendly environment, and explanation with reassurance all help build trust. Distraction with toys, blowing bubbles, reading, or story-telling is a very powerful tool.

Utilize non-pharmacological adjuncts such as limb immobilization for injuries or dressings for burns. Interventions such as subcutaneous lidocaine can decrease the pain of cannula insertion with no change in success rate or time to insertion. If time permits, topical anaesthesia such as EMLA (Fig. 2) or Ametop cream should be applied in children prior to cannulation. LAT (lidocaine, adrenaline and tetracaine) gel may be applied to open wounds.

The initial management of pain should be tailored to the level of the pain. Entonox provides strong immediate analgesia. For moderate and severe pain this should be followed by a rapidly acting strong analgesic such

as intravenous opiate (morphine sulphate). The dose should be titrated carefully to effect. The nasal route provides an initial 'needle-free' route for children.

Paediatric considerations

Nasal diamorphine (or fentanyl) is a fast-acting analgesic for the relief of moderate to severe pain in children and is the initial analgesia of choice for traumatic injuries, e.g. fractures, burns/scalds, finger tip injuries and suturing. Giving drugs by the nasal route has several advantages including rapid absorption without the need for an intravenous cannula.

Simple analgesia such as paracetamol (acetaminophen) and NSAIDs should be commenced for patients with mild pain and also for those requiring opiates. Ensure that an appropriate loading dose is given and that a regular ongoing prescription is written.

Oral opiates such as codeine or morphine or synthetic analgesics such as tramadol may be used for ongoing moderate to severe pain.

Early commencement of more advanced analgesic regimes such as patient-controlled analgesia should be considered for patients with injuries such as chest wall fractures where immobilization is not practical. Oral ketamine, gabapentin, amitriptyline or other centrally acting drugs may be useful on occasions.

Procedural sedation

Before deciding on sedation consider the optimal approach to pain

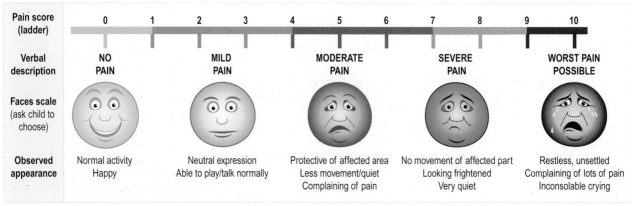

Fig. 1 **A universal assessment tool (PAT).**

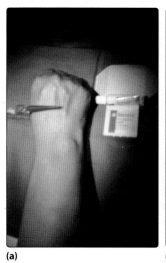 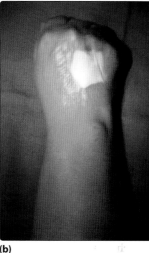

(a)   (b)

Fig. 2 **Application of EMLA cream over potential cannulation site.**

avoidance. Alternatives such as regional anaesthesia; nerve blocks, Bier's block or haematoma blocks should be considered. A combination of Entonox with either an opiate or local anaesthesia may be sufficient for very brief interventions. The risks and benefits of each option should be compared; often sedation with analgesia will provide the optimal environment for the procedure.

There are some rules to providing safe sedation in the emergency department.

- Avoid deep sedation (an unresponsive patient) and its loss of protective reflexes.
- Ensure a dedicated area or equipment for sedation.
- Ensure there is a nurse available for the entire procedure.
- Titrate opiate first followed by small amounts of sedative.

Always ensure adequate analgesia prior to administering sedative drugs. It is difficult to sedate when the patient is in pain. Sedation alone does not diminish thalamic stimulation and may lead to increased post-procedural pain.

Guidelines from the American College of Emergency Physicians suggest:

- Procedural sedation in the emergency department must be supervised by an emergency physician or other appropriately trained doctor.
- Perform a history and physical examination to identify medical illnesses, medications, allergies, and anatomic features that may affect procedural sedation and analgesia and airway management. This assessment must include a score of the patient's anaesthetic risk using a classification such as that from the ASA (Table 1).
- Recent food intake is not a contraindication for administering procedural sedation and analgesia, but should be considered in choosing the timing and target level of sedation.
- Oxygen, suction, reversal agents, and advanced life support medications and equipment should be available when procedural sedation and analgesia is used.
- Document vital signs before, during and after procedural sedation. Monitor the patient's appearance and ability to respond to verbal stimuli during and after procedural sedation. Pulse oximetry should be used.
- Drugs that can safely be used for procedural sedation in the emergency department include ketamine, propofol, or an opiate (fentanyl or morphine) and midazolam combination. Sedative agents should always be titrated to clinical effect. Ketamine can be safely administered to children for procedural sedation and analgesia in the emergency department.

Drugs

Fentanyl
A synthetic opioid, rapid onset, short duration. It is a pure analgesic.

Midazolam
A sedative, amnesic and anxiolytic with no analgesic properties. Can cause respiratory depression and hypotension. Commonly used with an opioid analgesic such as fentanyl or morphine.

Ketamine
Rapid acting dissociative anaesthetic that produces a profound analgesic effect. Given intravenously onset is 1 minute, duration 10–20 minutes; given intramuscularly, onset is 5 minutes, duration 15–45 minutes. It has a strong safety profile in children and is becoming popular in adults at a low dose. Side effects include vomiting, hypersalivation and emergence phenomenon/hallucinations.

Propofol
A general anaesthetic agent which at lower doses facilitates sedation and hypnosis. It has amnesic, anxiolytic, anti-emetic and anti-epileptic properties, but has NO analgesic effect. Propofol can cause profound respiratory depression, bradycardia and hypotension. Avoid with soya or egg allergies.

Discharge criteria

Recovery time depends on the drugs used. In general the patient should have returned to a pre-treatment level of verbalization, awareness and mobility, have normal vital signs and be able to take oral fluids.

Table 1 **American Society of Anesthesiologists (ASA) physical status classification**

I	Healthy patient
II	Mild systemic disease
III	Severe systemic disease – functional limitation
IV	Severe systemic disease with constant life threat
V	Moribund

> **Key points**
>
> - Avoid painful procedures where possible.
> - Give adequate analgesia first.
> - Use local anaesthesia where appropriate.
> - Provide procedural sedation not general anaesthesia – the patient should never be unresponsive.

Local anaesthesia

Local anaesthetic agents are commonly used in the emergency department and work by reversibly blocking nerve impulses.

There are two groups of local anaesthetic agents:

- amides – lidocaine, bupivacaine, prilocaine
- esters – procaine, cocaine, tetracaine, benzocaine.

A vasoconstrictive agent (adrenaline) may be mixed with the local anaesthetic to increase duration of action and aid in haemostasis. When performing digital nerve blocks it has previously been advised not to use adrenaline. The evidence to support this is poor, with increasing evidence to show that it is safe; though local policy should be followed.

Toxic side effects of local anaesthetics are dose related. In general, maximum doses are dependent upon the type of local anaesthetic, the route of administration, patient weight and concomitant use of a vasoconstrictor (Table 1).

Toxic effects usually manifest in the central nervous system (CNS) and, to a lesser degree, the cardiovascular and haematological systems.

CNS toxicity presents with three phases:

1. pre-excitation – circumoral paraesthesia, tinnitus, dizziness
2. excitation – muscle twitching, convulsions
3. depression – decreased level of consciousness, coma.

Cardiac toxicity leads to hypotension, bradycardia and cardiac arrest.

Methaemaglobinaemia is a process where iron in haemoglobin is altered, reducing its oxygen-carrying capability, which produces cyanosis and symptoms of hypoxia. Treatment of toxicity is supportive. Allergic reactions are rare, but more common in the ester group.

Local anaesthetics may be administered, topically (to the eye), locally (subcutaneous), intravenously (Bier's block), regionally (peripheral nerve blocks) or in the epidural and spinal spaces.

Topical anaesthesia

Topical anaesthetic eye drops are useful for assessing corneal pathology such as corneal abrasions and for removal of foreign bodies. Warn the patient that it will sting initially. They should not be used repeatedly as they impair healing.

Topical anaesthetic cream (such as EMLA cream) may be used to anaesthetize the skin to a depth of 3–5 mm. An anaesthetic depth of 3 mm is achieved after 60 minutes. It is often used for percutaneous procedures in children (venepuncture) and superficial dermal procedures. It should not be placed directly into an open wound.

Several local anaesthetic gels, for example tetracaine, adrenaline and cocaine (TAC gel) and lidocaine, adrenaline and tetracaine (LAT gel), have been created to insert directly into an open wound to allow cleaning and closure. They may need to be augmented with subcutaneous local anaesthetic.

Subcutaneous infiltration

Here local anaesthetic is injected directly into the wound and subcutaneous tissue. Several techniques are available to reduce patient anxiety and pain from a local anaesthetic injection:

- Keep the needle hidden when possible.
- Consider topical anaesthesia on its own or prior to infiltration.
- Warm the local anaesthetic to 37–42°C.
- Use buffered local anaesthetic (buffered with 8.4% sodium bicarbonate).
- Use a fine, long needle (27–30 gauge).
- Inject slowly.
- Use smallest volume necessary.
- Infiltrate through wound edges.
- Inject from 'looser' subdermal to 'tighter' dermal tissue.
- Block individual nerves.

Intravenous regional anaesthesia (Bier's block)

Intravenous regional anaesthesia is safe as long as due care is taken with the technique. Prilocaine is the local anaesthetic agent of choice. A Bier's block is used to anaesthetize a distal upper limb. Secure venous access in both arms. Ensure the tourniquet equipment is regularly maintained and in good condition; use a cuff of width 20% greater than the diameter of the arm; consider using a double cuff. Exsanguinate the affected arm by elevation, inflate the tourniquet to 300 mmHg and slowly inject the prilocaine.

Regional (peripheral nerve blocks)

Regional anaesthesia is excellent for pain relief; any peripheral nerve may be blocked, individually or as part of a plexus. The most serious risk is peripheral nerve injury; this occasionally results in long-term injury (1:5000) or transient injury (1:350). The two most commonly performed blocks in the emergency department are:

Table 1 **Comparison of different local anaesthetics**		
	Characteristics	Dose (subcutaneous injection)
Lidocaine (formerly known as lignocaine)	Rapid onset, but short acting (1 hour)	3 mg/kg 7 mg/kg with adrenaline
Bupivacaine	More potent than lidocaine, slower onset, more toxic, lasts 4–6 hours	2 mg/kg 2 mg/kg with adrenaline
Levobupivacaine	Less toxic than bupivacaine, equal potency lasts longer than bupivacaine, slower onset	2 mg/kg 2 mg/kg with adrenaline
Prilocaine	Rapid onset lasts slightly longer than lidocaine, very high clearance	6 mg/kg 9 mg/kg with adrenaline

- digital nerve block
- femoral nerve block.

Digital nerve block

There are two ways to block a digit. With the conventional 'ring' block each individual digital nerve is blocked, requiring two needle sticks. With the transthecal or modified transthecal block it is possible to block the whole finger with one injection (Fig. 1).

Conventional 'ring' block

Using a 3 mL syringe with small-gauge needle (25 to 30 gauge), insert the needle into the dorsolateral aspect of the proximal phalanx in the web space just distal to the metacarpophalangeal joint, advance the needle to the bone and inject 0.5 mL of anaesthetic. Withdraw the needle slightly and then advance it toward the volar surface and inject 1 mL of anaesthetic. Repeat the procedure on the opposite side of the digit.

Transthecal and modified transthecal block

A transthecal block is performed on the palmar surface at the distal palmar crease proximal to the metacarpophalangeal joint; the modification uses metacarpal crease at the base of the finger (Fig. 1). Supinate the hand and insert the needle in the midpoint of the metacarpal crease. Apply pressure with your non-dominant thumb proximal to the injection site; this directs the flow of the anaesthetic distally. Insert the needle through the flexor tendon until you feel bone, withdraw slightly and inject.

With both blocks wait 5 minutes to allow the block to reach full effect.

Femoral nerve block

A femoral nerve block is used in the emergency department for acute analgesia, and to facilitate placement of splints for femoral shaft fractures in adults and children. There are several methods of femoral nerve block.

'By feel'

Insert a needle 2 to 3 cm lateral to the arterial pulse and advance it until the fascia lata is pierced, at which point the tip should lie in close proximity to the nerve (Fig. 2). Inject long-acting local anaesthetic.

'Nerve stimulator'

Using a peripheral nerve stimulator, advance the needle until the

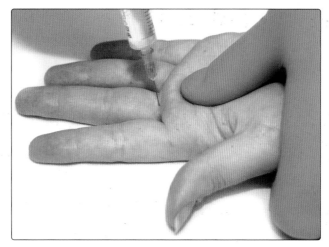

Fig. 1 **A modified transthecal digital nerve block.**

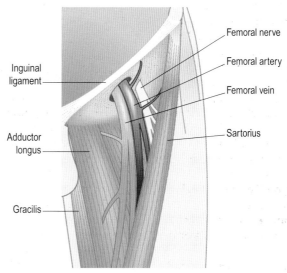

Fig. 2 **Anatomy of the femoral nerve;** note the femoral nerve emerges under the inguinal ligament and is lateral to the artery.

quadriceps muscle twitches and then inject the local anaesthetic.

'Ultrasound guidance'

It is possible to identify the femoral nerve and vessels with portable ultrasound to ensure accurate placement of the local anaesthetic.

Variations of the femoral nerve block include 3 in 1 block, where a larger volume of local anaesthetic is used and pressure is placed distally to direct fluid proximally to block the femoral nerve, lateral cutaneous nerve of thigh and the obturator nerve.

A fascia iliacus block relies on the fact that a large volume of anaesthetic solution injected immediately posterior to the fascia iliaca spreads along the inner surface of this fascia and contacts the femoral nerve, lateral cutaneous nerve, genitofemoral nerve and obturator nerve.

Epidural and spinal anaesthesia

Epidural and spinal anaesthesia is seldom used in the emergency department.

Key points

- Calculate doses carefully; toxicity is dose dependent (particular care is required in calculating appropriate doses in children).
- Local anaesthetic toxicity initially presents with signs of CNS excitation.
- Use the smallest needle possible and inject slowly.

Casts and splints

Casts or splints are applied for comfort, to prevent further injury and to immobilize an injured limb until healing occurs.

- A cast is a custom-made circumferential support, moulded around the injury, and made of either plaster of Paris (POP) or a synthetic material such as fibreglass.
- A splint may be custom-made, e.g. from POP for an acute injury; from plastic (thermally moulded) for a sub-acute injury; or may be an 'off the shelf' pre-made splint, such as a wrist or knee splint.

Due to the risk of further swelling following an acute injury, backslabs are often used initially in the emergency department (ED). A backslab is a half or three-quarter circumference plaster slab and is applied and held in place with a crepe bandage. This allows for swelling of the affected limb in the first 24 to 48 hours. A plaster backslab can fit any deformity, size or shape of patient (Fig. 1). If a backslab is applied in the ED, written plaster advice ought to be given (Table 1). It is essential to keep the cast or splint dry. Patients may simply elevate a limb out of the bath. Discourage wrapping the limb in a simple plastic bag and submerging the limb as plastic bags commonly leak. Commercially available covers are preferable and may enable the patient to swim or undertake hydrotherapy.

Different injuries require different casts or splints depending on the individual injury.

Most backslabs and plasters applied in the ED are with traditional plaster of Paris (Gypsona). It is heavier and takes longer to dry, but is easier to mould and apply on acute injuries. Synthetic casting materials continue to improve, come in several different colours (even glow in the dark); they are lighter and dry to full hardness very quickly. Soft Cast is a synthetic variant; it is more pliable than conventional synthetic casts and can be cut off by the parents with a pair of scissors, and it is very useful for stable paediatric injuries that simply need a little support while healing.

Increasingly, prefabricated splints and boots are being utilized; they often

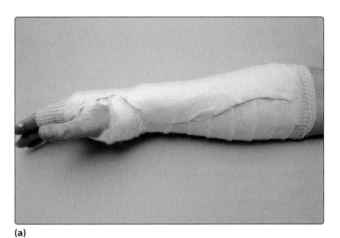

(a)

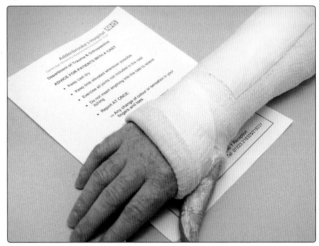

(b)

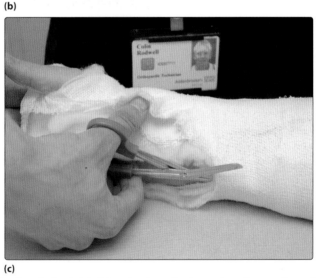

(c)

Fig. 1 **Application of a backslab. (a)** Apply a layer of ortho-wool evenly, normally overlapping each turn by half, leaving two layers of padding in total. The use of stockinette is optional (avoid using Tubigrip). Wet and apply a premeasured, precut backslab. **(b)** Secure the backslab with a crepe bandage and gently mould, depending on the fracture configuration, to provide three point fixation and then allow it to set. Always provide the patient with written plaster advice. **(c)** Ensure the plaster is not circumferential, allowing easy removal by cutting the ortho-wool and crepe with a pair of scissors.

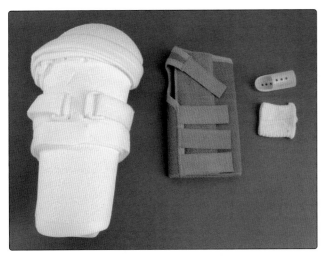

Fig. 2 **A selection of upper limb prefabricated splints:** humeral brace, Futuro wrist splint, mallet splint, Bedford finger splints.

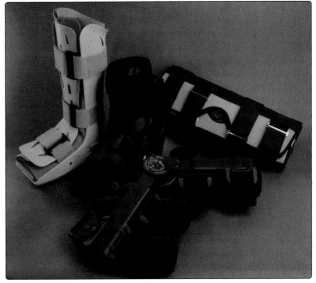

Fig. 3 **A selection of lower limb prefabricated splints:** foot and ankle, canvas knee splint, hinged knee brace.

Table 1 **Plaster advice**
■ Elevate your injured limb just above the level of your heart, to minimize swelling.
■ If the cast or backslab feels tight, elevate the affected limb.
■ If the limb becomes blue, swollen, increasingly painful, numb or you feel pins and needles, return to the ED.
■ Keep your plaster dry.
■ Don't put any objects like pens or knitting needles down the inside of the cast.
■ Contact plaster room if your cast becomes loose, tight, stained, wet, soft or cracked.

allow a little adjustment to fit individual patients. They are usually used for stable injuries that simply require support and protection while healing. Depending on the injury, they can be removed to bath/shower. It is possible for the splint/boot to be removed to allow the joint to move gently and avoid stiffness (Figs 2 and 3).

Upper limb splints

The mallet splint is used for mallet finger injuries (see 'Hand injuries' chapter). The cotton elastic double finger bandage (Bedford splint) is essentially neighbour strapping that is easier to remove and apply for stable finger and metacarpal injuries. Zimmer splints, or foam-covered aluminium splints, can be shaped for more

complex finger and metacarpal injuries. Futuro splints support the wrist and may be used in stable paediatric distal radial fractures, patients with a suspected scaphoid fracture and patients with minor ligamentous injuries to the wrist. The humeral brace is used for humeral shaft fractures. Traditionally a U slab was initially applied and converted to a humeral brace one to two weeks later. U slabs are notoriously difficult to apply and a humeral brace applied in the ED may be more comfortable.

Lower limb splints

Synthetic knee braces with hinges may be locked or adjusted to allow variable amounts of knee movement.

The 'Beckham' boot or Cam Walker is a very useful boot for stable ankle and foot injuries. It provides considerable support and can be simply removed for rehabilitation, bathing or showering. The Velcro and inflatable air cells allow the patient to control how tight the splint is and can be released if it feels too tight.

Casts

Certain injuries may benefit from a full circumferential cast initially. If

there is a risk of swelling, the cast should be split along opposite edges. Early review is recommended in this situation.

Paediatric considerations

■ Consider using a Futuro splint for unicortical (buckle) stable distal radial fractures.

■ Soft Cast, a form of synthetic cast, is very good for providing support to stable paediatric injuries and can be removed by the parents (unwrapped or simply cut off with scissors).

Key points

■ Half or three-quarter backslabs are applied initially to allow for swelling of the injured extremity.

■ Written advice on how to look after the injured limb and cast or splint should be given to the patient.

■ Traditional plaster of Paris (Gypsona) is very versatile and remains the most important casting material in the ED. However, modern synthetic casting materials and splints are playing an increasing role.

Central venous catheterization

Central venous catheterization (CVC) to obtain central venous access is an essential part of the management of many emergency conditions. The principal indications are provision of a route for delivery of caustic or critical medications or for the measurement of central venous pressure.

Contraindications for the placement of a CVC include infection over the target vein and thrombosis of the target vein; coagulopathy is a relative contraindication.

The procedure is associated with significant risks. These risks are increased in association with several characteristics:

- abnormal patient anatomy such as morbid obesity or local scarring
- the emergency clinical setting, for example patients receiving mechanical ventilation, in emergencies such as cardiac arrest
- co-morbidity (bullous emphysema, coagulopathy)
- inexperience of the operator.

The complications associated with attempted CVC insertion include arterial puncture, haematoma, pneumothorax, haemothorax, chylothorax, brachial plexus injury, arrhythmias, air embolus and catheter malposition. Complication rates have been reported to be as high as 10%, and failure to cannulate the vessel may occur in up to 20% of cases.

Landmark technique

CVC insertion has traditionally been performed 'blindly' using anatomical landmarks as a guide to vessel position. The commonest sites are the internal jugular vein (IJV), subclavian vein (SCV) and femoral vein (FV). As all these veins are in close relationship with other important structures such as arteries and nerves, accurate cannulation is essential to minimize the risk of accidental damage to adjacent structures. Anatomy may vary from patient to patient; the position of the internal jugular vein in relation to the common carotid artery provides a good example of this (Fig. 1).

Ultrasound guidance

Real-time ultrasound guidance of CVC insertion provides the operator with the added benefit of visualizing the

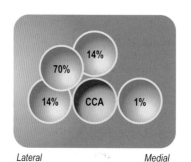

Lateral — Medial

Fig. 1 **Position of the internal jugular vein in relation to the common carotid artery in the population.**

target vein and the surrounding anatomic structures (Fig. 2), prior to and during insertion of the catheter (Fig. 3). The use of ultrasound significantly reduces complication and failure rates (Table 1).

Table 1 **A summary of the evidence for ultrasound-guided versus landmark technique for internal jugular vein access**

	Ultrasound-guided	Landmark
Ultimate success rate	100%	88–96%
Success on first attempt	73–82%	43–54%
Success on second attempt	14.5%	14–37%
Complication rate	1.4–2.3%	5.3–17%

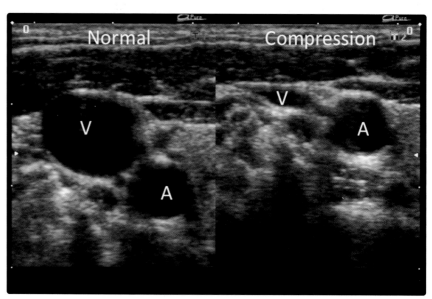

Fig. 2 **Ultrasound image of the right internal jugular vein (V) and common carotid artery (A) before and during compression** – note the compressibility of the vein.

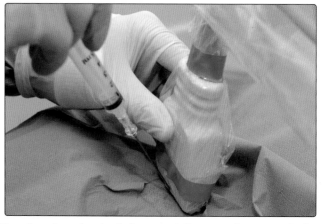

Fig. 3 **Position of needle and probe during cannulation** – note the steep angle of approach.

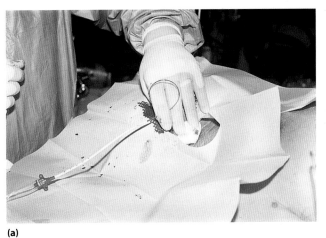 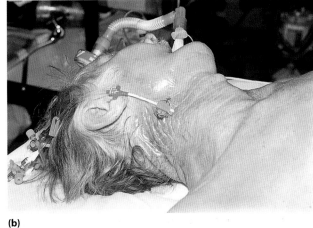

(a)   **(b)**

Fig. 4 **Central venous catheter insertion using the Seldinger technique. (a)** Catheter passes over guide wire. **(b)** Catheter in situ.

Portable ultrasound machines specifically designed for vascular access are available, though any standard ultrasound machine with a mid to high frequency linear array probe can be used. It is possible for a single user to operate the ultrasound and perform vascular access simultaneously.

The key steps in ultrasound-guided venous access are:

1. preparation of equipment
2. maintenance of aseptic technique (the gel-coated probe must be covered with a sterile sheath)
3. identification of vascular anatomy (including presence of thrombus, valves, strictures, and abnormal features)
4. confirming compressibility of veins as opposed to arteries (Fig. 2)
5. administration of local anaesthesia
6. placement of centre of ultrasound probe over centre of vein
7. skin puncture and visualization of needle-tip approaching and penetrating vein
8. confirmation of successful puncture by aspiration as well as visualization
9. completion of catheterization by Seldinger technique.

Seldinger technique

The Seldinger technique is a series of steps that can be followed to replace a needle in a vessel with a catheter (Fig. 4). Once the needle is in the vein, hold it carefully and disconnect the syringe. The tip of the guide wire is introduced into the needle and is advanced. Remove the needle, leaving the wire in place. Carefully maintain control of the wire, and make a 1–2 mm incision at the site of skin puncture. Advance a dilator over the guide wire, remove the dilator and thread the catheter over the wire and into the vessel. Then remove the guide wire, confirm blood return, flush, secure, and apply a sterile dressing.

To minimize central-line infections, ensure hand hygiene, barrier precautions, use of chlorhexidine, selection of an optimal catheter site, and remove when the catheter is no longer required.

Key points

- Routine use of ultrasound is indicated for central venous access.
- Ultrasound improves success and reduces complications.
- Always ensure that an aseptic technique is used.

Intercostal drain insertion

The indications for intercostal drain (ICD) insertion in the emergency department include:

- traumatic pneumothorax – a small traumatic pneumothorax with no other significant injury may occasionally be treated either conservatively or by aspiration (depends on size)
- traumatic haemothorax
- pneumothorax in a ventilated patient
- tension pneumothorax (after initial needle decompression)
- spontaneous pneumothorax that recurs or persists after simple aspiration
- spontaneous pneumothorax >2 cm in breathless patient over 50 years of age with underlying lung disease
- empyema
- complicated pleural effusion.

Procedure details

Ensure the patient does not have a bleeding disorder and is not on anticoagulants; if needed, check the coagulation profile and platelet count prior to ICD insertion. Obtain written consent if sedation is to be used. ICD insertion is a painful procedure: administer intravenous opiate analgesia and consider using sedation (e.g. low dose ketamine; see p. 33) but be very wary in patients with underlying lung disorders such as COPD.

Use a sterile technique with sterile gown, gloves, drapes and antiseptic solution. Check you have all the equipment and instruments available (Fig. 1).

Position the patient with hand behind their head or arm at their side with the elbow bent slightly and hand at side of the hip (Fig. 2).

Identify and mark the insertion point, the fourth or fifth intercostal space just anterior to the mid-axillary line. Ensure your entry point is at or above the nipple; the diaphragm comes up as high as the fifth intercostal space on full expiration (Figs 2 and 3). Bedside ultrasound should be used to confirm the optimal insertion point. Infiltrate

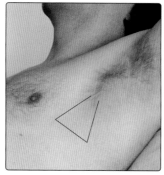

Fig. 2 **Insertion point of ICD in safe triangle;** a triangle bordered by the anterior border of the latissimus dorsi, the lateral border of pectoralis major muscle, a line superior to the horizontal level of the nipple, and an apex below the axilla.

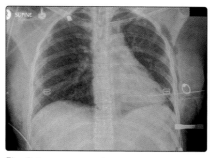

Fig. 3 **Incorrect ICD placement.** ICD too low. Note nipple ring in female; if the drain is placed below the nipple, there is a risk of diaphragmatic injury.

with local anaesthetic, remembering that the intercostal neurovascular bundles run along the inferior margin of the rib above, and infiltrate down to the pleura; the parietal pleura is very sensate.

Seldinger technique

Small gauge chest tubes may be inserted using the Seldinger technique over a guide wire. Use a needle and syringe to localize the position for insertion, identifying air or pleural fluid. Pass a guide wire through the needle, remove the needle, enlarge the tract using a dilator and then pass a small bore tube into the chest cavity.

Blunt dissection technique

If inserting a large bore ICD make an incision, slightly bigger than the width of your finger, in line with the fourth or fifth intercostal space at the superior margin of the rib below. Blunt dissect with a haemostat to the pleural cavity, slipping it just above the rib below. On puncturing the pleural cavity you feel a pop and might hear a small rush of air. Insert your finger through the hole and sweep it around to ensure no adhesions are present between the pleural lining and the underlying lung. Remove the trocar from the drain before insertion and using the haemostat at the tip of the drain, introduce the drain, aiming superiorly and posteriorly if air is being drained and inferiorly if fluid is being drained. Place it at least 5 cm deeper than the last hole in the side of the drain. Anchor the drain with a mattress suture, with the ends tied around the drain. Attach the drain to the underwater seal and cover the wound with a sterile dressing. Ensure the ICD is in the correct position by asking the patient to take a few deep breaths and cough: the water level in the tube should swing and bubbles appear. Listen for improved breath sounds (lung expansion). Obtain a chest x-ray to check the position.

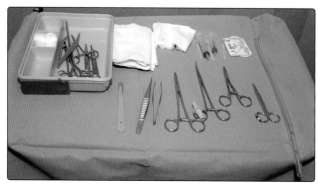

Fig. 1 **Chest drain insertion pack.** Antiseptic solution, sterile drapes, gauze swabs, syringes and needles, local anaesthetic, scalpel, suture for wound and drain, curved blunt haemostat for dissection, chest tubes of various sizes (trocar removed, 10–14 French for pneumothorax, 28–30 French for haemothorax), closed underwater drainage system (filled to correct level with sterile water), dressings.

> **Key points**
>
> - Do surgical checklist just prior to undertaking procedure: indication, bleeding disorder, consent, equipment and instruments, premedication, position, TIME OUT (confirm correct side).

Trauma

What we have to learn to do, we learn by doing

Aristotle

Initial approach to the trauma patient

When faced with a polytrauma patient it can be difficult to prioritize what needs to be done. One is often faced with multiple injuries, which on the surface all require immediate attention. The American College of Surgeons have developed an approach to such polytrauma patients, the Advanced Trauma Life Support® (ATLS®) system, the practice and principles of which have almost universally been accepted around the world. It provides a sound, safe approach to the multiply injured patient.

The underlying principle is to identify and treat life-threatening injuries in the order that they will kill a patient, i.e. airway and breathing problems will kill you before blood loss (circulation). It is divided into the primary and secondary surveys. Although described here in sequential order, in the setting of a team approach, each stage should happen in parallel. Prior to attending to a patient protect yourself, take universal precautions: wear gloves, mask, eye protection and a gown or apron.

Primary survey

A Airway (with cervical spine control)
B Breathing
C Circulation (with haemorrhage control)
D Disability (neurological evaluation)
E Exposure/environment but avoid hypothermia

Secondary survey

Focused history and a systematic detailed head-to-toe examination.

Primary survey

A: Airway with cervical spine control

Even once you have mastered the principles and theory of ATLS, it can be very daunting in the heat of the moment when a severely injured patient arrives. Essentially in the first few minutes there is one key question: 'Does this patient need to be intubated?' The simplest way to assess the airway is to ask the patient an open question; a talking patient has a patent airway. Assess the airway further by looking, listening and feeling for airflow. Next try simple airway manoeuvres like jaw thrust and chin lift. Be aware of the possibility of a cervical spine injury and protect the cervical spine with manual in-line immobilization or a cervical collar and three-point immobilization until the cervical spine can be cleared, either radiologically or clinically. If simple airway techniques are ineffective, or any of five indications for intubation are present (Table 1), secure a definitive airway (cuffed endotracheal tube).

B: Breathing

In all trauma patients give supplementary oxygen (high flow mask with reservoir bag) (Fig. 1). Feel for tracheal deviation (possible tension pneumothorax), expose the chest and look at the effort of breathing, chest wall movement (paradoxical breathing, flail segment), percuss the chest, checking for resonance (pneumothorax) and dullness (possible haemothorax), and listen for air entry bilaterally.

Treat life-threatening injuries as they are identified; for example, a tension pneumothorax (respiratory distress, tracheal deviation, hypotension, hyper-

---

Table 1 **Five indications for early intubation**

1. Respiratory failure
2. GCS <8
3. Cardiovascular instability
4. Mid-face fractures
5. The confused, agitated, uncooperative patient

---

resonance, no air entry on affected side) is a true emergency, so never waste time waiting for a chest x-ray; treat immediately with needle decompression in the second intercostal space in the mid-clavicular line. This is followed by insertion of an intercostal drain. If there is no ventilation or respiratory effort, secure a definitive airway and ventilate. Monitor the patient with pulse oximetry.

C: Circulation with haemorrhage control

First stop any ongoing external bleeding using simple pressure or limb elevation. Assessment and treatment should occur concurrently. Assess vital signs and general tissue perfusion (nature of pulse, peripheral vasoconstriction, capillary refill). Secure two large-bore intravenous cannulae and take blood for FBC, U&E, clotting, group and save, and βHCG in female patients. Administer one to two litres of crystalloid solution. Monitor the response to fluid challenges. Shock in the polytrauma patient should be considered to be haemorrhagic in the first instance and treated with fluid resuscitation. Look for the source of bleeding, 'One, on the floor, and four more' external blood loss, pelvis, long bones, chest, abdomen. A FAST scan is very useful in looking for fluid in the abdomen and chest (see 'Abdominal trauma' chapter). Haemorrhagic shock is classified into four groups (Fig. 2). Patients can compensate efficiently for blood loss and blood pressure

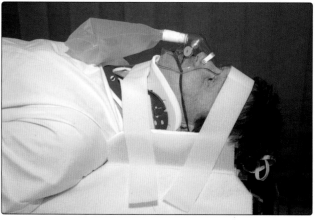

Fig. 1 **Administer high flow oxygen to all trauma patients using a mask with a reservoir bag.** Immobilize and protect the cervical spine till injury actively excluded.

commonly only falls after blood losses in excess of 1500 mL. The young and very fit compensate best, maintaining their blood pressure until extreme blood loss and then rapidly decompensate. The elderly have very low cardiorespiratory reserve and may be on medications such as beta-blockers that blunt any sympathetic response. While it is important to resuscitate with fluids and blood, it is of paramount importance to stop ongoing blood loss. If there is no head injury and massive blood loss into the abdomen, pelvis or chest, consider hypotensive resuscitation (systolic BP of 100 mmHg) and ensure treatment is instigated to stop the blood loss (angiography, surgery, stabilization of fractures).

D: Disability

Check the level of consciousness using the AVPU score or Glasgow Coma Scale (GCS). A patient with a GCS score of <8 is considered to be in coma

(see 'Head and spinal trauma' chapter). Examine briefly for any gross focal neurological abnormalities and examine the eyes for pupillary reflexes.

E: Exposure and environment

Expose the whole patient to ensure no missed major injuries; take due care to protect the patient's dignity and privacy. Avoid hypothermia; cover up the patient once the various body regions have been examined. Hypothermia significantly impacts on survival and morbidity from trauma, largely from promoting coagulopathy.

Adjuncts to primary survey

Consider the need for 'tubes and fingers in every orifice'. Perform trauma radiographs (chest and pelvis), blood pressure, pulse oximeter, ECG, urinary catheter, naso- or orogastric catheter, arterial blood gases, rectal and vaginal examination.

All unconscious trauma patients and all polytrauma patients should,

whenever possible, have a trauma CT scan (head to pelvis ± limbs). Ultrasound (FAST) scanning should be performed for unstable patients, or for high-risk patients when CT is delayed.

Secondary survey

Take a history according to the mnemonic: AMPLE (A, Allergies; M, Medication; P, Past medical history, Pregnancy; L, Last meal; E, Events).

Perform a thorough physical examination from top to toe to identify any further injuries not identified in the primary survey. Do not forget to look in the eyes and ears (contact lenses, retinal detachment, haemotympanum), log roll the patient and examine the back (Fig. 3), spine and back of head. Injuries are often missed in the primary and secondary survey; take your time and look carefully. Obtain radiographs of injured extremities and if required obtain imaging for spinal clearance.

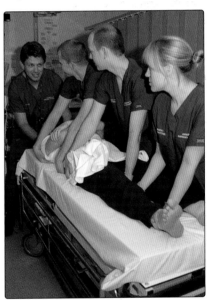

Fig. 3 **Demonstration of how to log roll a patient;** note three assistants looking at the head holder ready to roll together. Note positioning of assistants' hands to ensure roll is smooth and spine kept in alignment.

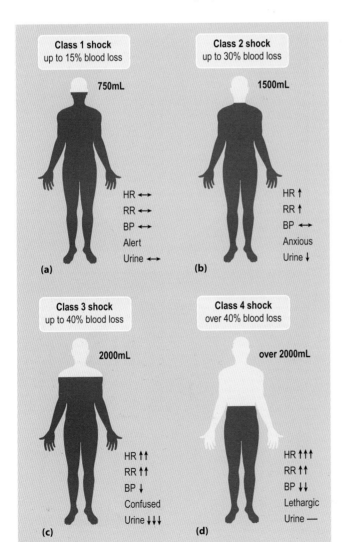

Class 1 shock up to 15% blood loss	Class 2 shock up to 30% blood loss
750mL	1500mL
HR ⟷ RR ⟷ BP ⟷ Alert Urine ⟷	HR ↑ RR ↑ BP ⟷ Anxious Urine ↓
(a)	(b)

Class 3 shock up to 40% blood loss	Class 4 shock over 40% blood loss
2000mL	over 2000mL
HR ↑↑ RR ↑↑ BP ↓ Confused Urine ↓↓↓	HR ↑↑↑ RR ↑↑ BP ↓↓ Lethargic Urine —
(c)	(d)

Fig. 2 **Classification of hypovolaemic shock;** note blood pressure only drops once >30% of circulating blood volume has been lost. (Calculations of blood loss based on 70 kg male.)

Key points

- Approach all trauma patients in a systematic manner.
- Use the ABCDE approach to identify and treat life-threatening injuries.
- Early comprehensive CT scanning should be considered.
- Hypotension in the trauma patient should initially be considered to be haemorrhagic.
- STOP THE BLEEDING.

Head and spinal trauma

Head trauma

Head injury is defined as head trauma with an associated loss of consciousness (LOC) or period of amnesia. While many head injuries are relatively minor with minimal or no long-term sequelae, occasionally neurological deterioration is possible following an apparent full recovery. Emergency management will depend upon the severity of the injury and is guided by a clinical risk assessment. The Glasgow Coma Scale (GCS) is often used to grade the severity of the injury: mild (GCS 13–15), moderate (GCS 9–12) and severe (GCS 3–8).

History

Ascertain the mechanism of injury, considering the amount of energy transferred. Determine the duration of LOC and also the degree of retrograde amnesia (amnesia before the injury) and anterograde amnesia (amnesia after the injury). Enquire about vomiting and headache. Vomiting, particularly repeated vomiting, is a highly significant symptom. Consider the social circumstances, and especially if considering discharging a patient, ensure a responsible adult will be available for the first 24 hours. Take a drug history, particularly noting the use of anticoagulant medication.

Examination

Assess the level of consciousness; AVPU or GCS (see 'Coma' and 'Coma and seizures in children' chapters). Check for signs of a basal skull fracture; examine for CSF otorrhoea or rhinorrhoea, the tympanic membranes looking for haemotympanum, look for bilateral periorbital haematoma (racoon/panda eyes) and check behind the ears for bruising over mastoid process (Battle's sign). Examine the pupils (size and reactivity) and carry out a neurological examination looking for any focal neurological signs. Examine and actively exclude an injury to the cervical spine.

Treatment

The management priority for moderate and severe head injuries involves the early detection of injuries requiring surgical intervention and the prevention of secondary brain injury. The primary brain injury is the injury resulting from the initial impact on the brain, the secondary brain injury results from subsequent insults to the already damaged brain such as hypoxia and hypotension. Approach as for all trauma patients (ABCDE), ensuring adequate oxygenation, ventilation and perfusion of the brain. Secure a definitive airway if the patient is unable to protect their own airway. Ensure adequate protection of the cervical spine until cleared radiologically and clinically. Arrange a head CT urgently (Fig. 1).

Treatment of minor head injuries is more controversial and practice may vary. Several guidelines exist for the investigation and treatment of mild head injuries. Clinical judgement is required when selecting which patients should undergo early CT scanning. There are several clinical prediction algorithms which help predict the need for imaging of the head such as the Canadian CT head rule (Table 1).

Consider observing a patient for 24 hours, if:

- CT head is indicated but not available
- abnormal CT head (always consult a neurosurgeon)

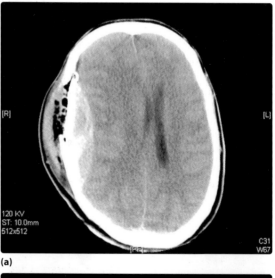

(a)

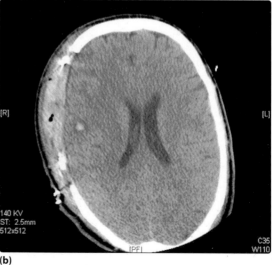

(b)

Fig. 1 **(a) CT scan showing depressed skull fracture and underlying extradural haematoma;** note compression of the ventricles and midline shift to the left. **(b) CT scan post partial craniectomy and evacuation of haematoma;** note restoration of ventricles and less midline shift.

Table 1 **Canadian CT head rule***
Computed tomography is required in patients with minor head injuries with any one of the following findings:
1. GCS score lower than 15 at 2 hours after injury
2. Suspected open or depressed skull fracture
3. Any sign of basal skull fracture (haemotympanum, racoon eyes, cerebrospinal fluid, otorrhoea or rhinorrhoea, Battle's sign)
4. Two or more episodes of vomiting
5. 65 years or older
6. Amnesia before impact of 30 or more minutes
7. Dangerous mechanism (pedestrian struck by motor vehicle, ejection from motor vehicle, fall of ≥3 ft or five stairs)

*The rule is not applicable if the patient did not experience a trauma, has a GCS score lower than 13, is younger than 16 years, is taking warfarin or has a bleeding disorder.

- depressed level of consciousness (GCS <15) with normal CT scan
- persistent vomiting, or severe headache, even if CT head is normal
- social issues, no responsible adult.

Spinal trauma

Assume all patients following trauma have a spinal injury until actively excluded. Spinal protection, rather than spinal clearance, is the priority when dealing with a polytrauma patient.

Patients are often transferred to hospital on a spinal board; this is good for transport, but the hard board may lead to pressure areas particularly in insensate skin (e.g. in an unconscious patient). Once in the emergency department, log roll the patient off the board onto a firm padded trolley or padded trauma board. Triple immobilize the cervical spine with hard collar, sandbags and tape and log roll at all times until a spinal injury has been excluded either clinically or radiologically.

The NEXUS study showed that it is possible to clinically exclude cervical spine injury as long as the following criteria are satisfied:

- no posterior midline cervical-spine tenderness
- no evidence of intoxication, alcohol or drugs (beware opioids given for other injuries)
- no decreased level of consciousness (GCS 15)
- no focal neurological deficit
- no painful distracting injuries (patient is able to concentrate on the neck).

If all five of the above criteria are satisfied, remove the collar and ask the patient to actively move the neck; if

there is no pain, no paraesthesia, and a full range of movement, the collar can safely be removed. Always evaluate the whole spine; log roll the patient, look for bruising, and feel for any areas of tenderness or steps in the cervical, thoracic and lumbar spine. Perform a thorough neurological examination, including a rectal examination for tone and perianal sensation. Patients with a neurological injury may have different motor and sensory levels, with the level varying from side to side. Document dermatomes and myotomes clearly using the MRC power grading (see 'Weakness and sensory loss' chapter).

Imaging of the spine in polytrauma patients

Traditionally imaging of the cervical spine has included trauma radiographs of the cervical spine (AP, lateral and open mouth), radiographs of the lumbar and thoracic spine (Fig. 2), followed by CT of any abnormal areas. Increasingly with modern multislice CT scanners, CT is being use as the primary imaging modality, particularly for the cervical spine. In moderate or high energy blunt trauma, it may be better in some patient groups (such as intubated head injured patients) to avoid using plain radiographs and proceed directly to CT. Similarly if a patient is having a chest and abdomen CT it is possible to reformat and produce reconstructions of the thoracic and lumbar spine removing the need for plain radiographs. MRI is very

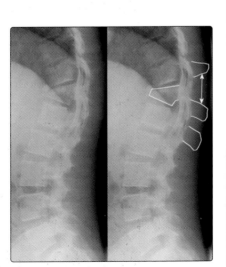

Fig. 2 **Plain radiographs of thoracolumbar spine.** The enhanced image on the right demonstrates not only the anterior wedging of T12, but also the widening of the interspinous distance posteriorly. This indicates a three-column unstable injury.

sensitive and would be considered the gold standard. However, it is often not immediately available and may not be appropriate for a potentially unstable trauma patient. It is not possible to absolutely exclude ligamentous injury of the cervical spine on plain radiographs and CT. Flexion and extension views and dynamic fluoroscopy have been used in the past to exclude ligamentous injury but these techniques have been surpassed by multislice CT and MRI. In a patient with an identified spinal injury there is a 10% risk of non-contiguous spinal injury, so if one injury is identified, actively look for another (the whole spine must be imaged).

Treatment of spinal injuries

Consider the stability of any bony injury and look for any evidence of neurological injury, determining if complete or incomplete (often only shown to be incomplete by evidence of sacral sparing). Spinal shock is the initial phase following a spinal injury, characterized by a flaccid paralysis, loss of reflexes and sensory loss. Spinal shock is a neurological phenomenon, not to be confused with neurogenic shock which is a cardiovascular phenomenon (hypotension resulting from venodilatation as a consequence of loss of sympathetic tone after a spinal cord injury). Spinal shock usually resolves within the first few days and is characterized by the return of spinal reflexes, the first being the bulbocavernosus reflex.

Web resource

http://www.asia-spinalinjury.org – the American Spinal Injury Association.

Key points
- Never assume a depressed level of consciousness is due to alcohol or drugs; actively exclude a significant head injury.
- In moderate to severe head injuries prevent hypoxia and hypotension to avoid secondary brain injury.
- Assume all trauma patients have sustained a spinal injury until actively excluded.
- Spinal protection is the priority, not spinal clearance.

Cardiothoracic trauma

Cardiothoracic trauma is one of the leading causes of death from trauma. The majority of cardiothoracic injuries can be managed with simple measures in the emergency department: oxygen, fluid resuscitation, analgesia and intercostal drain (ICD) insertion (see 'Intercostal drain insertion' chapter). Approach all trauma patients in a systematic manner (see 'Initial approach to the trauma patient' chapter). Acute life-threatening thoracic injuries must be identified in the primary survey:

- Airway obstruction
  Remove obstruction, if not responding to simple airway measures patient may require cricothyroidotomy (surgical airway).
- Tension pneumothorax
  Clinical diagnosis, perform needle decompression, mid-clavicular line, second intercostal space, followed by ICD insertion.
- Open pneumothorax
  Dress wound and seal three sides of dressing, followed by ICD insertion.
- Massive haemothorax
  Fluid resuscitation, ICD insertion, refer to cardiothoracic surgeon if initial chest drainage >1500 mL or ongoing loss >200 mL per hour.
- Flail chest
  Pain relief, ventilatory support/ intubation.
- Cardiac tamponade
  Needle pericardiocentesis and aspiration, followed by pericardial window or thoracotomy.

During the primary or secondary survey, other cardiothoracic injuries important to identify include haemothorax, pneumothorax, pulmonary contusion, blunt cardiac injury, tracheobronchial injuries, aortic rupture, diaphragmatic rupture and oesophageal injury.

History

The mechanism of injury is important (blunt or penetrating). A history of rapid deceleration should alert you to the possibility of an aortic rupture.

Examination

Perform a standard examination of the heart and lungs, paying particular attention to tracheal position (deviation), neck veins (distended, empty), chest expansion (asymmetrical, paradoxical, good, poor) heart sounds (murmurs, muffled, distant) and lung sounds; do not forget to examine the back. If injury is detected investigate further as appropriate with arterial blood gases, ECG, cardiac enzymes (troponin), chest radiograph, bedside ultrasound and contrast-enhanced CT chest scan. Depending upon the injury sustained, other possible investigations required include digital subtraction angiography of the aorta, bronchoscopy and thoracoscopy.

Aortic rupture

Traumatic aortic rupture may follow acute deceleration injury and is often fatal. A few patients develop a contained rupture and survive. A high index of suspicion, early diagnosis and treatment is essential. Several chest radiograph signs have been proposed, the best known being widening of the mediastinum >8 cm. Contrast-enhanced spiral CT scanning has been shown to be efficient and accurate at excluding major aortic rupture. Alternative investigations include transoesophageal echocardiography and digital subtraction angiography (DSA). Traditionally these injuries have all required surgical repair; recently some are being repaired using endovascular techniques (Fig. 1).

Pulmonary contusion

This is common, and potentially life-threatening. It is usually associated with other chest injuries. The patient becomes hypoxic, tachypnoeic and auscultation reveals decreased air entry. The hypoxia may lead to agitation and confusion. Radiographic changes may take time to develop showing a patchy parenchymal infiltrate; a chest CT will show the changes earlier (Fig. 2).

Treatment is supportive; avoid fluid overload and administer supplemental oxygen. Treat associated injuries. It is important to ensure adequate analgesia for rib fractures to allow patient to cough and breathe deeply.

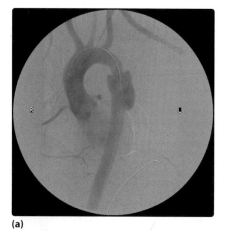

(a)

(b)

Fig. 1 **Acute traumatic aortic rupture.**
(a) Digital subtraction arch angiogram, showing aortic rupture distal to origin of left subclavian artery in region of aortic isthmus and contained pseudoaneurysm. **(b)** Post-endoluminal stenting; note stent bridging rupture, stopping before the origin of the left subclavian artery.

Blunt cardiac injury

Blunt cardiac injury can lead to myocardial contusion, cardiac chamber rupture, papillary muscle rupture or conduction system injury. Have a high index of suspicion for cardiac injury if the patient has a sternal fracture or fracture of the first or second ribs. Initial investigations include ECG, cardiac enzymes, chest radiograph, lateral sternal x-ray and bedside echocardiography. ECG abnormalities include multiple ventricular ectopics,

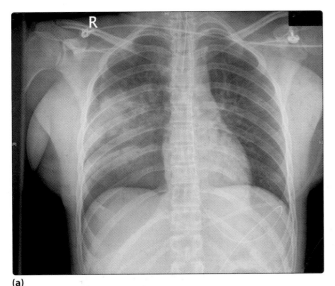

(a)

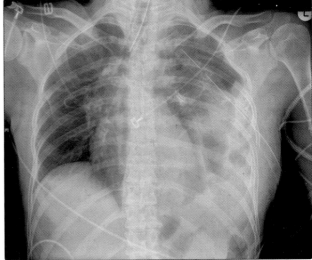

Fig. 3 **Chest radiograph showing ruptured left diaphragm;** note no distinct left hemidiaphragm, loculated air in left chest and continuation of bowel gas shadows into chest.

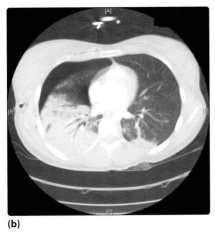

(b)

Fig. 2 **Pulmonary contusion. (a)** Chest radiograph showing right-sided pneumothorax and pulmonary contusion. **(b)** CT of same patient clearly showing pneumothorax and pulmonary contusion. Note how much clearer it is on the CT; chest radiograph changes may take a few hours to days to become fully visible.

sinus tachycardia, atrial fibrillation, new bundle branch block and non-specific ST segment changes. If any positive clinical findings or ECG abnormalities, consider continuous ECG monitoring for 24 hours post-injury. Cardiac rupture presents as an acute cardiac tamponade. Papillary muscle rupture presents with acute aortic or mitral valve regurgitation, with associated murmur and heart failure.

Traumatic diaphragmatic rupture

Diaphragmatic injury may be difficult to diagnose; have a high index of suspicion following penetrating or blunt trauma. The tear may initially be small and then enlarge over time (months to years), leading to herniation of abdominal contents into the chest. Diaphragmatic rupture is more common on the left as the liver protects the right side. Features on a chest radiograph suggesting diaphragmatic injury include loss of distinct diaphragmatic outline, an elevated hemidiaphragm, pulmonary effusion, mass-like density above the diaphragm and nasogastric tube above the diaphragm (Fig. 3). When inserting an intercostal chest drain always insert your finger first and sweep, feeling

for abdominal contents. If a large rupture is present the diagnosis may be easy. Be wary of small tears, particularly following penetrating injury.

Emergency department thoracotomy

Emergency department thoracotomy is only indicated in penetrating chest trauma where the patient either arrests in the emergency department or is pulseless for less than 5 minutes before arrival in the emergency department. Patients with prolonged arrest following penetrating chest trauma and those who arrest after blunt chest trauma are not candidates for resuscitative thoracotomy as the prognosis is universally dismal. By performing an emergency thoracotomy it is possible to release cardiac tamponade by evacuation of pericardial blood, control haemorrhage and repair cardiac or pulmonary injury, perform open cardiac massage and cross clamp the thoracic aorta, redistributing blood to brain and heart. Emergency thoracotomy may be performed via an anterior thoracotomy or median sternotomy, depending on which organ is most likely to be injured. Occasionally, bilateral anterior thoracotomies may be joined across the midline to form a 'clamshell' incision.

> **Key points**
> ■ Most cardiothoracic injuries can be dealt with in the emergency department with simple measures, fluid resuscitation, oxygen and intercostal drain insertion.
> ■ Have a high index of suspicion of contained aortic injury in rapid deceleration injuries, patients with first or second rib fractures, and actively exclude injury.

Abdominal trauma

Trauma to the abdomen is traditionally classified according to the mechanism, either blunt or penetrating injury. Blunt injury is commonly caused by road traffic collisions, whilst penetrating injury is generally caused by interpersonal violence, either stab wounds or gunshot injuries.

Anatomy

The abdominal cavity extends from the lower thorax down into the pelvis. In expiration the diaphragm extends as high as the fifth rib; lower thoracic injuries may injure intra-abdominal organs such as the liver on the right and spleen on the left side. Similarly, injury to the pelvis may involve damage to intra-abdominal organs such as the bladder, rectum and vagina. The solid organs (liver and spleen) are more commonly injured with blunt trauma, whilst with penetrating trauma the commonest organs injured are the liver (due to its size) and the small bowel (due to its central position).

Approach

The approach to a patient with abdominal injuries is a systematic structured approach involving a primary and a secondary survey. In the primary survey it is essential to identify catastrophic intra-abdominal haemorrhage. This is not always straightforward, especially in a patient with an altered mental state such as a patient with an associated head injury or an intoxicated patient. The abdomen is generally assessed as part of the circulation assessment ('C' in the ABCDE system), although in a stable patient it may be deferred until the secondary survey. In the context of trauma, if there is cardiovascular compromise it is likely that the shock is due to blood loss (hypovolaemic shock). Other causes of shock (cardiogenic, neurogenic, obstructive and septic) can occur in trauma but are uncommon. The site of the blood loss must be ascertained urgently. Failure to identify intra-abdominal haemorrhage is one of the leading causes of preventable trauma-related death. Urgent chest and pelvis x-rays can be helpful (Table 1). In a shocked trauma patient with a normal chest x-ray and normal pelvis x-ray, no obvious long bone fractures and no obvious bleeding from open wounds, the most likely source of the blood loss is intra-abdominal haemorrhage. In such a patient resuscitation, surgical involvement and often urgent laparotomy are indicated. Difficulty may arise where a patient has another possible explanation for blood loss, for example a pelvic fracture. Even in such a patient, if they are shocked and intra-abdominal haemorrhage is likely, urgent laparotomy is appropriate. Other tests may help such as ultrasound (FAST: focused assessment with sonography in trauma), diagnostic peritoneal lavage (DPL) and CT. DPL is very rarely undertaken, whilst FAST is being used increasingly (Table 2). Laboratory tests are less important in abdominal trauma. However, a raised amylase or liver transaminases should alert the clinician to the possibility of organ injury. Serial measurement of the haematocrit or haemoglobin, looking for blood loss, can aid conservative management of abdominal injury.

Management

The key to management of intra-abdominal trauma is to have a high index of suspicion. In a persistently shocked patient with a positive abdominal FAST scan (Fig. 1) or with likely intra-abdominal haemorrhage, urgent laparotomy is indicated, with CT scanning being reserved for more stable patients. CT will, however, clearly delineate the nature of the injuries and allow the surgical team to make a more informed management plan. CT is very good at identifying solid organ injury and free fluid but less good at early identification of hollow organ injury (Fig. 2). In countries where experience of managing penetrating injury is relatively rare, most penetrating injuries will require laparotomy. However, in countries where a substantial number of penetrating injuries are seen (e.g. South Africa) a more conservative course is often adopted for stab wounds and, increasingly, gunshot wounds to the abdomen. Solid organ injuries can be managed either surgically or conservatively. The decision lies with the senior surgeon caring for the patient.

Table 1 One of four or one on the floor

In a shocked trauma patient the chances are that the shock is haemorrhagic in nature and due to blood loss:

1. Into the chest: a chest x-ray will help to immediately identify significant intrathoracic blood loss (roughly 500 mL blood can be concealed in each hemithorax on a supine chest x-ray)
2. From a pelvic fracture: this can lead to damage to the presacral venous plexus and profuse haemorrhage. An AP pelvic x-ray will help identify a fracture
3. From long bone fractures: associated haemorrhage from long bones can be considerable, a fractured femur can cause up to 1500 mL of blood loss
4. Intra-abdominal haemorrhage: difficult to diagnose, blood loss is easily concealed. Ultrasound helps to identify significant haemorrhage
5. On the floor – haemorrhage from open wounds can be considerable

---

Table 2 Advantages of DPL, CT and ultrasound

	Advantages	Disadvantages
DPL	Sensitive	Invasive
	At bedside	Does not assess the retroperitoneum
		Not repeatable
		Makes subsequent imaging (ultrasound or CT) difficult to interpret
Ultrasound	At bedside	Sensitivity user dependent
	Reasonably sensitive	Does not assess the retroperitoneum
	Non-invasive	
	Repeatable	
CT	Very sensitive	Transfer required
	Good at assessing retroperitoneum	Stable patient required
		Radiation exposure

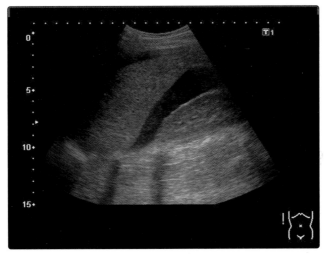

Fig. 1 **A positive FAST scan showing free fluid in the hepatorenal angle (Morrison's pouch).** The fluid appears black and can be seen to be collecting between the liver and the right kidney.

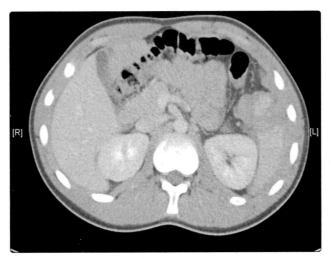

Fig. 2 **CT scan showing a splenic injury.**

Paediatric considerations

- The vast majority of abdominal injuries in children are managed non-surgically.
- If surgical intervention is required in children, it is best undertaken by either a dedicated paediatric surgeon or by an appropriate subspecialty surgeon.
- Always consider a possible non-accidental cause for abdominal injury, especially in younger children.
- An important cause of injury in children involves handlebar injury. As the child falls from the bike they sustain blunt trauma to the abdomen from the handlebars. The injury may take time to manifest fully and children sustaining this injury type generally require a period of observation.
- The ribs are more flexible in children and so provide less protection to the liver and the spleen than in adults. Similarly the bladder is higher in children and less well protected by the pelvis.
- Air swallowing, aerophagia, is a relatively common response to both fear and pain in children. Acute gastric distension can be dramatic causing abdominal distension and tenderness. If identified, the stomach can be decompressed using a nasogastric tube.
- DPL is rarely, if ever, appropriate in children.
- Rectal examination is distressing and rarely helpful in children with abdominal injury. If really felt to be absolutely necessary, it is best undertaken by the most senior surgeon available.

Key points

- Undiagnosed abdominal injury is a major cause of preventable trauma deaths.
- Have a high index of suspicion.
- Have a low threshold for imaging (CT in a stable patient) in suspected abdominal injury.

Lower limb and pelvic trauma

Lower limb and pelvic injuries may follow low or high energy trauma. A pubic ramus fracture may occur to an elderly osteoporotic patient after a fall from standing height or to a young motorcyclist thrown off at speed. Although in both cases a pubic ramus fracture has been sustained, associated injuries and definitive treatment may be very different. Similarly, an intracapsular femoral neck fracture in a 20-year-old is a totally different injury to that in an 80-year-old. Always consider the injury in the appropriate context.

Pelvic trauma

Major pelvic trauma usually becomes apparent when assessing C (circulation). Considerable blood loss may occur into the pelvis and abdomen often due to disruption of the presacral venous plexus. It is essential to stabilize an unstable pelvic injury to prevent continual disruption of the clot and allow formation of a stable clot.

There are essentially three mechanisms of injury that can lead to failure of a stable pelvic ring: anteroposterior compression injury, lateral compression injury and vertical shear injury. The history and pre-hospital information may give clues: a passenger in a car with a side impact is likely to sustain a lateral compression injury whereas a person who falls from a height and lands on one leg is likely to sustain a vertical shear type injury.

Initial assessment and management is by using the standardized structured ABCDE approach (see 'Initial approach to the trauma patient' chapter) with large amounts of cross-matched blood often needed. Specific treatment of the pelvic injury depends upon the pattern of injury. A lateral compression injury is stable and often requires no immediate treatment (Fig. 1). An anteroposterior compression injury (or open book type fracture – the pelvis opens up at the symphysis pubis, much like a book opens) requires a pelvic binder. This may be either a commercially available binder or, if not available, a folded bed sheet wrapped to bind the pelvis. This will help reduce the pelvic volume, stabilize the pelvis and allow a tamponade effect to enhance clot formation. In severe injuries, an external fixator might be applied in the ED by a suitably qualified orthopaedic surgeon (Fig. 2). Occasionally a vertical shear type injury may require a pelvic binder and leg traction on the affected side to stabilize the pelvis and help reduce the leg. If bleeding persists, emergency angiography with embolization may be life-saving. Alternatively a damage control laparotomy and packing of abdomen and pelvis may be required. Since the pelvis is a ring, it is not possible to fracture it in only one place; always check for an anterior injury (pubic symphysis and pubic rami) and posterior injury (sacrum and sacroiliac joints). The posterior injury is often only demonstrated on CT (Fig. 1b).

Lower limb trauma

Hip

Fractures of the neck of the femur are very common and usually occur in osteoporotic, elderly females following low energy injury. Patients present with

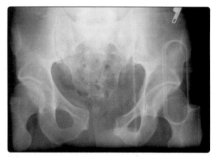

(a)

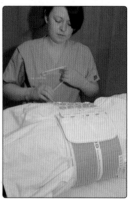

(b)

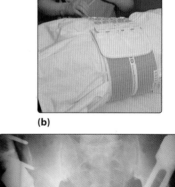

(c)

Fig. 2 **(a) Radiograph of antero-posterior compression injury;** note anterior injury with diastasis of pubic symphysis and posterior injury, opening of sacroiliac joint on the left. **(b) Application of commercially available pelvic binder** allows temporary stabilization of pelvis. **(c) Radiograph post application of anterior external fixator;** note reduction of the pubic symphysis and reconstitution of the pelvic ring.

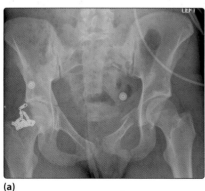

(a)

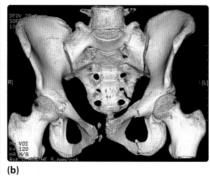

(b)

Fig. 1 **Lateral compression pelvic injury. (a)** AP radiograph of the pelvis showing a lateral compression injury with obvious fractures of the superior and inferior pubic rami on the left. **(b)** 3-D CT of the pelvis showing the superior and inferior pubic rami fractures on the left, an impaction fracture of the right superior pubic ramus; NOTE the posterior injury, impaction fracture of left sacral ali propagating through the sacral foramina.

pain and inability to bear weight; if displaced the patient's leg may be shortened and externally rotated. With impacted minimally displaced fractures, the hip movements may be good, but the patient will not be able to weight bear. If, following an injury, there is persistent hip pain and an inability to weight bear despite normal radiographs, an occult fracture is possible. Further investigation is warranted with a bone scan, CT scan or MRI depending on availability. Over 95% of femoral neck fractures will require operative intervention. Most patients are elderly and will have significant medical co-morbidity. Always consider the reason why the patient has fallen and arrange appropriate investigation. Hip fractures may be either intra- or extracapsular. Intracapsular femoral neck fractures in a young patient are an orthopaedic emergency and need urgent surgery to help minimize the chance of avascular necrosis.

Femur

It takes a considerable force to fracture a femur and it is possible to lose well over a litre of blood, placing a patient into class 1 or class 2 haemorrhagic shock (see Fig. 2 in 'Initial approach to the trauma patient' chapter). After basic resuscitative measures have been undertaken, specific treatment for a femoral shaft fracture includes analgesia, traction and splinting (e.g. with a Thomas splint). Analgesia is best achieved using a femoral nerve block which can be inserted either blind or ultrasound guided. Intravenous opiate analgesia is also required. The majority of femoral shaft fractures will be treated with an intramedullary nail. Always obtain a radiograph of the pelvis with good views of the femoral neck; ipsilateral

femoral neck fractures occur in up to 15% of cases.

Knee

Knee injuries are very common and most are simple sprains. The Ottawa knee rules (Table 1) can be used to predict if a radiograph is needed. It may be difficult to assess ligamentous stability in the acute setting. Treat symptomatically with analgesia, splint and crutches. Arrange follow-up for repeat examination a week later.

Patella dislocation may occur with relatively low energy. The patella always dislocates laterally and will usually reduce spontaneously with knee extension. A true knee dislocation (tibiofemoral joint) is an orthopaedic emergency with injury to the popliteal artery being relatively common.

Tibia

With all tibial shaft fractures consider the possibility of a compartment syndrome (see 'Compartment syndrome' chapter). Compartment syndrome can occur in a simple transverse fracture and in open fractures. Ensure there is adequate analgesia (intravenous opiate analgesia), place the leg in an above-knee backslab and make arrangements for admission and

observation. Definitive treatment depends largely on the fracture pattern and displacement.

Foot and ankle

Most foot and ankle injuries can be dealt with in the ED. The Ottawa ankle rules (Table 2 and Fig. 3) help to identify which patients require radiographs and if so which radiographs are required. If there is an obvious dislocation of the ankle (with or without fracture) and the foot or ankle is grossly deformed it is best to reduce the ankle acutely before radiographs as it is important to minimize skin tension and help prevent tissue necrosis (Fig. 4).

Table 2 **Ottawa ankle rules** (see Fig. 3)
An ankle x-ray is indicated if there is any pain in the malleolar zone and any of these findings:
bone tenderness at A
bone tenderness at B
inability to weight bear both immediately and in the ED
A foot x-ray is indicated if there is any pain in the midfoot zone and any of these findings:
bone tenderness at C
bone tenderness at D
inability to weight bear both immediately and in the ED

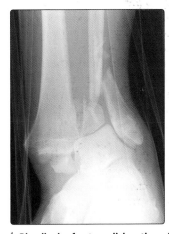

Fig. 4 **Bimalleolar fracture dislocation of the ankle;** note how the skin is tented over the medial side. This ankle should have been reduced prior to the radiograph with simple inline traction ('making a leg look like a leg').

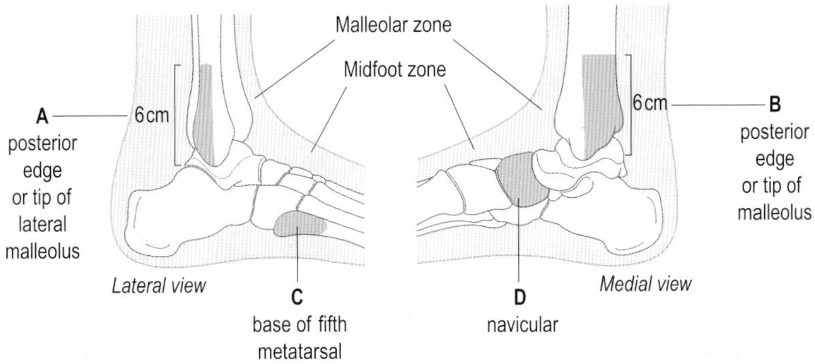

Table 1 **Ottawa knee rules**
A knee x-ray is indicated following knee injuries in patients with any of these findings:
age 55 or over
isolated tenderness of the patella (no bone tenderness of the knee other than the patella)
tenderness at the head of the fibula
inability to flex to 90°
inability to weight bear both immediately and in the casualty department (4 steps – unable to transfer weight twice onto each lower limb regardless of limping)

Malleolar zone

Midfoot zone

A — 6 cm
posterior edge or tip of lateral malleolus

Lateral view

C
base of fifth metatarsal

6 cm — B
posterior edge or tip of malleolus

D
navicular

Medial view

Fig. 3 **Ottawa ankle rules** (see Table 2).

Key points

- Resuscitate appropriately with high energy injuries and consider the reason for the fall in elderly patients.
- Pelvic injuries and femoral shaft fractures can be the source of considerable blood loss.
- Reduce any grossly deformed lower limbs with simple inline traction before obtaining a radiograph.

Upper limb trauma

Upper limb injuries, from the clavicle to the hand, can be caused by a variety of mechanisms and can lead to pain and loss of function if not treated correctly. Adopt a consistent approach with all patients; identify the injury, note the mechanism of injury and the amount of energy the arm has absorbed (fall from standing height as opposed to being thrown from a motorcycle). Establish the patient's functional demands, dominant arm, occupation, sports or hobbies as well as the patient's general health and medical history.

Examine the whole arm; a fall on the outstretched arm may fracture the distal radius at the wrist and injure the radial head at the elbow due to the force being transmitted up the arm. Perform a thorough neurological examination of the arm to exclude brachial plexus or peripheral nerve injury. Obtain adequate x-rays of affected areas, being sure to examine thoroughly the joint above and the joint below any identified injury. If there is any swelling or tenderness obtain an x-ray of the adjacent joints: see Monteggia and Galeazzi fractures (in 'Forearm' section below). Injuries may be bony (fractures) or soft tissue (ligaments, tendons, muscles).

Sternoclavicular joint

Sternoclavicular joint injuries are rare. The joint may dislocate, either anteriorly or posteriorly. Imaging the sternoclavicular joint with plain radiographs is difficult and if an injury is suspected a CT scan will delineate it better. Posterior dislocations may impinge on neurovascular structures in the root of the neck; urgent reduction is required in theatre.

Clavicle

Fractures of the clavicle are very common, the majority being fractures of the middle third. Traditional treatment has been non-operative but consider referral in displaced comminuted fractures. Lateral third clavicle fractures may be displaced or undisplaced. Most are treated non-operatively but some patients with displaced lateral third fractures may benefit from surgery. Acromio-clavicular joint (ACJ) dislocations are common, usually following a fall onto the point of the shoulder. Patients have point tenderness over the ACJ and depending on the severity of the injury, may have a prominence at the ACJ. Treatment is usually non-operative, unless there is dramatic superior or posterior displacement of the clavicle in relation to the acromion. Conservative treatment for both clavicle fractures and ACJ injuries involves a broad arm sling and analgesia followed by gentle mobilization.

Shoulder

Dislocations of the shoulder are very common and the majority of these are anterior dislocations. Posterior dislocations may occur following high energy trauma, seizures and post electrocution. Obtain good quality x-rays including an axillary view if a posterior dislocation is suspected; posterior dislocations are missed due to inadequate x-rays. Reduce the dislocation using gentle traction or a standard manoeuvre such as Milch or Kocher. Sedation may be required. Always obtain post-reduction x-rays.

Fractures of the proximal humerus may be simple (two-part) or complex (four-part). In four-part fractures the vascularity of the head is compromised and patients may require a hemiarthroplasty (shoulder replacement). Beware of soft tissue injuries around the shoulder; if the x-rays are normal and the patient is unable to actively move the arm they may have torn their rotator cuff. Rotator cuff injuries are easily overlooked. Timely repair improves outcome so ensure that the patient has adequate follow-up. Rupture of the long head of biceps leads to a popeye sign. Often this occurs in elderly men and treatment is usually expectant; the deformity does not improve, but shoulder and arm function is usually good.

Humerus

Most humeral shaft fractures will heal with non-operative treatment (Figs 1 and 2). Carefully examine the function of the radial nerve as it may be injured in the spiral groove. Place in a 'U' slab or humeral brace. The patient should be advised to sleep sitting upright for the first 10–14 days as it is often more comfortable. Distal humeral fractures may be extra-articular (supracondylar) or intra-articular. Always examine carefully for neurovascular injury.

Elbow

The elbow is a fairly unforgiving joint; bony and soft tissue injuries often lead to stiffness. Elbow dislocations may be simple or complex (associated with fractures). Carefully assess the distal neurovascular status before reduction. Rupture of the distal tendon of biceps is not uncommon and occasionally missed as the bicipital aponeurosis may remain intact and the patient is still able to flex the elbow. Biceps is only one of a number of elbow flexors, its main function being supination. Early repair improves outcome; delay leads to the potential need for an interposition tendon graft. Triceps

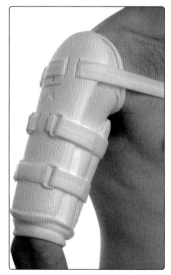

Fig. 1 **Demonstration of humeral brace, used for humeral shaft fractures.**

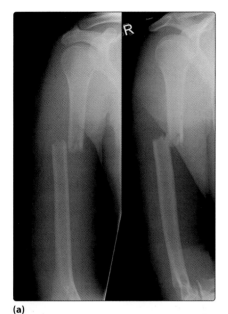

(a)

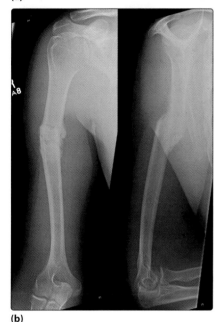

(b)

Fig. 2 **(a) AP and lateral radiographs of humerus showing displaced transverse fracture** – treated non-operatively in humeral brace. **(b) Follow up radiographs at 3 months** demonstrating bony union.

rupture is rare and occasionally missed as gravity extends the elbow. Ensure the patient can actively extend the elbow against gravity. The most common fracture around the elbow is of the radial head. Most radial head fractures are undisplaced or minimally displaced simple fractures. Comminuted and displaced fractures that limit pronation and supination may require repair. Displaced olecranon fractures require fixation to restore the integrity of the extensor mechanism.

Forearm

The forearm can be considered as a joint that allows pronation and supination. In adults an anatomical reduction is required. If both forearm bones are fractured, open reduction and internal fixation is usually required. Undisplaced isolated ulnar shaft fractures (night stick) may be treated non-operatively. Monteggia fractures, a fracture of the ulna with dislocation of the proximal radioulnar joint at the elbow, requires operative repair. A Galeazzi fracture is a fracture of the radius and dislocation of the distal radioulnar joint and also requires operative repair. Examine the patient closely to ensure they are not developing compartment syndrome (see 'Compartment syndrome' chapter).

Wrist

Fractures of the distal radius may have volar or dorsal displacement and be either extra- or intra-articular. Treatment depends upon fracture displacement and the patient's functional demands. Generally, volar displaced and displaced intra-articular fractures require surgical treatment. Dorsally angulated extra-articular fractures of the distal radius ('Colles fracture') are manipulated in the emergency department. If a satisfactory position is obtained, follow-up is arranged in one week to ensure no re-displacement. Check for median nerve compression.

The most commonly injured carpal bone is the scaphoid. Patients present following a fall onto the outstretched hand with tenderness in the anatomical snuffbox. The initial radiographs, which should include scaphoid views, may be normal. Further imaging is required to rule out a scaphoid fracture. Depending on local availability, an MRI, spiral CT or bone scan may give an immediate answer. Alternatively, patients with a possible scaphoid fracture may be placed in a futura splint and reviewed at 2 weeks. If tenderness persists repeat x-rays will be required. Ligamentous injuries around the wrist include scapholunate dissociation, which may be subtle and require stress x-rays to demonstrate. Carpal

dislocation most commonly involves the lunate and usually follows a high energy injury (Fig. 3). Check for median nerve injury. These injuries require urgent reduction.

Hand

See 'Hand injuries' chapter.

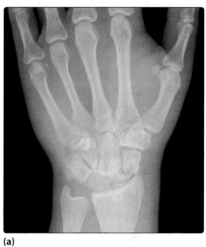

(a)

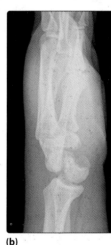

(b)

Fig. 3 **Trans-scaphoid perilunate dislocation. (a)** AP view; note scaphoid fracture. **(b)** Lateral view; note dorsal translation of carpus and empty lunate.

Key points

- The aim of treating upper limb injuries is prompt, safe return of maximum function.

- Examine the whole upper limb, particularly the joint above and below any injury.

- Examine the peripheral nerves carefully.

- Do not forget in the absence of a bony injury the potential for soft tissue injuries.

- Never accept suboptimal x-rays.

Hand injuries

Hand injuries are common yet very important presentations to the emergency department. Prompt, accurate evaluation and appropriate treatment will limit disability from the injury.

Take a thorough history, noting:

- mechanism of injury; if caused by glass consider radiograph for retained foreign body
- time since injury
- patient's functional demands (occupation and hobbies)
- dominance (remember the non-dominant hand is also important, it holds the thing the dominant hand is working on)
- significant medical history (diabetes, allergies).

Examination

Basic nomenclature: name the digits (thumb, index, long, ring, little) do not number them. It is permissible to number the metacarpals. Avoid using medial and lateral, use radial and ulnar. Avoid anterior and posterior, use palmar (or volar) and dorsal.

Examine the hand carefully, noting resting posture of the hand, site of wounds, swelling or tenderness. Document perfusion; palpate the radial and ulnar arteries. The ulnar artery is usually the dominant artery but may be congenitally absent (Allen's test); check capillary refill, normally under 2 seconds.

Test sensation with light touch and two-point discrimination (use paper clip): Abnormal if >6 mm on static testing and >3 mm on moving two-point discrimination. Use other fingers or the opposite hand to compare.

When testing the motor component of the nerve supply to hand, remember that there is some crossover of supply between the ulnar and median nerves.

For ulnar nerve function, test the intrinsic muscles of hand, test and palpate first dorsal interosseous muscle in the first web space. For median nerve motor function at the wrist level, it is best to test abductor policis brevis (APB); with hand flat on table palm up, ask patient to push thumb away from palm towards the ceiling.

Fingertip injuries

Crush injuries to the fingertip are very common. They range from a simple subungual haematoma to fingertip amputations. Trephine (drain) subungual haematomas that are very painful; it is still permissible to trephine a subungual haematoma in the presence of a tuft fracture of the distal phalanx. When the nail has been avulsed from the nail bed it is important to reduce it back under the nail fold. Nail bed lacerations should be repaired using 6-0 or 7-0 absorbable suture or glue; replace the nail to splint the nail bed. Open fractures of the distal phalanx require prophylactic antibiotics. Fingertip pulp injuries with minimal or no bone exposure can be treated conservatively using serial non-adherent dressings, allowing the wound to heal by secondary intention. Fingertips contain no muscle and so can tolerate longer periods of ischaemia, approximately 8 hours for warm ischaemic time and 30 hours for cold ischaemic time. Wrap the amputated part in sterile gauze moistened in normal saline, place in a sterile plastic bag, then place the sealed bag in a mixture of ice and water to keep cold. This avoids freezing and soaking the affected part. Consider all fingertip amputations for replantation, particularly thumb amputations where digit length is very important.

Penetrating injuries to the hand and wrist

A thorough knowledge of hand and wrist anatomy is needed to exclude injury to vital structures of the hand and wrist. Identify the location/trajectory of the wound, consider and actively exclude injuries to the underlying structures. Beware of partial tendon injuries. If the injury was caused by glass, obtain a radiograph to look for foreign bodies.

Closed tendon injuries

It is possible to avulse tendons from bone, e.g. mallet finger. The flexor and extensor tendons of the hand have unique anatomy leading to certain specific injuries. Clinical examination needs to test all the tendons and their components.

Relevant anatomy

Extensor tendons. The index and little fingers have two extensor tendons; the other fingers only have one. All the tendons form an extensor tendon hood at the level of the finger. A central slip inserts into the base of the middle phalanx, two lateral bands travel alongside the central slip, joining together in the midline distally as they insert into the base of the distal phalanx.

Flexor tendons. The thumb has one long flexor; the fingers have two flexor tendons, flexor digitorum profundus (FDP) and flexor digitorum superficialis (FDS). FDS inserts via two slips into the volar aspect of the middle phalanx; FDP travels deep to FDS and emerges between the two slips of FDS to insert into the base of the distal phalanx. Hence in penetrating injuries it is important to test independently both FDS and FDP to all the fingers.

Mallet finger

Usually caused by a direct blow to the tip of the finger, e.g. while catching a ball or tucking in bed sheets, causing forced flexion to the distal interphalangeal joint (DIPJ). The extensor tendon is avulsed from the distal phalanx, resulting in drooping of the distal phalanx with loss of active extension. Full passive extension is still possible. It is important to obtain a radiograph to exclude a bony mallet; occasionally a bony flake may be avulsed and if it constitutes >30% of the joint surface area, or if the joint is subluxed, surgical treatment should be considered (Fig. 1). Standard treatment is with a mallet splint, holding the DIPJ continuously in extension for 6 weeks (Fig. 2).

Central slip extensor tendon injury

This occurs when the proximal interphalangeal joint (PIPJ) is forcibly flexed during active extension. Volar

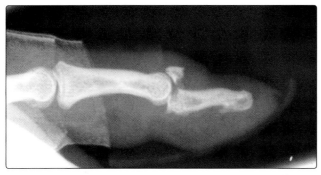

Fig. 1 **X-ray of a bony mallet injury.** Note the joint is subluxed in the mallet splint and the fragment is 30% of the joint surface; these injuries require surgical treatment.

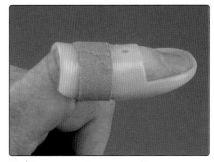

Fig. 2 **Mallet splint.** Note position of strapping; the PIPJ is left free to allow flexion of PIPJ.

dislocation of the PIPJ may also cause central slip tendon rupture. Look for tenderness over the dorsal aspect of the middle phalanx. Perform Elson's test: place the finger over the edge of a table, with PIPJ flexed to 90° and ask patient to extend finger against resistance. Weakness of resisted extension of the PIPJ and hyperextension of the DIPJ occurs if the central slip is ruptured. Treatment involves splinting the finger in full extension for 6 weeks. A delay in treatment may lead to a Boutonnière deformity.

Rugger jersey finger

The FDP tendon is avulsed from the base of the distal phalanx, commonly involving the ring finger. Test for active flexion of DIPJ and obtain a radiograph looking for a flake of bone attached to the end of the avulsed tendon. This is best seen on the lateral radiograph. These injuries may require surgical repair.

Fractures and dislocations

When dealing with any fracture of the fingers or metacarpals ensure there is no rotational deformity by looking at the orientation of the nails with the fingers held straight (Fig. 3a). Ask the patient to flex the fingers (make a fist) to see if they cross over each other, ensuring all the fingers point towards the base of the scaphoid (Fig. 3b). Refer all fractures with an unstable fracture pattern and with rotational deformity to a hand surgeon.

Dislocations of the interphalangeal (IP) joints are usually reduced with in-line traction. Test stability of joint post reduction, particularly the stability of the collateral ligaments. Palmar dislocations are best immobilized with the IP joints in extension, using a

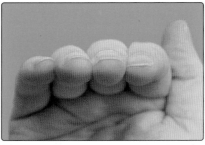
(a)

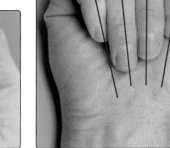
(b)

Fig. 3 **With phalangeal and metacarpal injuries it is important to exclude rotational deformity. (a)** Look at fingers end on, noting orientation of nails. **(b)** Flex fingers into palm; in general they should all point towards the base of the scaphoid bone.

Zimmer splint (Fig. 4). Dorsal dislocations if unstable should be immobilized in slight flexion. It is best to use a dorsal blocking splint, allowing active flexion but limiting extension.

Metacarpophalangeal joint (MCPJ) dislocations may be difficult to reduce. They are best pushed back into place rather than simply pulled with in-line traction. Particularly in complex dislocations of the thumb MCPJ, traction may further entrap the head of the proximal phalanx.

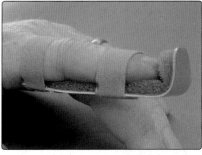

Fig. 4 **Demonstration of Zimmer splint immobilizing IP joints in extension;** note the splint is not folded around the tip of the finger. The perfusion of the finger may easily be assessed.

> ### Key points
>
> - Most hand injuries are fairly simple and can be managed in the emergency department.
> - It is important to have a thorough knowledge of hand anatomy and function.
> - Inappropriate treatment and missed injuries will often significantly compromise outcome.
>
> - Beware of partial tendon injuries.
> - With metacarpal and phalangeal fractures, ensure that there is no rotational deformity.

Maxillofacial trauma

The primary concern in a patient with a maxillofacial injury is airway management.

With respect to the injury, the face can be divided into three parts:

- the upper face; fractures involve the frontal bone and frontal sinus
- the midface, fractures involve the nasal bones, nasoethmoidal complex, zygomaticomaxillary complex, or the orbital floor
- the lower face, fractures are isolated to the mandible.

In mid-third facial fractures, the need for definitive airway protection should be assessed as early as possible, as swelling and oedema can quickly cause airway compromise. Examine the mouth and oropharynx, remove any avulsed teeth, dentures or denture fragments and gently aspirate any blood or saliva under direct vision. If able to, allow the patient to hold the suction catheter to clear out their own mouth.

The facial bones and soft tissue have a rich blood supply and can bleed profusely. Control bleeding from mucosal and facial lacerations by suturing wounds. It can be difficult to control the bleeding before bony stability is achieved. Reduce displaced fractures and teeth where possible. Epistaxis is common even following minor trauma (see 'Ear, nose and throat, and facial emergencies' chapter).

Beware of associated injuries. Have a high index of suspicion and actively exclude cervical spine injury, which occurs in up to a fifth of patients with serious facial injuries (see 'Head and spinal trauma' chapter). Ocular injuries are commonly seen with frontal bone fractures. Examine the eyes carefully, particularly the cornea, visual acuity, visual fields and eye movements. Check for intraocular foreign bodies, globe rupture, hyphaema, vitreous haemorrhage and retinal detachment.

Mandible dislocation/ subluxation

This can follow a direct blow to the chin while the mouth is open but often occurs spontaneously while yawning. Patients present with an open mouth, with the jaw jutting forward, and they are unable to close their mouth. In the setting of trauma, obtain radiographs to exclude a fracture of the mandible. Reduce the jaw by placing your thumbs over the lower molars pushing the mandible down and back. Sedation may help relax the jaw. Patients with connective tissue disorders (Marfan's syndrome, Ehlers–Danlos syndrome) may have recurrent dislocations.

Mandibular fractures

Ask the patient if their teeth fit together properly, and check for abnormal dental occlusion and for steps or gaps between the teeth. Look inside the mouth to identify missing or loose teeth, dento-alveolar fractures, and presence and extent of mucosal lacerations (see 'Dental emergencies' chapter). Patients with mandibular fractures commonly have sublingual haematomas. Mental nerve paraesthesia may be associated with displaced fractures. Treatment depends on the fracture pattern and displacement. Undisplaced fractures may be treated non-operatively with analgesia and soft diet. If displaced or mobile they are best treated with open reduction and internal fixation. A soft cervical collar can be used to support midline mandibular fractures in the short term.

Maxillary fractures

Maxillary fractures are normally caused by high energy trauma. Examine carefully to exclude injury to underlying vessels, nerves (facial nerve), and the lacrimal and parotid ducts. Midface fractures are characterized by symmetrical facial swelling, bilateral periorbital ecchymosis and subconjunctival haemorrhage. Test mobility of the maxilla by stabilizing the patient's head with one hand; using the thumb and forefinger of the other hand, grasp the anterior maxillary ridge and push pull the midface. Palpate the forehead, orbital rims and zygoma for steps.

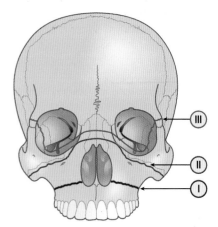

Fig. 1 **Le Fort classification of mid-third facial fractures.**

Exclude a frontal sinus fracture in patients with deep lacerations to the lower forehead, particularly if they have other midface fractures. Look for signs of base of skull fracture such as CSF rhinorrhoea.

Mid-third facial fractures are classified according to the Le Fort classification (Fig. 1):

- I: Low level above the nasal floor (swelling of upper lip)
- II: Subzygomatic (massive swelling or ballooning of face)
- III: Suprazygomatic (massive swelling of face and CSF rhinorrhoea).

Most mid-third fractures are treated by open reduction and internal fixation.

Zygomatic (malar) fractures

These are commonly caused by a punch to the face. Patients may notice their face swells after blowing their nose. Bony tenderness or flattening of the zygomatic arch with a palpable step suggests a fracture of the zygomatic arch. Examine the eye and periorbital region carefully for lateral subconjunctival haemorrhage, eye movements and diplopia. Diplopia, particularly on upward gaze, may occur in orbital blow-out fractures, where the rectus muscle becomes trapped (Figs 2 and 3). Test sensation below the eye as infraorbital nerve injury may occur. Undisplaced, uncomplicated fractures require no active treatment. Depressed and complicated fractures require elevation and internal fixation. All patients must be advised not to blow their nose, as increased pressure in the maxillary antrum causes air to leak into the soft tissues of the face through the fracture.

Nasal complex

Evaluate the nose for symmetry and mobility. Stand behind and above the seated patient and look down the length of the nose to look for asymmetry. Look in each nostril to localize bleeding areas or haematomas, particularly in the area of the nasal septum. A septal haematoma devascularizes the underlying septal cartilage and may lead to cartilage necrosis with resulting septal perforation. Refer nasal fractures with a septal haematoma immediately (Fig. 4). If the nose is too swollen to assess for underlying deformity, then review in outpatients within a week, once the swelling has diminished. Displaced asymmetrical nasal fractures should be reduced within 2 weeks. Radiographs of the nasal complex are not indicated.

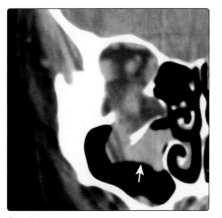

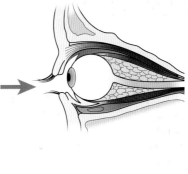

Fig. 2 **A coronal CT scan showing an extensive orbital blow-out fracture.** Notice how the soft tissue of the orbit (rectus muscle) has extruded into the roof of the maxillary antrum.

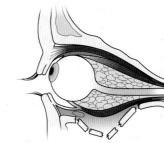

Fig. 3 **Orbital blow-out fracture.**

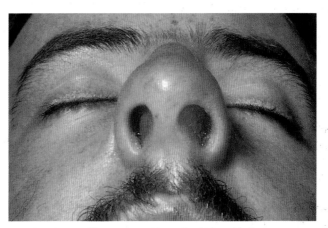

Fig. 4 **A post-traumatic septal haematoma.** Notice the thickened bulky septum encroaching on the nasal airways. The external nose is also swollen.

> ### Key points
>
> - There is significant risk to airway patency in mid-third facial fractures; intubate early.
>
> - Facial trauma may bleed profusely; reduce teeth and fractures, temporarily stabilize the jaw and suture lacerations.
>
> - Beware of associated injuries to cervical spine and eyes.

Burns

The majority of patients presenting to the emergency department (ED) with a burn will have a minor burn that can be easily dealt with in the ED. Major burns require prompt resuscitation. After initial resuscitation and management, patients with major burns should be transferred to a specialist centre (Table 1).

In the management of multiply injured patients complicated by burns it is important to initially stabilize the patient and consider the other injuries prior to transfer to a burns unit.

Initial management

If not already performed, the burn needs to be cooled by irrigation or immersion in tepid water. This is effective in limiting further injury for up to 20 minutes after the injury. In children be very careful when cooling large burns as cooling may cause hypothermia. In chemical burns never neutralize an acid with alkali or vice versa. Irrigate with copious amounts of water to dilute and remove the chemical. Remove any loose skin and dress wound, once the total burnt surface area (TBSA) and depth have been estimated. Always consider the need for analgesia; large burns commonly require opiate analgesia. Assess the need for tetanus immunization.

Assessment of burns

When assessing a patient with a burn it is essential to consider the age, co-morbidity and social circumstances.

Locally important factors to assess are:

- burn depth
- total burnt surface area (TBSA).

Table 1 Burns centre referral/transfer criteria

- Full thickness burns in any age group
- Partial thickness burns greater than 10% (TBSA) adult, 5% (TBSA) child
- Burns involving face, hands, feet, genitalia, perineum or major joints
- Circumferential burns to chest, torso or limb
- Electrical burns, including lightning injury
- Chemical burns >5% TBSA (hydrofluoric acid burn >1%)

Burn depth

Burn depth is important since the deeper the burn the longer it will take to heal. In general aim for a burn to heal within 3 weeks.

Burns can be classified into three groups according to the depth of the burn (Fig. 1).

- Superficial (epidermal) – the burn affects the epidermis but not the dermis, e.g. sunburn.
- Partial thickness burns (dermal) – the burn does not extend through all skin layers. Partial thickness burns are further divided into:
  superficial partial thickness (dermal) – the burn extends through the epidermis into the upper layers of the dermis and is associated with blistering
  deep partial thickness (dermal) – the burn extends through the epidermis and into the deeper layers of the dermis but not through the entire dermis.
- Full thickness burns – the burn extends through all skin layers into the subcutaneous tissue.

The estimation of burn depth can be very difficult, especially in fresh burns. It is important to look at several elements when trying to decide the depth.

- Bleeding on needle prick (21-gauge needle) – no bleeding suggests a full thickness burn.
- Sensation – diminished pain perception with needle prick suggests a deep dermal injury, full thickness burns are insensate.
- Appearance and blanching on pressure – the simple appearance of a burn can be deceptive. Apply pressure using a sterile cotton bud (microbiology swab), and assess

capillary refill. A red, moist burn that obviously blanches and then rapidly refills is superficial. A pale, dry but blanching burn that regains its colour slowly is superficial dermal. Deep dermal injuries have a mottled cherry red colour that do not blanch. Full thickness burns are dry, leathery or waxy and do not blanch.

Total burnt surface area (TBSA)

When assessing the TBSA do not include areas with simple erythema. There are three ways of estimating burn area.

1. Palmar surface: the palmar surface area (including fingers) is roughly 0.8% of body surface area.
2. Rule of nines: the body is divided into areas of 9%. Useful for medium size burns in adults, but is not very accurate in children (Fig. 2).
3. Lund–Browder chart: this is the most accurate method of calculating the TBSA (Fig. 3).

Fluid resuscitation

Patients with burns can lose excessive volumes of fluid from the burn. Adults with a TBSA >15% and children with a TBSA >10% require fluid resuscitation. The important principles of fluid resuscitation of burns patients are:

- TBSA is area where the burn is partial thickness or deeper; do not include areas of simple erythema.
- Use the time of burn, not time of admission when calculating fluid administration.
- All formulas are a guide; the end point is adequate tissue perfusion, as indicated by a urine output of 0.5–1.0 mL/kg/hour in adults and 1.0–1.5 mL/kg/hour in children.

The Parkland formula is commonly used and is relatively straightforward to use:

- For the first 24 hours use a crystalloid, e.g. 0.9% saline (normal saline).
- Total fluid requirement in 24 hours = 4 mL × (TBSA as percentage) × (body weight in kg)

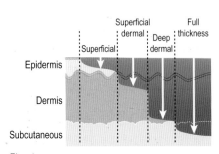

Fig. 1 **Depth of burn.**

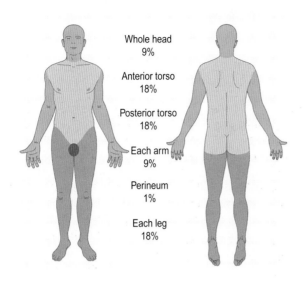

Fig. 2 **Wallace rule of nines.**

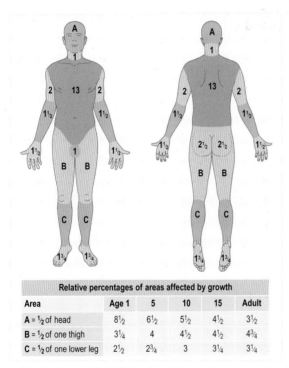

Relative percentages of areas affected by growth					
Area	Age 1	5	10	15	Adult
A = ½ of head	8½	6½	5½	4½	3½
B = ½ of one thigh	3¼	4	4½	4½	4¾
C = ½ of one lower leg	2½	2¾	3	3¼	3¼

Fig. 3 **Lund–Browder chart to calculate TBSA.**

- If the wound is likely to heal by secondary intention within 3 weeks continue with dressings (see below specialist dressings).
- If likely to take longer than 3 weeks to heal refer to a plastic surgeon/ burn service.

Depending on how healing is progressing, change the dressing every 2 to 5 days. Dressings should be changed earlier if the wound becomes painful or smelly or the dressing becomes soaked.

Specialist dressings

- Silver sulfadiazine cream (Flamazine) – effective against Gram-negative bacteria.
- Hydrocolloid occlusive dressing (Granuflex) – adhesive and waterproof.
- Non-adhesive silicone dressing (such as Mepitel) – easy removal.

Paediatric considerations

- Beware hypothermia if cooling large surface area.
- Refer to burn centre if TBSA >5%.
- Institute fluid resuscitation if TBSA >10%.
- TBSA estimation – rule of nines is less reliable; use Lund–Browder chart or palm of hand.
- Add maintenance fluid to resuscitation fluid, aim for urine output >1.0– 1.5 mL/kg/hour.
- Use non-adhesive silicone dressings since they are less adherent to wounds.

- 50% given in first 8 hours, 50% given in next 16 hours (times since burn).
- This volume is in addition to maintenance fluid.

If there is muscle damage, then aim to achieve a higher urine output (1.5–2 mL/kg/hour) to help prevent rhabdomyolysis.

Dressings

Initially, it is easiest to dress the wound with simple clingfilm. The commercially available roll is essentially sterile if the first few centimetres are discarded. Lay the clingfilm on the wound and avoid creating a constricting circumferential dressing. If the patient is not being transferred use simple paraffin gauze (Jelonet) with dressing gauze, adding a layer of absorbent gauze or wool and firm (not tight) crepe bandage. Silver sulfadiazine cream (Flamazine) is a good dressing. In general, however, it is best to avoid topical ointments initially since they make burn depth estimation difficult. Review the burn in 24 hours when burn depth and size can be more accurately assessed. A decision needs to be made at this stage:

Key points

- With all burns assess the depth and area of the burn.
- Consider the need for transfer to a specialist burn centre.
- Assessment of depth of burn may be misleading in the first 24 hours.

Wound management

The ultimate goal with all wound management is reconstitution of the integrity of the skin and underlying structures in a safe, efficient manner with minimal residual scarring. Optimal wound healing conditions involve maintenance of a moist, warm environment until epithelialization occurs, followed by avoidance of UV light exposure for up to 6 months.

History

When taking a history consider both the wound and the general condition of the patient.

- Wound. What caused the wound? Was it a sharp or blunt injury? If involving broken glass, consider retained foreign bodies. Clean knife or rusty nail? How long is it since the wound occurred (greater or less than 6 hours)?
- Patient. Consider anything that may impair wound healing or predispose to infection; for example diabetes, immunocompromise for any reason, medication (steroids, immunosuppressive agents, anticoagulants), allergies (local anaesthetic, latex, antibiotics, iodine), prosthetic heart valve (need for antibiotic prophylaxis). Always establish tetanus immunization status.

Examination

Assess and document the dimensions, and level of contamination of the wound. If overlying a joint, move the joint through a full range of motion while examining the wound. Examine neurovascular status before using any local anaesthetic; check light touch and two-point discrimination. Actively exclude tendon injury and beware of partial tendon lacerations.

Obtain an x-ray if an underlying fracture is possible, e.g. crush injuries or lacerations with heavy objects (axe/sword), or to look for radio-opaque foreign material. Wounds with high suspicion for retained foreign bodies should be further investigated with radiographs. If concern for radiolucent foreign bodies exists consider an ultrasound or CT.

Treatment

Cleaning the wound is the most important aspect of initial wound treatment. The volume of solution used is more important than the type. Avoid antiseptic solutions as they are tissue toxic. Irrigate under clean tap water if possible and remove all foreign material. Excise obvious non-viable tissue, being careful not to excise normal tissue, especially on the hands or face. Remove all grit and gravel to prevent permanent tattooing. Clip or comb hair away from a wound rather than shaving the skin.

Methods of wound closure (Figs 1 and 2):

- Primary closure. The wound edges are approximated after thorough debridement and cleaning of the wound at the time of initial presentation. There are several methods of wound edge approximation (Table 1).
- Delayed primary closure. Consider if the wound is at increased risk of complications; for example, a grossly contaminated wound or wound greater than 6 hours old. Simply wash out, debride and dress the wound. If the wound remains clean and not infected, close the wound 2 to 5 days later.
- Secondary intention. Consider for very small wounds, bites or contaminated wounds not suitable for delayed primary closure. Apply repeated dressings, allowing the wound to heal on its own. It usually takes a lot longer for a wound to heal by secondary intention and leaves a less cosmetic scar, but is safer than closing a contaminated/infected wound.

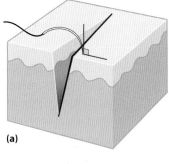

(a)

Insert needle through the skin with the point at right angles to the skin

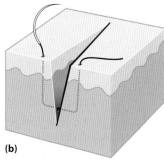

(b)

Symmetry is important, ensure the entry and exit points are equidistant from the wound edges, and ensure depth of tissue bite on both sides is similar

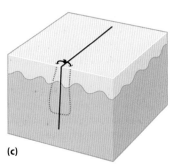

(c)

With suture knotted approximate wound edges, everting slightly if possible, try not to invert wound edges (leads to more cosmetic wound)

Fig. 1 **Technique for a simple suture. (a)** Insert needle through the skin with the point at right angles to the skin. **(b)** Symmetry is very important; ensure the entry and exit points are equidistant from the wound edges, and ensure depth of tissue bite on both sides is similar. **(c)** With suture knotted, approximate wound edges, everting slightly if possible, try not to invert wound edges (eversion leads to more cosmetic wound).

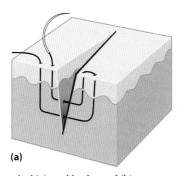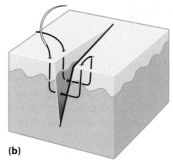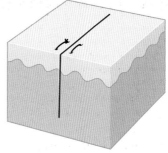

(a)   (b)

Fig. 2 **A vertical (a), and horizontal (b) mattress suture.** Vertical and horizontal mattress sutures are used for deeper wounds and help evert wound edges.

Table 1 **Methods for primary skin closure**		
Method of closure	**Advantages**	**Disadvantages**
Steristrips	No needles needed. Quick and easy to apply Useful for skin lacerations in elderly skin	Realistically not possible to close large deep wounds that are under tension, if gets wet Steristrips flake off
Tissue glue	No needles needed. Quick and easy to apply Cosmetically similar to sutures in wounds <4 cm. Produces a waterproof seal and is possible to get wet, sloughs off spontaneously, no need for removal. Cheaper than sutures	Not good for wounds over or around joints Becomes brittle on drying and cracks Not good for large wounds or wounds under tension; however, can be used in conjunction with deep absorbable sutures
Sutures	Very versatile, using absorbable and non-absorbable sutures	Requires local anaesthetic with or without procedural sedation Non-absorbable skin sutures require removal
Staples	Very quick and easy to use	More painful to remove than conventional sutures

- Plastic surgical techniques. Large wounds with tissue or skin loss may require plastic surgical input for a skin graft or soft tissue flap.

Special types of wound:

- Puncture wounds – clean thoroughly and prescribe prophylactic antibiotics.
- Pre-tibial wounds – in elderly or patients on steroids. Approximate (not necessarily close) the wound edges with Steristrips, and apply a non-adherent dressing.
- Fingertip injuries – see 'Hand injuries' chapter.
- Animal bites – generally, animal bites are best not sutured. Seek specialist opinion for deep lacerations on the hand or face. Give prophylactic antibiotics (co-amoxiclav) if the wound is deep, or on the hands or face. Universal prescription of prophylactic antibiotics for all bite wounds is not indicated. Check tetanus status.
- Human bites – human bites are more likely to become infected than dog bites. Remember to assess the risk for transmission of blood-borne viral infections (hepatitis, HIV). Beware of the 'fight bite', where a patient punches someone in the

mouth and a tooth lacerates the knuckle; this wound commonly involves the extensor tendon and the MCP joint. The cut may be deceptively small but requires aggressive, active treatment to avoid infection of the MCP joint. Clenched-fist human bite wounds are at highest risk for infection and mandate prophylactic antibiotic therapy; refer to a hand surgeon for surgical debridement.

Wounds that require referral to a plastic surgeon:

- anatomically complex wounds (eyelids, nasal septum, lips)
- suspected associated nerve or tendon injury
- extensive soft tissue loss
- retained foreign bodies
- pretibial lacerations with extensive skin loss
- 'fight bite' – tooth injury to MCP joint
- high pressure jet injuries.

Tetanus immunization

A total of five doses of tetanus vaccine are considered to provide lifelong immunity. This is usually achieved by

a primary three-dose course in infancy, followed by school entry and school-leaving boosters; or as a primary course at any time, followed by a booster 10 years later and a further booster 10 years after that. Treatment depends on the patient's immunization status and whether the wound is clean or tetanus prone.

Tetanus prone wounds include:

- wounds or burns sustained more than 6 hours before surgical treatment
- wounds with a significant degree of devitalized tissue (crush wounds)
- puncture-type wounds
- contact with soil or manure likely to harbour tetanus organisms
- clinical evidence of sepsis.

Thorough surgical debridement and irrigation of the wound is essential whatever the tetanus immunization history. Specific tetanus prophylaxis should be administered.

Paediatric considerations

It is important to consider the rapid healing potential of children. Most small (<4 cm) clean wounds may be simply glued together with tissue adhesive. Similarly, for deep wounds consider using deep absorbable sutures with glue for the skin; it provides a waterproof seal and obviates the need for later suture removal. It is, however, important to ensure the wound is thoroughly cleaned; this may require the administration of local anaesthetic (see 'Pain management and procedural sedation' and 'Local anaesthesia' chapters).

Key points

- Wound irrigation and cleaning are key.
- Primary closure is the preferred approach.
- Ensure that underlying structures have been assessed thoroughly before wound closure.

Compartment syndrome

Compartment syndrome occurs when the pressure within a closed osseofascial compartment becomes raised sufficiently to impair capillary blood flow. This impairment of capillary blood flow leads to tissue ischaemia and ultimately cellular hypoxia. There are several reasons why the pressure within a particular osseofascial compartment may increase (Table 1). Compartment syndrome may develop anywhere, the commonest sites being the lower leg and the forearm, and the commonest cause is a long bone fracture.

Symptoms and signs

The diagnosis of a compartment syndrome is largely a clinical one and it is essential to have a high index of suspicion. The cardinal symptom of a compartment syndrome is pain and the cardinal sign is pain on passive stretch. The pain experienced is severe and unrelenting and may be out of proportion to the clinical signs. The affected compartment may feel tense and may be tender to touch. With advanced tissue ischaemia, paraesthesia, pulselessness and pallor may be present; but these are late signs. Paraesthesia suggests nerve ischaemia which has been present for at least one hour. Pulselessness is a very late sign; the capillary microcirculation is interrupted at a much lower pressure, long before the pressure rises enough to limit arterial blood flow. It is imperative to diagnose compartment syndrome before these late signs are present.

Investigations

The diagnosis is largely clinical; further investigation is only required where the diagnosis is in doubt and in patients with an impaired level of consciousness. In these circumstances compartment pressure monitoring may help to confirm or exclude the diagnosis. Several commercially available compartment pressure monitors are available but it is possible to use a pressure transducer to make a compartment pressure monitor (Fig. 1). Ideally a side-ported 18-gauge needle should be used since using a standard hypodermic needle tends to overestimate the pressure. For fractures, the highest pressure is usually at, or near, the fracture site. Measure the pressure near the fracture. If this is normal also, measure 5 cm proximal and 5 cm distal to the fracture. Measure the pressure in all the compartments of the affected area. An absolute pressure of 30 mmHg or a pressure difference (diastolic pressure – compartment pressure) less than or equal to 30 mmHg is indicative of a compartment syndrome. It is important to interpret the reading in the clinical context and if needed consider continuous pressure monitoring or repeat the measurements, e.g. intubated patients.

Treatment

The definitive treatment of a compartment syndrome is fasciotomy. A fasciotomy is the surgical release of all the compartments in the area involved (Fig. 2).

Simple measures may help to minimize ischaemia while awaiting definitive surgery.

1. Elevation to the level of the heart or just above; avoid extreme elevation since this reduces the inflow pressure.
2. Split circumferential dressings or casts down to the skin.
3. For circumferential burns perform an escharotomy (longitudinal incision through burnt tissue, releasing constricting burnt tissue).
4. For patients with a bleeding disorder, correct any coagulation abnormalities.

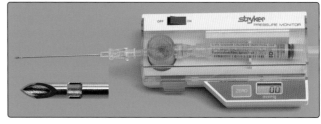

Fig. 1 **Commercially available pressure monitor;** note inset photo a side-ported needle; standard 18-gauge needles tend to overestimate the pressure.

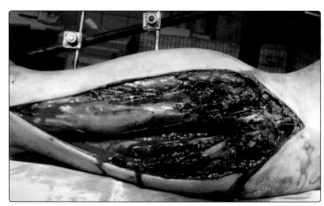

Fig. 2 **Fasciotomy of the lower leg for compartment syndrome.**

Table 1 **Causes of compartment syndrome for patients presenting to the emergency department**
■ Trauma with either fracture or soft tissue injuries
■ Circumferential dressings or plaster cast
■ Coagulation abnormalities with haematoma formation
■ Prolonged sustained pressure in an obtunded patient
■ Circumferential burns

Key points

■ Compartment syndrome is a clinical diagnosis; have a high index of suspicion at all times, not only in severe bony injuries.

■ Increasing severe pain and pain on passive stretch are important signs and symptoms. Beware the unconscious or intubated patient; if in doubt obtain senior input and measure compartment pressures.

Emergency presentations

What we see depends mainly on what we look for

Sir John Lubbock

Chest pain

Introduction

Chest pain is the second most common reason for attendance to an emergency department (ED), accounting for 3% of visits. Cardiac conditions are the commonest cause of chest pain in the ED population but the underlying diagnosis can vary from life-threatening conditions such as myocardial infarction, through to the trivial such as chest wall pain due to simple musculoskeletal strain. Between these extremes lie many varied diagnoses, providing a challenge for the emergency physician who has the task of recognizing and selecting those patients at high risk of serious disease.

As with most emergency conditions, making an accurate diagnosis of chest pain depends upon focused points in the history of the illness as well as a careful examination and appropriate investigations. When compiling a differential diagnosis for chest pain, consider the different organs and systems present in the upper torso which are the likely sources of the patient's pain (Fig. 1). Pain may be classified as visceral, somatic or referred. Visceral pain originates from the affected organ such as the heart, lungs or oesophagus and can be difficult to differentiate. Somatic pain arises from chest wall structures and can often be localized. Referred pain is commonly from abdominal pathology.

Differential diagnosis and key diagnostic points

In the ED it may be more useful to categorize chest pain diagnoses into *life-threatening* (Table 1) and *non-life-threatening* (Table 2). The *life-threatening* diagnoses are those which, if missed or managed inappropriately, are likely to lead to serious morbidity or mortality. These conditions must be recognized or excluded, whether by a history and examination focusing on recognized discriminating points, or by obtaining investigations to exclude the suspected diagnosis. Once the life-threatening diagnoses have been excluded, the *non-life-threatening* diagnoses can be considered.

Emergency management

On presentation to the ED, any patient complaining of ongoing chest pain should be triaged as high priority to a monitored area, where they should receive high flow oxygen and soluble aspirin (usually 300 mg). Vital signs should be measured and cardiac monitoring and pulse oximetry applied, a 12-lead electrocardiogram (ECG) should be obtained and an intravenous cannula sited. This should take no more than 10 minutes. The urgency of this approach is important, not only because of the seriousness of some of the potential differential diagnoses, but also because of the need for rapid intervention in conditions such as ST-elevation myocardial infarction.

Following this initial triage, a focused primary survey (ABCDE) is completed, followed by a focused history of the presenting problem and relevant past history. Early administration of analgesia is important for patients with chest pain. Not only does it relieve their suffering, it also decreases sympathetic drive, with potential benefits for several of the life-threatening diagnoses, e.g. myocardial infarction (MI), acute coronary syndrome (ACS) and aortic dissection. If MI or ACS is suspected, buccal or sublingual nitrate is appropriate. Careful titration of an intravenous opiate (e.g. morphine sulphate) is administered.

Emergency treatment is then initiated if one of the life-threatening diagnoses has been identified or is likely.

Appropriate investigations must be arranged urgently to determine the actual diagnosis. Resuscitative measures and treatment of ongoing symptoms must continue while waiting for tests.

Some life-threatening conditions cannot be excluded in the time available in the ED. If symptoms or signs suggest that such a diagnosis is a possibility, then the patient must be admitted for further investigations. This is commonly practised for the exclusion of ACS, where serial cardiac markers up to 12 hours after the pain's onset may be indicated.

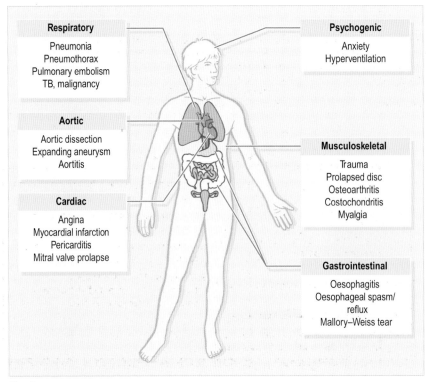

Respiratory
Pneumonia
Pneumothorax
Pulmonary embolism
TB, malignancy

Aortic
Aortic dissection
Expanding aneurysm
Aortitis

Cardiac
Angina
Myocardial infarction
Pericarditis
Mitral valve prolapse

Psychogenic
Anxiety
Hyperventilation

Musculoskeletal
Trauma
Prolapsed disc
Osteoarthritis
Costochondritis
Myalgia

Gastrointestinal
Oesophagitis
Oesophageal spasm/
reflux
Mallory–Weiss tear

Fig. 1 **Causes of chest pain.**

Table 1 Life-threatening causes of chest pain

Diagnosis	Key points: history	Key points: examination	Key points: investigations	Key points: emergency treatment
Acute MI/STEMI	Somatic cardiac pain – central chest pain/heaviness/pressure Radiation – jaw, neck, shoulder Duration – sustained (often longer than 30 minutes) Associations – dyspnoea, sweating Risk factors – previous CAD, smoking, DM, age, HT, obesity, FH	No findings specific to AMI Often signs of sympathetic activity	12-lead ECG – look for ST changes (elevation or depression), new bundle branch block (QRS widening), T-wave inversion Serial cardiac markers Urgent angiography (if available)	Oxygen Aspirin/antiplatelet Nitrates Analgesia Reperfusion therapy – thrombolysis – PCI
ACS/Angina	ACS – similar to AMI Angina – similar to ACS but duration shorter. Often brought on by exercise. Relieved by rest or nitrate	No findings specific to ACS/angina	12-lead ECG – look for ST changes (elevation or depression), new bundle branch block (QRS widening), T-wave inversion Serial cardiac markers	Oxygen Aspirin/antiplatelet Nitrates Analgesia Anticoagulation
Aortic dissection	Abrupt onset of pain Severe/worst ever Tearing/ripping in character Pain in chest/back History of hypertension Syncope	Hypertension (occasionally hypotensive) Aortic insufficiency murmur Unequal blood pressure/pulse deficit in upper limbs Focal neurological signs	ECG – may show ischaemic changes CXR – may show widened mediastinum etc. (see Fig. 3 in 'Aortic, vascular and hypertensive emergencies' chapter) Bedside ultrasound may show pericardial effusion/dilated aortic root Contrast CT or TOE most reliable available tests	Consider the diagnosis Control blood pressure and heart rate – beta blockade initially Type A – surgical repair/stenting Type B – medical therapy +/– surgical repair/stenting
Pulmonary embolism	Sharp/pleuritic pain Breathlessness Syncope Haemoptysis Risk factors include – previous DVT/PE, recent surgery or pregnancy, immobility, cancer, strong family history Often no risk factors	Tachycardia (50%) Tachypnoea Hypoxaemia Added respiratory sounds (crepitations, pleural rub) Signs of DVT Fever	A pre-test probability score (e.g. Wells score) should precede investigations D-dimer – a negative test rules out in a low risk patient V/Q scan or CTPA Bedside ultrasound may show right heart strain and dilatation in the shocked patient	Anticoagulation Consider: Thrombolysis in cardiac arrest or hypotensive patient Surgical thrombectomy if available and compromised patient
Pneumothorax	Unilateral pleuritic type pain Breathlessness May follow trauma Risk factors – smoking, asthma/COPD, tall/thin body habitus	Decreased breath sounds on affected side Hyper-resonance to percussion Tachypnoea Trachea deviated in tension pneumothorax	Clinical diagnosis for tension pneumothorax CXR Bedside ultrasound or CT for supine patients	Urgent needle thoracocentesis for tension pneumothorax Aspiration for small to medium simple pneumothorax Thoracostomy tube (chest drain) for large or recurrent pneumothoraces
Pneumonia	Pleuritic type pain Breathlessness Cough, fever or other signs of sepsis	Fever, tachypnoea, tachycardia Focal chest signs including crepitations, wheeze, increased vocal resonance	CXR Arterial blood gases (hypoxaemia) Full blood count (leucocytosis)	Oxygen/ventilatory support Early fluid resuscitation Early cultures and antibacterial therapy
Oesophageal rupture	Rare diagnosis Severe progressive central chest pain Preceded by vomiting or oesophageal instrumentation	Progressive signs of infective mediastinitis – tachycardia, fever, Hamman's sign (crunching noise synchronous with heart sounds)	CXR – may show pneumomediatinum or pneumothorax CT scan, gastrograffin swallow or endoscopy	Vigorous fluid resuscitation Early antibiotics Early surgical repair
Pericardial tamponade	Rare diagnosis Breathlessness or weakness often preceded by chest pain	Classically (though uncommon): Beck's triad – muffled heart sounds, distended neck veins and hypotension Tachycardia Pulsus paradoxus	Bedside ultrasound/echocardiography – demonstrates pericardial fluid with collapse of right heart in diastole ECG – may see low amplitude complexes or electrical alternans (variable size complexes)	Volume resuscitation initially Pericardiocentesis

If life-threatening causes have been excluded, or are thought to be very unlikely, the doctor should try to identify if there is a non-life-threatening cause which can be treated.

Table 2 Non-life-threatening causes of chest pain (by organ)

Organ	Diagnosis
Heart	Pericarditis
	Valvular disease
Lungs	Bronchitis
	'Pleurisy'
GI tract	Oesophagitis/GORD/PUD
	Gallstones
Chest wall	Costochondritis
	Musculoskeletal
	Cutaneous: herpes zoster

Key points and red flags

- Patients with chest pain should be triaged to a high priority and receive early monitoring, early 12-lead ECG and early treatment.
- Cardiac ischaemia is common and must be considered in all patients presenting with chest pain.
- AMI does not always present with classical type pain.
- A normal ECG does not exclude ACS/AMI.
- Relief of chest pain by a specific treatment does not validate a specific diagnosis, e.g. relief of pain by an antacid does not confirm dyspepsia.
- Chest wall tenderness does not rule out serious diagnoses.
- Cardiac markers should be performed at the appropriate intervals.
- Always consider all the major life-threatening diagnoses before labelling a patient with 'non-cardiac' pain.

Acute coronary syndromes

An acute coronary syndrome (ACS) is a set of signs and symptoms, usually a combination of chest pain and other features, resulting from cardiac ischaemia. The most common cause for an ACS is the disruption of atherosclerotic plaque in a coronary artery. The subtypes of acute coronary syndrome include unstable angina (UA) with no rise in cardiac markers, and two forms of myocardial infarction (MI), in which heart muscle is damaged and a rise in cardiac markers is detectable. MI can be subdivided by the appearance of the electrocardiogram (ECG) as non-ST segment elevation myocardial infarction (NSTEMI) and ST segment elevation myocardial infarction (STEMI) (Fig. 1).

ACS should be distinguished from stable angina, which occurs during exertion and resolves with rest. Unstable angina occurs suddenly, often at rest or with minimal exertion, or at lesser degrees of exertion than the individual's previous angina (crescendo angina). New onset angina is also considered unstable angina, since it suggests a new problem in a coronary artery.

Many patients with ACS will benefit from early revascularization of their obstructed coronary artery. This can be achieved by primary coronary intervention (PCI), or by thrombolysis where PCI is unavailable. PCI involves coronary angiography and where appropriate an intervention such as angioplasty or placement of a coronary stent.

ST-elevation acute coronary syndrome (STEMI)

In the setting of acute onset of ischaemic chest pain lasting greater than 20 minutes, ECG changes suggestive of myocardial infarction include:

1. ST segment elevation >1 mm in contiguous limb leads (II, III or aVF) or >2 mm in contiguous chest leads (V_1–V_6).
2. New left bundle branch block (LBBB).
3. ST depression in V_1–V_3 with dominant R wave suggesting a posterior myocardial infarction. True posterior myocardial infarction in isolation is rare; it is normally associated with either inferior or lateral infarction.

If the above criteria are fulfilled emergency PCI should be undertaken (Fig. 2) or a thrombolytic agent administered. The decision whether to proceed with PCI or thrombolysis should be based on local protocol. Where the local protocol advocates thrombolysis every effort should be made to thrombolyse eligible patients within 30 minutes of arrival at hospital. Prior to administration a rapid assessment and establishment of contraindications for thrombolysis is necessary (Table 1). Diagnosis of MI on the ECG can be difficult and there are several pitfalls (Table 2).

Non-ST-elevation acute coronary syndrome (NSTEMI and UA)

This is defined by a typical history with ST depression or T wave changes during the pain; or ECG changes other than those defined above (non-specific changes) along with a typical history; or nitrate-reversible ST segment elevation if none of the other criteria for infarction are fulfilled.

These patients are still high risk, and urgent treatment is required, but they are not eligible for thrombolysis. The initial management of ACS is

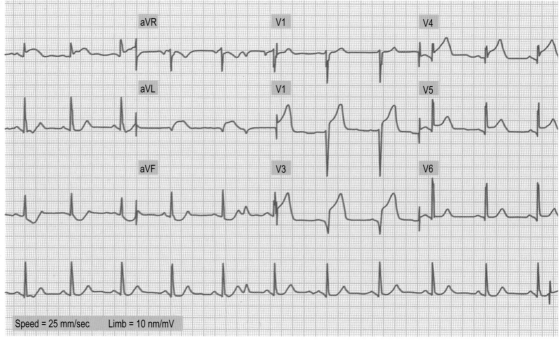

Speed = 25 mm/sec   Limb = 10 nm/mV

Fig. 1 **ECG showing an acute anterior myocardial infarction.**

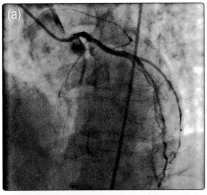

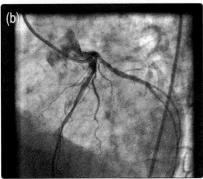

Fig. 2 **Occlusion of the left anterior descending artery (a) and reperfusion following PCI (b).**

treatment with aspirin, heparin (usually a low-molecular weight heparin such as enoxaparin), beta blockade and clopidogrel, together with intravenous glyceryl trinitrate and opioids if the pain persists. Nitrates have no prognostic benefit but are used for symptom relief.

Cardiac markers, such as troponin, are measured 8 to 12 hours after onset of the pain. A rise indicates myocyte damage. Completion of a risk assessment such as a TIMI score predicts likelihood of future cardiac events (Table 3). In higher risk patients

PCI is performed on an urgent basis. If the troponin is negative, an exercise stress test may be performed since UA has not been ruled out (Fig. 3).

Table 1 Contraindications to thrombolysis (emergency PCI needs to be considered)

- Major surgery within 1 month
- Previous haemorrhagic stroke (at any time)
- Any stroke in past 3 months
- Active peptic ulceration or internal bleeding
- Pregnancy or recent postpartum
- Hypertension >180/110 mmHg (use nitrates to control prior to thrombolysis)
- Traumatic cardiopulmonary resuscitation

Table 2 Difficult ECG diagnoses in ACS

Sgarbossa criteria for diagnosis of AMI in the presence of LBBB	1 mm inappropriate concordance of ST segment
	ST segment depression of ST in V_1–V_3
	ST segment elevation >5 mm
	NB: Most MIs with LBBB will not show this
Right ventricular wall MI	Consider if ST elevation is greater in lead III than in lead II
	Diagnose by right ventricular leads on ECG
	Avoid nitrates
Posterior MI	ST depression in V_1–V_3
	Associated inferior infarction
	Dominant R wave in V_1
	ST elevation in posterior leads (V_7 and V_8 inferolateral and inferior to lower pole of scapula)
	Treat as STEMI
Brugada syndrome	Down-sloping ST elevation (transient)
	Genetic abnormality of sodium transport in myocardium
	Associated with arrhythmias (e.g. VT)
	Treat with implantable cardioverter defibrillator (ICD)

Table 3 TIMI score

Score 1 point for each of the following:

- Age ≥65 years
- ≥3 risk factors for coronary artery disease (CAD); family history, hypertension, hypercholesterolaemia, smoker or diabetes
- Known CAD
- Aspirin use in past 7 days
- Severe angina >2 episodes in past 24 hours
- ST segment deviation
- Positive cardiac marker (such as troponin)

Risk of death, MI or requiring urgent PCI in next 14 days

Score	Risk
0/1	4.7%
2	8.3%
3	13.2%
4	19.9%
5	26.2%
6/7	40.9%

Fig. 3 **Management of acute coronary syndromes.**

- Symptoms suggestive of ACS/myocardial ischaemia
  - oxygen
  - aspirin 300mg
  - 12-lead ECG
  - IV access

- No → Symptoms suggestive of serious non-cardiac diagnosis
  - follow appropriate algorithm

- Stable chronic angina with no ECG changes
  - outpatient management

- ECG showing ST elevation or new LBBB
  - No → ACS risk assessment (TIMI or other)
    - Low: TIMI 0–2
    - Intermediate: 3–4
    - High: 5–7
  - Yes → Reperfusion therapy
    - thrombolysis
    - PCI

- High or intermediate risk

- Antiplatelet agent (e.g. clopidogrel) / Beta blockade / Anticoagulation (LMWH) / Nitrates / ACE inhibitor / Statin

- Positive
  - cardiac markers
  - ECG changes
  - No → Low risk / Negative cardiac markers / No ECG changes

- Yes → Consider early cardiac catheterisation

- Positive stress test
  - Yes → Consider early cardiac catheterisation
  - No → Outpatient management

- Yes → Outpatient management

Key points

- Consider ACS as a possible diagnosis in all patients with chest pain.
- Perform an early ECG and repeat if pain persists.
- Risk stratify all patients accurately.
- Measurement of cardiac markers does not rule out UA.

Breathlessness (1)

Breathlessness (dyspnoea) is a feeling of difficulty in breathing. It is a common presentation and can result from disease processes of many systems. An acutely breathless patient may have an acute cardiorespiratory cause, an acute exacerbation of a chronic cardiorespiratory disorder, disorders of the blood, such as anaemia, metabolic problems such as acidosis, sepsis, pregnancy, neurological disorders such as Guillain–Barré syndrome, MS and MND, or psychological problems.

Principles of management

Use the established ABC approach for assessment and emergency treatment. The goal is to establish a patent airway; ensure adequate ventilation and oxygenation while rapidly assessing the patient for reversible causes for the breathlessness. Only after the adequacy of ventilation has been established and emergency treatment initiated should the differential be broadened beyond the immediately life-threatening causes.

Oxygen: Patients who present acutely with breathlessness will have varying requirements for oxygen therapy depending on the underlying cause of their symptoms. A proportion of patients with acute breathlessness will have COPD. A number of these COPD patients will require controlled oxygen therapy because they are at risk of carbon dioxide retention and respiratory acidosis. In general the breathless patient should receive high flow oxygen unless known or suspected to have COPD. The oxygen delivery system in COPD patients who are thought to have lost their hypoxic drive should be adjusted to maintain a saturation of 90–92%.

Treating the underlying condition

Rather than initially treating all known causes of breathlessness simultaneously, the primary survey and initial assessment should give some indication as to the underlying aetiology.

First line treatments may include nebulized beta-2 agonists (salbutamol) for asthma and COPD, sublingual or buccal nitrates for left ventricular failure, or a procedure such as needle thoracocentesis for tension pneumothorax.

If the patient is hypoxic despite oxygen therapy, non-invasive ventilation or even endotracheal intubation and ventilation may be required urgently.

After initial therapy, the continuously breathless patient should have a chest radiograph and arterial blood gas performed. Further tests such as peak expiratory flow rate (PEFR) measurement may be appropriate. The underlying cause should guide further management. Continuous SpO_2 monitoring is essential until stability is reached.

Respiratory failure

Respiratory failure is defined as a failure to maintain adequate gas exchange and is characterized by abnormalities of arterial blood gas tensions.

Type I respiratory failure is defined by a PaO_2 of <8 kPa with a normal or low $PaCO_2$. Type II respiratory failure is defined by a PaO_2 of <8 kPa and a $PaCO_2$ of >6 kPa.

Respiratory causes

Asthma

Asthma is a chronic inflammatory disorder of the airways, causing recurrent episodes of wheezing, breathlessness, chest tightness and coughing, particularly at night or in the early morning. The airflow obstruction is caused by mucosal inflammation and associated bronchoconstriction.

Initial assessment involves a rapid ABC assessment and risk assessment. This includes a PEFR measurement (if possible) and key points in the history such as frequency of previous attacks, hospital admissions, ICU admissions/ventilation, and use of steroids.

A life-threatening attack in an adult is indicated by any one of:

- PEFR <33% of predicted/best
- silent chest/cyanosis
- bradycardia, dysrhythmia or hypotension
- exhaustion, confusion or coma
- SpO_2 < 92%, PaO_2 < 8 kPa, *normal* or raised pCO_2.

A severe attack is indicated by any one of:

- inability to complete sentences in one breath
- respiratory rate >25
- tachycardia of >110.

Initial treatment

Administer high flow oxygen (>40%) and follow with continuously nebulized beta-2 agonist (salbutamol). A nebulized anticholinergic (ipratropium) should be added. Steroids should be given early either orally (prednisolone) or, if unable to take orally, intravenously (hydrocortisone). Consider starting intravenous crystalloid fluids.

Initial investigations

A chest x-ray should be performed if there is clinical suspicion of pneumothorax or pneumonia, or if there is no initial improvement. Arterial blood gas analysis should be performed if there is no initial improvement and in life-threatening cases.

The mainstay of treatment is continued administration of beta-agonists. Adjuncts include magnesium (IV or nebulized); and adrenaline (epinephrine) if allergy/anaphylaxis is possible. Consider early administration of antibiotics if infection suspected.

Involve the intensive care team in life-threatening cases and severe cases when there is no improvement.

Chronic obstructive pulmonary disease (COPD)

COPD is characterized by limitation of airflow in the airway that is not fully reversible. COPD is an umbrella term for chronic bronchitis, emphysema and a range of other lung disorders. It is most often due to tobacco smoking but can be due to other airborne irritants such as coal dust, asbestos or solvents, as well as congenital conditions such as alpha-1-antitrypsin deficiency.

Acute exacerbations of COPD are common, with patients presenting with an abrupt increase in symptoms of shortness of breath and/or wheezing, often associated with increased production of purulent sputum. The patient's exercise tolerance is also often reduced.

Initial management
The principles of management are similar to asthma, but with a cautious approach to oxygen administration due to the dependency of many patients on their hypoxic respiratory drive. Acute exacerbations are treated with controlled oxygen, inhaled beta-2 agonists, inhaled anticholinergics, antibiotics and corticosteroids. Theophyllines may be considered in patients who do not respond to other bronchodilators. Antibiotic therapy is directed at the most common pathogens, including *Streptococcus pneumoniae*, *Haemophilus influenzae* and *Moraxella catarrhalis*. Sputum cultures should be obtained.

Hospitalization is required if the symptoms are severe. Non-invasive ventilation may be indicated for patients with significant type II respiratory failure and acidosis (Table 1 and Fig. 1). If symptoms are milder, discharge with appropriate follow-up is possible. Acute respiratory teams can assist with this goal.

Pneumonia/lower respiratory tract infection
Pneumonia is inflammation of lung tissue and consolidation of alveoli (Fig. 2). Pneumonia can result from a variety of causes, including infection with bacteria, viruses, fungi or parasites, and chemical or physical injury to the lungs. Typical symptoms include cough, chest pain, fever and breathlessness. Patients may present in septic shock, or with confusion. Common organisms include *Streptococcus pneumonia* (50%), *Haemophilus influenzae*, atypical organisms such as *Legionella*, and *Mycoplasma*, and viruses such as influenza and varicella. Always consider tuberculosis and pneumocystis pneumonia (PCP) in immunocompromised patients (e.g. HIV).

Initial assessment should focus on a general assessment of the patient looking for signs of shock, as well as a thorough respiratory assessment. Early antibiotics are indicated and local guidelines should be followed. Amoxicillin is often sufficient for mild cases of community-acquired pneumonia. For more severe cases, broader cover with a cephalosporin and macrolide combination may be given.

Severity can be assessed using the 'CURB-65' score from the British Thoracic Society: 1 point is given for each of confusion, elevated urea >7 mmol/L, respiratory rate >30, low blood pressure (systolic <90 or diastolic <60 mmHg) and age >65 years. A score of 2 or more warrants hospital admission.

Pleural effusion
Pleural effusion is excess fluid in the pleural cavity. Serous effusions are classified into transudates (low protein) and exudates (high protein). Other causes include blood (haemothorax), chyle (chylothorax) or pus (empyema).

Clinical signs include dullness to percussion over the fluid and diminished breath sounds. An erect chest x-ray (Fig. 3) can detect 300 mL of fluid, whereas 50 to 100 mL can be detected by CT or ultrasound.

A sample can be obtained by pleural aspiration (under ultrasound guidance if available). CT scanning can help differentiate between benign and malignant disease.

Treatment depends on the underlying cause of the pleural effusion. Therapeutic aspiration may be sufficient; larger effusions may require insertion of a chest drain.

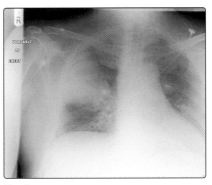

Fig. 2 **A chest x-ray showing pneumonia.**

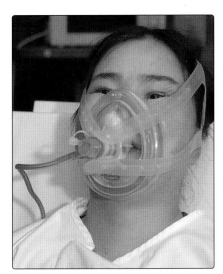

Fig. 1 **Non-invasive ventilation by facemask** (CPAP/BIPAP on a patient).

Table 1 **Indications and contraindications for non-invasive ventilation (NIV) and continuous positive airway pressure (CPAP) in the emergency department**

Indications	
CPAP	Cardiogenic pulmonary oedema
	Type I (hypoxaemic) respiratory failure
	Community-acquired pneumonia
	Lung contusion
	Acute respiratory distress syndrome (ARDS)
	Consider as a holding measure in type II respiratory failure, if NIV not available and if 'not for intubation'
NIV (BiPAP)	Type II (hypercapnic) respiratory failure
	Acute exacerbation of COPD
	Thoracic wall deformities
	Acute respiratory failure in obesity hypoventilation syndrome
	Chronic respiratory failure
	Immunocompromised patients
	As a ceiling therapy in patients 'not for intubation'
Contraindications	
CPAP/NIV	Need for immediate intubation and ventilation
	Recent facial or upper airway surgery, burns or trauma
	Upper airway obstruction
	Inability to protect the airway
	Vomiting/copious respiratory secretions
	Life-threatening hypoxaemia
	Coma/confusion/agitation
	Bowel obstruction
	Pneumothorax (a chest drain should be inserted before commencing NIV)

Breathlessness (2)

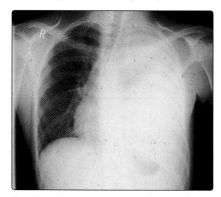

Fig. 3 **A chest x-ray showing a large left pleural effusion.**

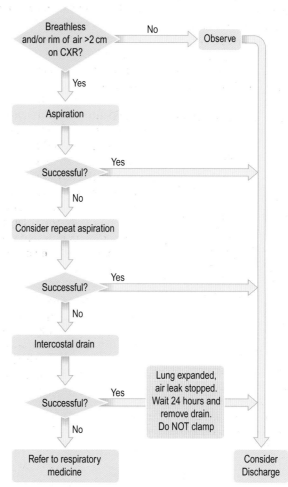

Fig. 4 **Pneumothorax algorithm.** CXR, chest x-ray.

Pneumothorax

Pneumothorax is air in the pleural space; between the lung and the chest wall. In spontaneous pneumothorax there is no apparent precipitating event. A pneumothorax may be either primary or secondary. A secondary pneumothorax is a pneumothorax that is associated with an underlying lung disease. Risk factors for primary pneumothorax include smoking and height in male patients. The size of a pneumothorax may be 'small' or 'large' depending on the presence of a visible rim of <2 cm or >2 cm between the lung margin and the chest wall.

Lateral chest x-ray, CT and ultrasound can aid diagnosis. Treatment is by observation, aspiration or chest drain insertion based on size and symptoms (Fig. 4).

Tension pneumothorax

This results from the operation of a one-way valve system, drawing air into the pleural space during inspiration and not allowing it out during expiration. It is associated with a sudden deterioration in the cardiopulmonary status of the patient related to impaired venous return, reduced cardiac output, and hypoxaemia.

Treatment is with high concentration oxygen by mask, and immediate needle decompression with a cannula in the second anterior intercostal space mid-clavicular line. This is followed by placement of a chest drain. Needle decompression can be life-saving.

Non-respiratory causes

Heart failure

Heart failure is a syndrome and not a single pathological process. There are many different ways to categorize heart failure, including:

- low-output heart failure versus high-output heart failure (e.g. thyrotoxicosis)
- left heart failure versus right heart failure
- systolic dysfunction versus diastolic dysfunction
- the degree of functional impairment conferred by the abnormality (as in the NYHA classification).

Heart failure is common and presents with symptoms of breathlessness and exhaustion at rest or with less than the normal degree of exertion.

Heart failure may be acute or chronic. Acute heart failure has a dramatic presentation with dyspnoea and hypoxia; oedema, either pulmonary or peripheral; organ underperfusion; and tachycardia and diaphoresis (sweating). Chronic heart failure may be more insidious with chronic exercise limitation, orthopnoea, paroxysmal nocturnal dyspnoea (PND), ankle swelling, anorexia and weight loss.

Assessment of the patient with suspected heart failure

Severity of breathlessness graded according to New York Heart Association (NYHA) class:

NYHA I: Impaired LV function but no symptoms

NYHA II: Breathless on vigorous exertion, e.g. walking briskly, walking uphill

NYHA III: Breathless during everyday activities, e.g. walking around the house

NYHA IV: Breathless at rest

Acute heart failure/cardiogenic pulmonary oedema

Increased pulmonary venous pressure results in accumulation of alveolar fluid and decreased oxygen transfer from air to capillary.

Causes include congestive heart failure, myocardial infarction with left ventricular failure, arrhythmias, pericardial effusion with tamponade and fluid overload, e.g. from renal failure.

The initial management for acute heart failure is as follows:

- Sit the patient up and administer high concentration oxygen.
- Attach cardiac monitoring and treat arrhythmias if present.
- Vasodilator therapy – buccal nitrate or intravenous nitrate (GTN) decreases preload and afterload and can be immediately effective.
- Intravenous diuretic (furosemide 40–80 mg) has both venodilator and diuretic effects.
- Continuous positive airway pressure (CPAP) has been shown to reduce the requirement for ventilation and can effect a rapid improvement in symptoms (see below).
- Intravenous opiate analgesia may be considered if the patient is anxious. Caution is required as this may reduce ventilatory effort.
- Intubation, ventilation or inotropes (dobutamine) may be required in hypotensive shocked patients: consider the need for urgent angiography with or without a balloon pump in this setting.
- Consider the need for specific therapies such as dialysis in renal failure or blood transfusion in severe anaemia.
- Initial investigations should include chest x-ray, ECG to identify the need for urgent reperfusion therapy, urinalysis, and if available, a focused echocardiogram to identify any pericardial effusion or left ventricular dysfunction. Blood tests include FBC, electrolytes, urea, LFTs, and cardiac enzymes.

Non-cardiogenic pulmonary oedema/acute respiratory distress syndrome (ARDS)

There is an acute onset of symptoms with bilateral infiltrates on chest radiograph and lack of clinical evidence of left ventricular failure.

Causes include inhalation of toxic gases, severe infection, pulmonary contusion, neurogenic causes, medications and aspiration.

Management is provision of supportive care with oxygen, ventilation, fluid restriction and treatment of the underlying condition.

Pericardial disease

The pericardium is a thin sac that surrounds the heart and the large blood vessels closely associated with the heart. Pericarditis is a condition in which the pericardium becomes inflamed (often following a viral illness). In pericarditis, the amount of pericardial fluid may increase causing a pericardial effusion which can restrict the motion of the heart. If the onset is rapid or if the volume of the pericardial effusion is large, cardiac tamponade can occur. Other causes of tamponade include penetrating trauma, malignancy and ventricular wall rupture.

Pericardial effusion/tamponade presents with dyspnoea and tachycardia. The classic findings of muffled heart sounds, jugular venous distension and low blood pressure are known as Beck's triad. Pulsus paradoxus may be present, with an elevation of the JVP on inspiration (Kussmaul's sign).

Initial assessment and treatment

Definitive diagnosis is made by bedside echocardiography (Fig. 5). Physical examination for the above signs, ECG and chest x-ray for a globular enlarged heart may raise the initial suspicion of the diagnosis.

The initial treatment is administration of high flow oxygen, boluses of IV fluids to increase preload followed by urgent pericardiocentesis to reduce intrapericardial pressure. Effusions without tamponade should

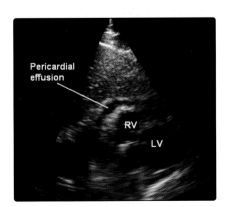

Fig. 5 **A bedside emergency echocardiogram showing a pericardial effusion.**

be referred to cardiology for further management. In trauma, urgent surgical release of the haemopericardium may be indicated (see 'Cardiothoracic trauma' chapter).

Pulmonary embolism

This condition should always be considered in the breathless patient, especially if there is no other apparent cause (see 'Thromboembolic disease' chapter).

Non-invasive ventilation and CPAP

Non-invasive ventilation (NIV) is the provision of *ventilatory support* using a mask. Continuous positive airway pressure (CPAP) is application of positive airway pressure using a facemask (Fig. 1). Technically, CPAP does not provide ventilation and as such is not true NIV.

Bilevel positive airway pressure (BiPAP) is a system of NIV in which two levels of airway pressure are applied: expiratory positive airway pressure (EPAP) and inspiratory positive airway pressure (IPAP).

The two main conditions for which NIV is considered in the emergency department are COPD and pulmonary oedema.

NIV should be considered in patients with an acute exacerbation of COPD with type II respiratory failure in whom a respiratory acidosis (pH <7.35) persists despite maximum medical treatment on controlled oxygen therapy.

Continuous positive airway pressure (CPAP) is effective in patients with cardiogenic pulmonary oedema who remain hypoxic despite maximal medical treatment. NIV (BiPAP) should be reserved for patients in whom CPAP is unsuccessful (Table 1).

Web resource

http://www.brit-thoracic.org.uk

Key points

- Always use the ABC approach for a breathless patient.
- Early intervention is often necessary and can be life-saving.
- Oxygen is important, but be cautious in COPD.

Thromboembolic disease

Venous thrombosis occurs when blood clots in a vein. Deep venous thrombosis (DVT) is the formation of a blood clot (thrombus) in a deep vein commonly affecting the deep leg veins, such as the femoral or popliteal veins, or the deep veins of the pelvis. Thrombus may also develop in other veins; for example, the axillary vein causing an axillary vein thrombosis, the mesenteric veins causing mesenteric venous thrombosis, and the intracerebral venous sinuses causing cerebral venous thrombosis. If a section of thrombus breaks off, it may be carried in the circulation and lodge in a branch of the pulmonary artery causing a pulmonary embolus (PE). Untreated, approximately one-third of patients who survive an initial PE will die of a future embolic episode.

Deep vein thrombosis

Patients with a DVT typically present with a painful swollen calf, with no history of trauma. Symptoms and signs may be minimal. DVT is an important diagnosis to consider in any patient with atraumatic lower leg pain. The assessment of the patient with a suspected deep vein thrombosis must include an assessment of the patient's risk. This risk may be assessed by using a scoring system (Table 1). A risk score together with a D-dimer allows a decision to be made as to whether further investigation is warranted. D-dimer is a protein degradation product that can be measured by assay. An elevated D-dimer is relatively non-specific; the real value of a D-dimer is in its negative predictive value. Trauma, recent surgery, haemorrhage, malignancy, sepsis and pregnancy may all cause an elevated D-dimer. In a patient who is low risk and has a negative D-dimer, a DVT is very unlikely. If, however, the D-dimer is elevated, or the patient is moderate or high risk, then imaging is required. First line imaging for DVT involves an ultrasound scan of the deep veins. If thrombus is identified, the patient will require anticoagulation. In most patients this will be with warfarin, but where there are problems with compliance or monitoring, for example with intravenous drug abusers, this may be with low molecular weight heparin (LMWH).

Pulmonary embolus

This life-threatening condition is often overlooked and needs to be considered in any patient with breathlessness. Breathlessness is the commonest presenting problem for patients with PE. Other presentations include pleuritic chest pain, haemoptysis and syncope.

Important clinical signs are tachypnoea, pleural rub, an elevated JVP, tachycardia and signs of a DVT; however, there may be no apparent diagnostic signs. As with a DVT it is essential to assess the patient's risk and this may be achieved by using a scoring system (Table 2). A D-dimer may be helpful, but again, its value is its high negative predictive value in a low risk patient. Patients with moderate or high risk, or those with an elevated D-dimer, require further imaging. Other initial investigations that may be helpful are a chest x-ray, ECG and arterial blood gases. The main role of the chest x-ray is to exclude other pathology such as pneumothorax or pneumonia, although certain signs such as lobar collapse, elevated hemidiaphragm, and basal atelectasis can be suggestive of PE. The most common ECG findings with a pulmonary embolism are sinus tachycardia and non-specific ST-T wave abnormalities. The 'classic' PE finding of S1Q3T3 (S wave in lead 1, Q wave in lead 3 and an inverted T wave in lead 3) is unusual and non-specific. Arterial blood gases may be helpful but again are neither sensitive nor specific. In larger PEs there may be hypoxia or slight hypocapnia from hyperventilation, whereas with smaller PEs the arterial blood gases are often normal. In a patient with a suspected PE that warrants further investigation, it is appropriate to administer a dose of LMWH prior to completion of investigations. Further investigation is commonly with either a ventilation-perfusion lung scan (V-Q scan) or a CT pulmonary angiogram (CTPA). A V-Q scan is limited by the availability of isotope. If the chest x-ray is abnormal or in patients with COPD interpretation of V-Q scans is difficult and in these cases a CTPA is recommended. Traditionally V-Q scans are reported as being normal, low, intermediate or high probability. A normal V-Q is sensitive at ruling out a PE and a high probability makes the diagnosis of PE very likely. Difficulty arises in the interpretation of low and moderate probability scans. Here the clinical context is important and alternative imaging may be required. A CTPA involves a large radiation dose but is often more readily available and may identify an alternative diagnosis such as consolidation, a pneumothorax or aortic dissection. CTPA is

Table 1 **The Wells scoring system for pre-test probability of DVT**	
Clinical parameter	**Score**
Active cancer (treatment ongoing, or within 6 months or palliative)	+1
Paralysis or recent plaster immobilization of the lower extremities	+1
Recently bedridden for >3 days or major surgery <4 weeks	+1
Localized tenderness along the distribution of the deep venous system	+1
Entire leg swelling	+1
Calf swelling >3 cm compared to the asymptomatic leg	+1
Pitting oedema (greater in the symptomatic leg)	+1
Previous DVT documented	+1
Collateral superficial veins	+1
Alternative diagnosis (as likely or greater than that of DVT)	−2

Total score:
3 or more indicates high probability.
1 or 2 indicates moderate probability.
0 or less indicates low probability.

Table 2 **The Wells scoring system for pre-test probability of PE**	
Clinical parameter	**Score**
Clinical signs of DVT	+3
Alternative diagnosis less probable than PE	+3
Heart rate >100/minute	+1.5
Immobilization or surgery <4 weeks ago	+1.5
Previous DVT or PE	+1.5
Haemoptysis	+1
Cancer	+1

Total score:
<2 indicate a low probability of PE.
2–6 indicates a moderate probability of PE.
>6 indicates a high probability of PE.

increasingly becoming the favoured investigation (Fig. 1). Treatment of PE involves anticoagulation initially with LMWH and warfarin, and then warfarin alone once therapeutic levels are reached. In massive PE, with hypotension (systolic blood pressure < 90 mmHg) and signs of right heart failure on echocardiography, thrombolysis should be considered. If thrombolysis is contraindicated, then consideration needs to be given to surgical thrombectomy. Patients with recurrent thromboembolic episodes despite anticoagulation, or those with a contraindication to anticoagulation, may be suitable for an inferior vena cava filter device (Fig. 2).

Thromboembolic disease in pregnancy

Thromboembolic disease remains the leading cause of maternal death in the UK. Successive reports into maternal death have identified shortcomings in both the diagnosis and management. Pitfalls in pregnancy include false positives with D-dimer and a hesitancy to consider the diagnosis or investigate appropriately. Pregnant patients should be fully investigated for thromboembolic disease, and if identified, anticoagulated with LMWH for the duration of the pregnancy.

Web resources

1. British Thoracic Society guidelines for the management of PE: http://www.brit-thoracic.org.uk
2. Royal College of Obstetrics and Gynaecologists guidelines for the management of thromboembolic disease in pregnancy: http://www. rcog.org.uk

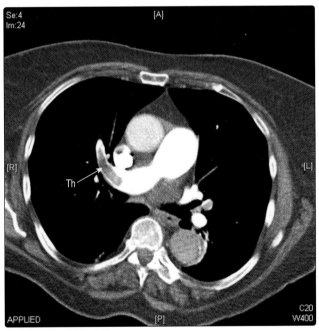

Fig. 1 **CTPA showing filling defect in the right pulmonary artery due to thrombus (Th) characteristic of pulmonary embolus.**

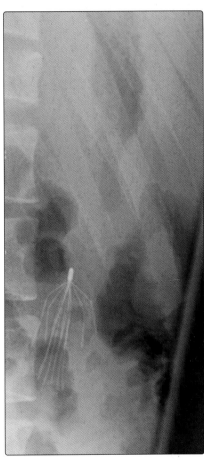

Fig. 2 **IVC filter device seen on X-ray.**

Key points

- Always consider the possibility of DVT in any patient with leg pain without a history of trauma.
- Always consider the possibility of PE in any breathless patient.
- The assessment of a patient with suspected DVT or PE must include an assessment of the risk by calculating the pre-test probability.
- D-dimer is only of value in ruling out PE and DVT in lower risk patients.

Blackouts and syncope

Patients commonly present as an emergency having collapsed with a period of loss of consciousness, i.e. a blackout. Although there are many potential causes, the most common are seizures and syncope. Syncope is defined as a transient loss of consciousness due to inadequate cerebral perfusion. It can be challenging to differentiate benign from serious causes and to decide which patients require admission for observation and urgent investigation.

Causes

Common causes

Generalized seizures can occur at any time and may be preceded by an aura such as a smell or taste. The patient commonly goes stiff, followed by jerking for 2–3 minutes. There is then a slow recovery and the patient is often sleepy and confused for an hour or two. Stigmata of a seizure include tongue biting and incontinence of urine, although these can occur with syncope. Continuous seizure activity or intermittent seizures without full recovery lasting for more than 30 minutes is defined as status epilepticus and is an emergency (see 'Seizures' chapter).

Syncope can be divided into neurally mediated, orthostatic or cardiac syncope (Table 1). Cardiac syncope carries a one-year mortality of 20–30%. Patients usually feel light-headed and sweaty, look pale and then fall or slump down. Any loss of consciousness is brief and there may be twitching for a brief period.

Neurally mediated syncope involves an acute vasodilatation with bradycardia. All types of neurally mediated syncope are due to inappropriate reflexes and many have specific triggers. Vasovagal faints are usually triggered by emotions such as fear or anxiety.

Other rarer causes

- Subarachnoid haemorrhage may present as sudden headache with a blackout (see 'Headache' chapter).
- Hypoglycaemia causes light-headedness and sweating and may cause a collapse, especially in elderly patients or those with autonomic neuropathy. A capillary glucose measurement is vital in any patient presenting with a collapse.
- Transient ischaemic attacks (TIAs) present as sudden loss of focal neurological function due to a vascular cause; they very rarely cause loss of consciousness, although a fall

may occur from acute ataxia or weakness.
- Narcolepsy is a tendency to fall asleep suddenly, often associated with emotional stress. It is rare and has no known cause.

Key diagnostic points

History: Obtain a clear detailed patient (and witness) description of the blackout. Important points include details of the activity being undertaken prior to the collapse, presence of any warning, any precipitating factors and how the patient felt afterwards (Fig. 1).

Most neurally mediated syncope has a clear vagal prodrome with nausea, sweating and light-headedness. Cardiac syncope tends to be sudden in onset with very little warning. Occasionally palpitations or chest pain occur; if present they are very suggestive of a cardiac cause. A collapse occurring with

Table 1 **Causes of syncope**
Neurally mediated syncope
■ Vasovagal
■ Cough syncope
■ Micturition syncope
■ Hyperventilation or Valsalva induced
Orthostatic syncope
■ Lack of intravascular volume
■ Autonomic failure
Cardiac
■ Arrhythmias such as VT, SVT
■ Mechanical obstruction as with aortic stenosis, pulmonary emboli or cardiomyopathy

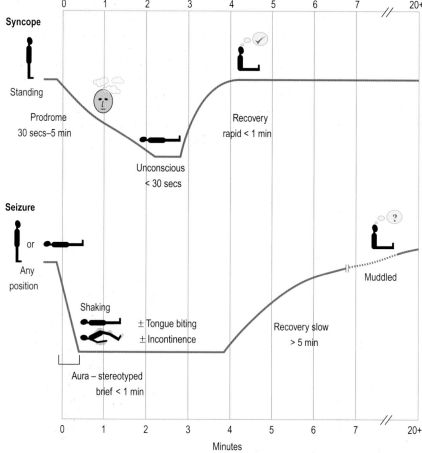

Fig. 1 **Features of syncope.**

exercise is also suggestive of a cardiac cause. Patients commonly make a rapid recovery after a syncopal episode. Symptoms of an aura, fitting for longer than one minute and slow recovery with a period of confusion and lethargy are more consistent with a seizure.

Examination is usually normal after a blackout, especially if due to syncope. After a seizure the patient may be hyper-reflexic with upgoing plantar reflexes for an hour or so. Examine for focal neurology and cardiovascular abnormalities including pulse, murmurs, signs of heart failure, and supine and erect blood pressure.

Emergency investigations for all patients presenting to the emergency department with a blackout should include an ECG and a measurement of blood glucose. A pregnancy test is imperative in all females of childbearing age. Further investigations depend upon the history. For syncope, these may include a 24-hour tape (Fig. 2), an echocardiogram or tilt table testing (Fig. 3). The detection rate of cardiac arrhythmias from a single 24-hour period is often very low and increasing use is made of more sophisticated devices. An echocardiogram detects structural lesions, such as aortic stenosis and tilt tables are used to investigate abnormal neuro-cardiac reflexes. After a seizure further investigations may include a CT head scan and electroencephalogram (EEG). An urgent CT head scan is appropriate if there are signs of focal neurology or continued depressed conscious level. New onset epilepsy in an elderly person is often due to a structural brain lesion such as a cerebral infarct. EEGs are often normal during inter-ictal periods although they can be useful in the emergency diagnosis of herpes encephalitis or non-convulsive status epilepticus.

Red flags for syncope

The following features suggest significant cardiac cause or higher short-term mortality:

- elderly
- known ischaemic heart disease
- low blood pressure on arrival to emergency department
- heart murmur
- syncope occurring during exertion
- syncope preceded by palpitations or chest pain
- abnormal ECG.

If multiple risk factors are present, the patient should be admitted for continuous cardiac monitoring and urgent cardiac investigations.

Emergency department management

If a patient has made a complete recovery from a probable syncope episode no treatment is required. The key decision in the emergency setting is to make an assessment of the patient's risk of having a serious underlying cause. This in turn determines whether the patient can be allowed home or should be admitted. The above 'flags' are the parameters associated with a poor short-term outcome and can be used as a guide to decide on admission.

Cases of hypoglycaemia need to be treated with oral glucose preparations (GlucoGel/Hypostop) or concentrated (10 or 50%) intravenous glucose, and any diabetes medications should be reviewed.

All patients with a blackout must be advised about the regulations for driving as well as general lifestyle advice about avoiding high risk situations such as swimming alone. It is a doctor's responsibility to make a patient aware of the local driving regulations and to advise the patient to contact the Driving and Vehicle Licensing Authority (DVLA) in the UK or equivalent. Following a seizure the driving licence is usually revoked for one year. A provoked seizure (e.g. secondary to hypoglycaemia or alcohol intoxication) is dealt with on an individual case basis. Following a transient ischaemic attack, the patient is allowed to drive after a 1-month period. There are no driving restrictions when a diagnosis of vasovagal or simple faint is made.

> **Key points**
>
> - Taking a thorough history is the most useful step in establishing a diagnosis.
> - Witness accounts are invaluable.
> - Risk stratification is important to determine who gets admitted or investigated urgently.
> - Any driving restrictions should be explained to the patient and documented.

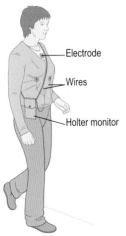

Fig. 2 **Holter monitor for 24-hour ECG recording.**

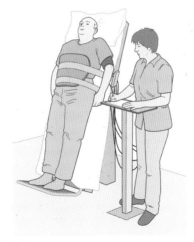

Fig. 3 **Tilt table test.**

Aortic, vascular and hypertensive emergencies

Abdominal aortic aneurysm

An abdominal aortic aneurysm (AAA) is a dilatation of the aorta so that the external diameter is greater than 3 cm. With increasing diameter there is an increasing risk of rupture. Once the diameter is greater than 5.5 cm, the risks of elective repair become less than the risk of surveillance. There is evidence that a structured national screening programme using ultrasound would be beneficial but this has not been implemented in many countries. As a result many patients have undiagnosed AAAs and may present to the emergency department as an acute leak or rupture.

Occasionally an aneurysm may become symptomatic prior to rupture; symptoms are thought to be due to a stretching of the aortic wall. The classic presentation of a ruptured aortic aneurysm is of collapse with sudden onset abdominal pain and a palpable pulsatile epigastric mass. However, the pain may be referred to the back or to the groin, or there may be no cardiovascular collapse, especially if the leak is contained and only involves a small volume of blood. Consider the possibility of a ruptured aneurysm in anyone over 50 years presenting with sudden onset abdominal, back or loin pain. Ruptured aneurysms are often misdiagnosed as renal colic; be cautious of diagnosing a first episode of renal colic in anyone over 50 years. Detection of AAA by palpation is notoriously unreliable and if AAA is suspected, then imaging with either ultrasound or CT is required. Bedside ultrasound is reliable for identifying the presence of an aneurysm (Fig. 1) but not at identifying rupture. CT is more reliable at identifying rupture and is essential prior to endovascular repair (Fig. 2). Permissive hypotension is acceptable so long as the patient is talking. Trying to normalize a hypotensive patient who is alert may result in dislodgement of clot and exsanguination. Repair may be either by open surgery or increasingly by using endovascular stenting techniques.

Aortic dissection

Aortic dissection occurs when there is a tear in the intima of the aorta with blood stripping along the media for a variable distance. Risk factors for aortic dissection include hypertension, Marfan's syndrome and other connective tissue disorders such as Ehlers–Danlos syndrome. Typically patients present with chest pain which is of sudden onset and may radiate to the back. The nature of the pain is important, with patients describing it as tearing or shearing. Signs suggestive of a dissection include a difference in blood pressure measurements between the right and left arm of greater than 20 mmHg, absent pulses or a disparity of pulses (e.g. strong radial but weak femoral pulses). If the dissection is of the proximal aortic arch there may be signs to suggest a pericardial effusion such as muffled heart sounds or Kussmaul's sign (elevation of the JVP on inspiration). If the dissection involves the carotid arteries, neurological signs may be present. A chest x-ray may show a widened mediastinum (Fig. 3), loss of aortic knob, left pleural effusion or deviation of the trachea to the right, but is normal in approximately 20% of patients. The most reliable method of diagnosis is a contrast-enhanced thoracic CT. Echocardiography, aortogram and increasingly magnetic resonance angiography (MRA) are alternative imaging modalities that can be utilized; MRA is useful in patients who are allergic to contrast media. Dissection can be divided into two types depending on the site of the dissection (Fig. 4). Type A generally requires surgical repair and type B is managed medically with optimization

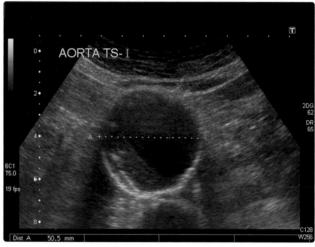

Fig. 1 **Ultrasound image of a 5 cm aortic aneurysm.** Fluid (such as blood) tends not to reflect ultrasound waves and so appears blacker. Note the thrombus visible in the lumen.

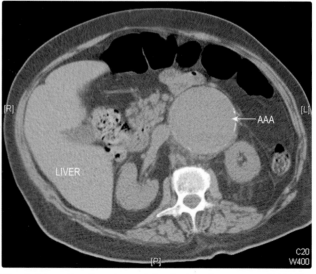

Fig. 2 **CT of the abdomen showing a large abdominal aortic aneurysm (AAA).** The right renal artery can be seen to be arising from the aneurysm sac.

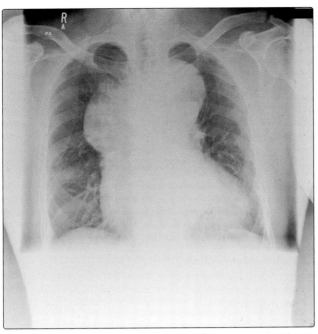

Fig. 3 **Chest x-ray showing widened mediastinum in patient with aortic dissection.**

Type A
Involves the
aortic arch

Type B
Starts distal to the
left subclavian artery

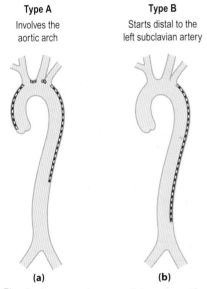

(a) **(b)**

Fig. 4 **The two main types of thoracic aortic dissection, type A and type B.**

of blood pressure control and attention to other risk factors. Endovascular techniques are being developed for treatment of thoracic aortic dissection.

The acutely ischaemic limb

This is caused by either thrombosis of a diseased vessel or by an arterial embolism from a distant site. Distinguishing between the two causes can be difficult but clues are often present. Acute upper limb ischaemia is unusual but when it occurs it is more likely to be embolic. The heart is the most likely source of the embolism with thrombus having formed in the left atrial appendage due to atrial

fibrillation. Lower limb ischaemia may be caused by embolism from the heart or from a proximal aneurysm (either aortic or popliteal). More commonly lower limb ischaemia is caused by thrombosis. In this case the contralateral limb may well have diminished or absent pulses suggesting established arterial disease in both legs. The most important symptom of an acutely ischaemic limb is pain. On examination the acutely ischaemic limb will be cool with absent pulses. The symptoms and signs can be remembered as the 5 'P's – pulseless, painful, perishing cold, paraesthesia and paralysis. Diagnosis is by angiogram and treatment is either with surgical embolectomy, bypass or by endovascular technique.

Bleeding varicose veins

People can die as a result of haemorrhage from varicose veins. Minor trauma may cause bleeding from where the varicosed vein has eroded through the skin. Bleeding can always be stopped with gentle pressure and elevation. It is prudent to place a suture through the vein. Patients will require referral to a vascular surgeon for consideration of varicose vein surgery to prevent a recurrence.

Hypertensive emergencies

As a general rule, hypertension (raised blood pressure; >140/90 mmHg) detected in the emergency department

should not be treated aggressively. The exception to this statement is in the rare case of a true hypertensive emergency, also known as malignant hypertension.

A hypertensive emergency is severe hypertension with acute impairment of an organ system with the possibility of irreversible organ damage. Systems affected are the central nervous system, the cardiovascular system and the renal system.

The measured blood pressure is usually greater than 220/140 mmHg. Cardiac presentations are angina, myocardial infarction and pulmonary oedema. Neurological presentations include occipital headache, cerebral infarction or haemorrhage, visual disturbance, or hypertensive encephalopathy (a symptom complex of severe hypertension, headache, vomiting, visual disturbance, mental status changes, seizure, and retinopathy with papilloedema). Blood pressure should be checked in both arms to assess for aortic dissection or coarctation. If coarctation is suspected, blood pressure also should be measured in the legs.

With a hypertensive emergency, the blood pressure should be lowered over minutes to hours with an antihypertensive agent such as intravenous labetalol. Hydralazine is reserved for pregnant patients, while phentolamine is the drug of choice for a phaeochromocytoma crisis. Blood pressure should be lowered smoothly and to a safe level; patients with chronic hypertension may not tolerate a 'normal' blood pressure.

Treatment of severe hypertension in the setting of stroke or intracranial haemorrhage is difficult and should be done with specialist neurological consultation.

Key points

- Always consider the diagnosis of AAA in elderly patients with collapse, abdominal pain or back pain.

- Aortic dissection cannot be ruled out by a normal chest x-ray, or by physical signs and symptoms.

- Patients with atrial fibrillation are at increased risk of embolic arterial occlusion leading to stroke, ischaemic bowel or acute limb ischaemia.

- Hypertension should not be rapidly lowered in the emergency department unless there is evidence of acute end-organ damage.

Acute abdominal pain

Patients with abdominal pain commonly present to the emergency department. While many will have serious underlying pathology, in up to half, no underlying pathology will be found. It is useful to think about the various causes in terms of the body system affected (Table 1).

History

Concentrate on taking a clear history of the pain, in particular the abruptness of onset, the site and the nature of the pain.

Abruptness of onset

A sudden onset suggests a potentially catastrophic event such as a perforated viscus or a leaking aortic aneurysm.

Site

The exact site of pain gives clues to the likely cause of the pain. Try to envisage which organs are situated under where the patient is complaining of pain; this will give an idea of the likely possible causes of the pain, e.g. right iliac fossa pain in a female may arise from the appendix, right fallopian tube or ovary (Fig. 1).

Nature of the pain

Broadly speaking there are two types of pain to consider; colicky pain, or constant pain caused by peritoneal irritation. A colicky pain is caused by the peristaltic action of the smooth muscle of a tube trying to overcome a blockage. Typically the pain comes and goes in waves with the patient feeling alternately in considerable pain and relatively well. The patient with colicky pain often moves around and is unable to get comfortable. Common causes of colicky pain are renal colic, biliary colic and bowel obstruction. In contrast, with peritoneal irritation, the pain is constant. The pain may get progressively worse but is persistent and constant. Typically a patient with peritoneal irritation lies still since any movement will exacerbate the pain (Fig. 2).

Examination

Pay attention to vital signs, particularly temperature, pulse and blood pressure. Any patient with abdominal pain warrants a thorough systematic examination including cardiorespiratory examination. Examination of the abdomen must be methodical and start with observation. If the patient is in pain, where is the pain located? Palpate gently at a site distant to the site of the pain and palpate in a clockwise fashion with the site of the pain last. Any tenderness is significant, but examine closely for any signs of peritoneal irritation. Involuntary guarding and rebound tenderness are both indicative of peritoneal irritation (peritonitis) and must never be ignored. Percuss for excess dullness, for the tympanic sound of pressurized gas and for percussion rebound tenderness. Lastly, auscultation for bowel sounds may be helpful. Bowel sounds may be absent in peritonitis with an associated ileus but will be more frequent and higher pitched 'tinkling' in bowel obstruction.

Investigations

Urine

- Urinalysis – may suggest a urinary tract infection (positive for nitrites, leucocytes, haematuria and protein);

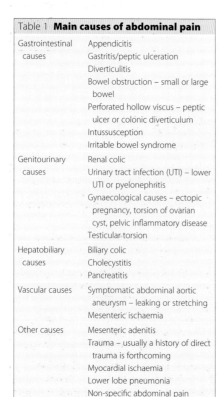

Table 1	**Main causes of abdominal pain**
Gastrointestinal causes	Appendicitis
	Gastritis/peptic ulceration
	Diverticulitis
	Bowel obstruction – small or large bowel
	Perforated hollow viscus – peptic ulcer or colonic diverticulum
	Intussusception
	Irritable bowel syndrome
Genitourinary causes	Renal colic
	Urinary tract infection (UTI) – lower UTI or pyelonephritis
	Gynaecological causes – ectopic pregnancy, torsion of ovarian cyst, pelvic inflammatory disease
	Testicular torsion
Hepatobiliary causes	Biliary colic
	Cholecystitis
	Pancreatitis
Vascular causes	Symptomatic abdominal aortic aneurysm – leaking or stretching
	Mesenteric ischaemia
Other causes	Mesenteric adenitis
	Trauma – usually a history of direct trauma is forthcoming
	Myocardial ischaemia
	Lower lobe pneumonia
	Non-specific abdominal pain

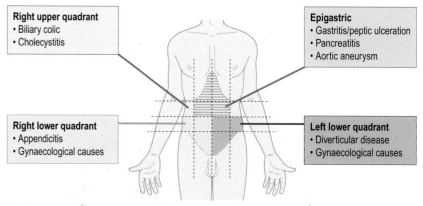

Right upper quadrant
- Biliary colic
- Cholecystitis

Epigastric
- Gastritis/peptic ulceration
- Pancreatitis
- Aortic aneurysm

Right lower quadrant
- Appendicitis
- Gynaecological causes

Left lower quadrant
- Diverticular disease
- Gynaecological causes

Fig. 1 **Schematic picture of abdomen with sites of pain relating to anatomical structure.**

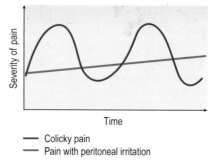

Colicky pain
Pain with peritoneal irritation

Fig. 2 **Schematic graph of pain against time, demonstrating the difference between colic pain and peritoneal irritation.**

microscopic haematuria occurs in renal colic (approximately 95% sensitivity). Be aware that inflammation adjacent to the renal tract can cause false positives.

- Urinary βHCG – test in all females of childbearing age. The safest policy is to make no exceptions – nuns and young teenagers all require a pregnancy test. In this way no one is offended: you cannot afford to miss an ectopic pregnancy.

Blood tests

- Venous blood gas – gives information of the acid–base status (pH, bicarbonate) as well as other parameters depending on the machine used (haemoglobin, lactate, potassium, sodium, glucose).
- Biochemistry – renal function tests, liver function tests, amylase, C-reactive protein.
- Haematology – full blood count, coagulation screen if you suspect liver impairment, the patient is on warfarin or you are suspicious of a coagulopathy.
- Transfusion – group and save if patient unwell, if you suspect patient has intra-abdominal bleeding, if the patient is anaemic or likely to require a major procedure.

Imaging

- Chest x-ray – ideally erect, to look for free air under the diaphragm (Fig. 3); however, the sensitivity for free air on an erect chest X-ray is less than 50%.
- Abdominal x-ray – main value is for looking at bowel gas pattern, particularly with obstruction.
- Ultrasound – is useful for the diagnosis of AAA, gallstones, fluid collections and pelvic pathology.
- CT scan of the abdomen – this is becoming increasingly available and has shown to be of value in the early assessment of acute abdominal pain. Perform urgently in systemically unwell patients.

Other investigations

- ECG – to look for myocardial ischaemia.

Emergency management

- Initial resuscitation, if the patient is unwell using the structured approach of ABCDE.
- Analgesia – if in pain a patient must receive adequate analgesia. An intravenous opiate, such as morphine, is the drug of choice. There is excellent evidence that administration of opiates does not significantly alter subsequent assessment of a patient with abdominal pain and there can never be any justification in withholding analgesia from a patient with abdominal pain. There is no convincing evidence to suggest that prophylactic anti-emetics reduce the incidence of emesis associated with opiates. The use of anti-emetics ought to be reserved for patients with nausea, those who have vomited or in trauma patients who have their spine immobilized.
- Fluid resuscitation – many patients with abdominal pain will be fluid depleted. This may be from reduced fluid intake but also from increased losses into extravascular spaces.
- Surgical opinion – have a low threshold for obtaining a surgical opinion. There is a case for admitting all patients with persistent unexplained abdominal pain and tenderness for a period of observation. This is especially true at the extremes of age.

Paediatric considerations

- Consider intussusception if the pain is intermittent. Intussusception can occur at any age but is most common in children under 3 years. Bilious vomiting is a significant symptom and the child may pass blood in the stool. Classically this is described as a 'redcurrant jelly' like stool. In an infant, bilious vomiting and intermittent pain are enough to justify a period of observation.
- Appendicitis can occur at any age.
- Mesenteric adenitis – enlargement of the mesenteric lymph nodes – may follow a viral illness in children.

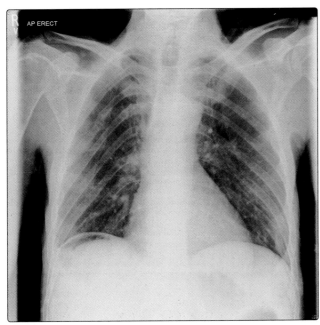

Fig. 3 **Erect chest x-ray showing free air under the right hemidiaphragm,** in this case from a perforated colonic diverticulum.

Key points

- Pregnancy test in any female of childbearing age.
- Consider obtaining an amylase in anyone with abdominal pain; pancreatitis may present in many subtle ways.
- Never ignore rebound tenderness, this is a sign of peritoneal irritation.
- Be very cautious about diagnosing renal colic in a patient who has no microscopic haematuria.
- Elderly patients may present atypically and there is a much higher incidence of significant pathology in elderly patients.
- Always consider the possibility of an abdominal aortic aneurysm (AAA).

Jaundice and hepatic disorders

When assessing a patient with liver disease in the emergency department there are two important considerations: first to consider the underlying cause of the liver disease; and second to identify and initiate treatment for any potentially life-threatening complications.

Life-threatening complications include:

- ascending cholangitis
- hepatic encephalopathy
- bleeding oesophageal varices
- spontaneous bacterial peritonitis.

Ascending cholangitis

This is a bacterial infection of the biliary tract. There is usually an abnormality of the biliary tract such as presence of gallstones or a stricture. Charcot's triad of jaundice, right upper quadrant pain and fever suggests ascending cholangitis.

Hepatic encephalopathy

Seen in patients with cirrhosis and shunting of the portal blood into the systemic system.

Oesophageal varices

These occur in patients with chronic liver disease which is commonly alcohol related. Portal hypertension causes dilatation of the venous network at the distal oesophagus.

Spontaneous bacterial peritonitis

This is an important complication of patients with ascites. It presents with abdominal pain and signs of sepsis.

Jaundice

Many patients with liver disease either present with jaundice or have established jaundice. The causes of jaundice are best classified as pre-hepatic, hepatic and post-hepatic (Fig. 1).

History

Enquire about:

- Associated pain: painless jaundice is generally considered to be more sinister with an increased possibility of it being due to malignant disease.
- Alcohol intake.
- Sexual history: unprotected intercourse or sexual partner from high risk group, for example an intravenous drug user (risk of hepatitis B or C).
- Recent tattoos, body piercing or blood transfusion (risk of hepatitis B or C).
- Recent travel abroad (risk of hepatitis A or E).
- Occupational exposure to hepatotoxic chemicals.
- Complete drug history: common hepatotoxic drugs include paracetamol, non-steroidal anti-inflammatory drugs, amiodarone and aspirin.
- History of pelvic inflammatory disease: possible Curtis–Fitz-Hugh syndrome, a perihepatitis caused by spread of chlamydial infection. The perihepatitis is generally not sufficient to cause jaundice but does cause right upper quadrant pain and abnormal liver function tests.

Examination

Jaundice will normally only become evident clinically when the bilirubin level exceeds 25 mmol/L (Fig. 2). Examine for general features of chronic liver disease (spider naevi, palmar erthythema, gynaecomastia, testicular atrophy). Palpate for an enlarged liver, spleen or for a gallbladder. Courvoisier's law states that in the presence of jaundice a palpable gallbladder is unlikely to be due to stones. The explanation of this is that with gallstones the diseased gallbladder is fibrotic and non-distensible and will not be palpable. In malignant disease (most commonly a carcinoma of the head of the pancreas compressing the common bile duct)

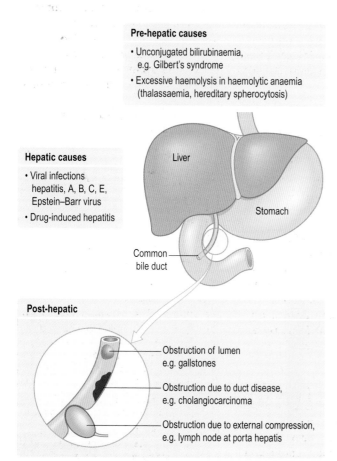

Pre-hepatic causes

- Unconjugated bilirubinaemia, e.g. Gilbert's syndrome
- Excessive haemolysis in haemolytic anaemia (thalassaemia, hereditary spherocytosis)

Hepatic causes

- Viral infections hepatitis, A, B, C, E, Epstein–Barr virus
- Drug-induced hepatitis

Liver

Stomach

Common bile duct

Post-hepatic

- Obstruction of lumen e.g. gallstones
- Obstruction due to duct disease, e.g. cholangiocarcinoma
- Obstruction due to external compression, e.g. lymph node at porta hepatis

Fig. 1 **Common causes of jaundice.**

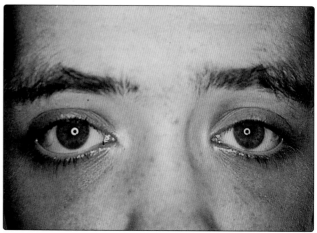

Fig. 2 **Patient with clinically obvious jaundice.**

the gallbladder will be distensible and may be palpable.

Murphy's sign is positive if tenderness over the gallbladder (tip of the right ninth costal cartilage) halts deep inspiration, without similar findings on the left. It is suggestive of cholecystitis. Look for signs of encephalopathy, confusion and liver flap (also known as asterixis, a low frequency flap of the hands when wrists held in full extension). Examine for signs of infection and possible ascending cholangitis.

Investigations

Liver function tests assess whether there is predominantly a hepatitic picture (raised transaminases such as alanine transaminase; ALT) or a cholestatic picture (raised alkaline phosphatase; ALP).

- Glucose: acute liver failure may cause hypoglycaemia
- Albumin: synthesized by the liver and long half-life makes it a good marker of chronic liver impairment.
- Hepatitis screen for hepatitis A, B and C, Epstein–Barr virus, and an autoimmune screen: often not analysed as an emergency test but important to initiate early.
- Renal function tests: to identify hepatorenal syndrome; renal impairment secondary to liver failure.
- Coagulation screen: essential in any jaundiced patient. Vitamin K dependent coagulation factors are synthesized in the liver and liver impairment will result in a reduction of their production with a consequent prolongation of the prothrombin time.
- Blood cultures: if cholangitis is suspected.
- Ultrasound: other than liver function tests this is the most important early investigation. The texture of the liver can be assessed, as well as the size of the common bile duct (greater than 6 mm is considered dilated, but may be normally slightly larger in the elderly or post cholecystectomy). A dilated common bile duct suggests an obstructive (cholestatic) cause for the jaundice. Abnormal masses may also be identified.

Treatment

Treat any life-threatening complication:

- Cholangitis: fluid resuscitation and antibiotics.
- Encephalopathy: lactulose reduces ammonia absorption from the gut.

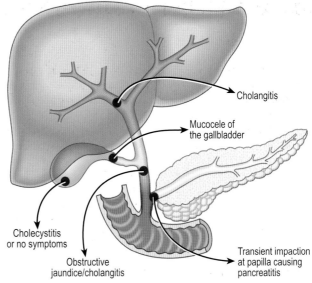

Fig. 3 **Gallstones and the conditions they cause** (after Rhodes).

Neomycin destroys ammonia-producing gut flora.
- Oesophageal varices: resuscitation, transfusion, fresh frozen plasma, octreotide or terlipressin (if known to have varices), urgent gastroscopy for injection or banding. In dire situations where the bleeding is torrential a Sengstaken–Blakemore tube may be utilized.
- Spontaneous bacterial peritonitis: resuscitate, aspirate and culture ascitic fluid, and administer antibiotics.
- Alcohol abuse: thiamine, benzodiazepine (chlordiazepoxide or diazepam) if withdrawal anticipated or already symptomatic (see 'Alcohol and drug-related problems' chapter).

Gallstones

Acute complications of gallstones include biliary colic, cholecystitis, obstructive jaundice, pancreatitis, gallstone ileus and cholangitis (Fig. 3). Approximately 10% of gallstones are radio-opaque; ultrasound is the imaging of choice to identify gallstones. The character of the pain, a positive Murphy's sign and the presence of any infective symptoms or elevation of infective markers (white cell count and CRP) can help to distinguish cholecystitis from biliary colic (inflammatory markers may be normal in the early stages of cholecystitis).

Pancreatitis

Typically presents with persistent epigastric pain, though atypical presentation is common. Consider in any patient presenting with abdominal pain. The pain is often severe and requires opiate analgesia. There is generally an elevation in the serum amylase but this may not be the case in patients with chronic pancreatitis. Serum lipase is an alternative marker enzyme that is more likely to be elevated in patients with chronic pancreatitis. Important causes of pancreatitis include gallstones, alcohol, drugs (azathioprine, NSAIDs, corticosteroids, furosemide), trauma (direct trauma to the upper abdomen) and iatrogenic induced post ERCP. Emergency department treatment is largely supportive with early assessment of the severity (Table 1). All patients with severe pancreatitis require management on either a high dependency unit or intensive care unit.

Table 1 **Assessing the severity of pancreatitis**
Age >55 years
Albumin <32 mmol/L
PO$_2$ on air <8.6 kPa
Calcium <2 mmol/L
Blood glucose >10 mmol/L
Lactate dehydrogenase >600 u/L
Urea >16 mmol/L
WBC >15×10^9/L
Three or more of the above in the first 48 hours suggests severe pancreatitis.

Key points

- In patients with liver disease, always consider the possibility of a life-threatening complication such as bleeding varices, encephalopathy or ascending cholangitis.

- The two most common causes of pancreatitis are alcohol and gallstones.

- Patients who have severe pancreatitis require admission to either a high dependency or intensive care unit.

Gastrointestinal bleeding

Bleeding can occur acutely from several sites in the gastrointestinal (GI) tract (Fig. 1). Bleeding is divided into upper GI and lower GI bleeding. This distinction is important, not least since it is common practice for the surgical team to look after patients with a lower GI bleed and physicians to look after those with an upper GI bleed. The distinction is made initially on clinical grounds depending largely on which symptoms the patient has.

Upper GI bleeding

Effective medical treatment to reduce acid production in the stomach first with H2 antagonists and subsequently proton pump inhibitors has led to a reduction in the incidence of upper GI bleeds in recent years. The development of minimally invasive techniques means that it is very unusual for a patient presenting with an upper GI bleed to require an emergency surgical procedure.

History

Occasionally identifying a patient with an upper GI bleed may be challenging, though most patients present with either haematemesis or melaena, making the diagnosis more straightforward. Bleeding may initially be concealed and it is important to consider the possibility of GI bleeding in any collapsed patient, especially if there are risk factors (history of alcohol abuse, NSAID ingestion, dyspeptic symptoms).

Mallory–Weiss tears occur at the distal oesophagus after repeated vomiting. The history is characteristic, with the patient having vomited several times with no blood in the vomit before vomiting fresh, bright red blood.

Reflux oesophagitis results in damage to the oesophageal mucosa which may be sufficient to cause bleeding. Patients with reflux oesophagitis commonly experience other symptoms such as acid reflux or retrosternal pain that is worse with bending forward. Non-steroidal anti-inflammatory or aspirin usage suggests a possible gastric or duodenal origin for bleeding.

Alcohol is a potent gastric and duodenal erosive agent and a causative factor for ulceration. It is essential to consider the possibility of bleeding oesophageal varices in any heavy drinker, especially if there are signs of chronic liver disease (see 'Jaundice and hepatic disorders' chapter). In any patient who has undergone previous aortic surgery the possibility of an aorto-enteric fistula must be considered, although this is extremely rare.

Examination

A drop in systolic blood pressure on standing can be caused by depletion of the intravascular volume. If feasible measure a lying and standing blood pressure in any patient with a possible GI bleed. Look for signs of chronic liver disease such as spider naevi. Examine for scars suggestive of previous aortic surgery.

Investigations

Oesophago-gastro-duodenoscopy (OGD) is the most helpful early investigation after initial resuscitation has been undertaken. The procedure is not purely diagnostic; there are numerous therapeutic techniques available such as injection sclerotherapy. Varices can be injected with a sclerosant, or banded. If the lesion is actively bleeding and cannot be dealt with endoscopically, then angiography and coiling of the bleeding vessel may be possible.

Emergency management

Resuscitate appropriately; ensure there is adequate venous access and that cross-matched blood is available. Check the coagulation profile and full blood count in all patients. Elevated urea may indicate an upper GI bleed since blood in the colon presents a significant nitrogen load to the gut. If an upper GI bleed occurs in a patient with known varices, then either intravenous terlipressin or octreotide (both vasoconstrictors) is indicated. In a patient with torrential bleeding from an upper GI bleed where oesophageal

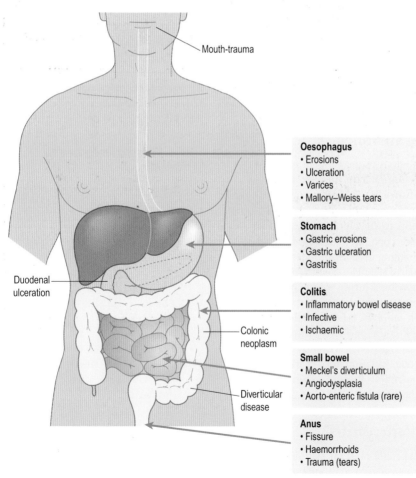

Mouth-trauma

Oesophagus
- Erosions
- Ulceration
- Varices
- Mallory–Weiss tears

Stomach
- Gastric erosions
- Gastric ulceration
- Gastritis

Colitis
- Inflammatory bowel disease
- Infective
- Ischaemic

Small bowel
- Meckel's diverticulum
- Angiodysplasia
- Aorto-enteric fistula (rare)

Anus
- Fissure
- Haemorrhoids
- Trauma (tears)

Duodenal ulceration

Colonic neoplasm

Diverticular disease

Fig. 1 **Sources of gastrointestinal haemorrhage.**

varices are suspected, a balloon device such as a Sengstaken–Blackmore tube may be life-saving in the emergency situation. The tube is placed blindly into the oesophagus and balloons dilated in either or both the stomach and oesophagus. This is a temporary life-saving measure and is only very rarely undertaken (Fig. 2). In patients with bleeding oesophageal varices there is evidence that administration of antibiotics reduces the incidence of further bleeding.

Lower GI bleeding

Lower GI bleeding may result from pathology in the colon (neoplasm, inflammatory bowel disease, diverticular disease) or the rectum and anus (anal fissure, haemorrhoids, trauma).

History
The nature of the blood, either fresh or altered, and whether mixed with stool or separate, are important aspects of the history. Unless the bleeding is very brisk, the fresher the blood the more distal the lesion is likely to be. If there is formed stool with separate blood it is more likely that the lesion is distal. Pain with defecation suggests a local cause such as an anal fissure. Any history of instrumentation of the anus or rectum either medically or recreationally is important to elicit. Significant trauma to the rectal mucosa can follow insertion of an object. A huge variety of foreign bodies have been inserted into the rectum; mobile phones are commonly hidden in the rectum by prisoners. Consider the possibility of sexual assault in any age or sex.

Examination
Local examination may reveal a fissure. Rectal examination may palpate a malignancy. Proctoscopy looking at the anus and very distal rectum and rigid sigmoidoscopy may identify a distal cause. More proximal endoscopy (flexible sigmoidoscopy or colonoscopy) may be appropriate if no satisfactory explanation is found.

Investigations
In most people it is possible to visualize the whole of the lower GI tract to the ileo-caecal valve with endoscopy and in the majority of patients this will identify the likely source of bleeding. Angiography may be helpful in patients who continue to bleed, making visualization with an endoscope difficult or impossible. Angiography is not only diagnostic in terms of identifying the bleeding vessel, but also therapeutic since it may be possible to stop the bleeding by coiling the vessel (Fig. 3). CT scanning may also be helpful in identifying the bleeding source.

Emergency management
Resuscitation and early involvement of specialty teams: Endoscopy may help to identify the site and the cause. If bleeding is brisk, views may be poor. Angiography or emergency surgery are alternative options.

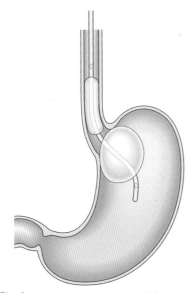

Fig. 2 **Position of Sengstaken–Blackmore tube.**

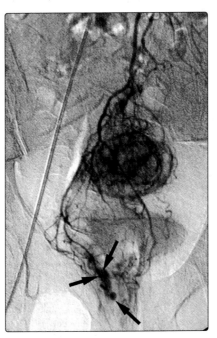

Fig. 3 **Selective angiography of inferior mesenteric artery** showing active bleeding from a haemorrhoidal artery.

> ## *Paediatric considerations*
>
> A Meckel's diverticulum with ectopic gastric mucosa may very rarely cause GI bleeding in children.

> ### Key points
>
> - Be alert to the possibility of concealed GI bleeding in a compromised patient with no melaena or haematemesis.
> - Consider the possibility of a variceal bleed in any patient with alcohol abuse who presents with haematemesis.
> - Left-sided colonic or rectal malignancy needs to be considered and excluded in all patients presenting with rectal bleeding.

Vomiting and diarrhoea

From personal experience we can all appreciate that vomiting is an extremely unpleasant act. It is therefore not surprising that vomiting is a relatively common primary presenting symptom to the emergency department. Diarrhoea is a much less common primary presenting complaint; when patients do present with diarrhoea it is normally in association with other symptoms.

Vomiting

Causes

The commonest cause of vomiting is infective gastroenteritis. It is essential that other causes of vomiting are considered and excluded since vomiting can be the primary presentation in a diverse number of conditions. Be very cautious about diagnosing gastroenteritis in a patient with vomiting but who has no diarrhoea (Table 1).

History

With gastroenteritis the history is often relatively short (less than 12 hours) and there is commonly a history of ingestion of a suspicious meal. Friends or family members may be affected. Diarrhoea is associated with the majority of common causes of gastroenteritis. Always consider other important causes for vomiting and enquire about associated symptoms.

Examination

With gastroenteritis there may be slight tenderness on abdominal examination but never signs of peritoneal irritation such as rebound tenderness or guarding. Always check for hernias, especially femoral hernias, and examine for other signs to suggest abdominal obstruction such as distension.

Investigations

If abdominal pain is prominent, pancreatitis needs to be excluded and an amylase or lipase obtained. Obtain a urinary pregnancy test in any woman of childbearing age (Fig. 1). Check blood glucose to exclude diabetes. Urea and electrolytes are important if the vomiting is profuse to ensure there is no electrolyte disturbance or renal impairment. Losing hydrochloric acid from the stomach leads to a metabolic alkalosis. In an attempt to preserve hydrogen ions the kidney exchanges potassium in preference to hydrogen ions and this leads to hypokalaemia. Hypokalaemia is the commonest electrolyte abnormality with persistent vomiting. Loss of large volumes of fluid can lead to renal impairment, especially if associated with diarrhoea and an inability to rehydrate orally because of persistent vomiting or nausea. If the patient is dehydrated the urea is elevated proportionally more than the creatinine. If an intracranial pathology is suspected then obtain a CT scan of the head (Fig. 2).

Emergency management

Rehydration and anti-emetics are the mainstay of initial management. Rehydration can be either orally or with intravenous fluids.

Diarrhoea

Causes

Diarrhoea is the passage of frequent loose stools. The causes of diarrhoea can be divided into infective and inflammatory. The commonest cause for patients presenting to the emergency department is infective. Increasingly it is important to consider *Clostridium difficile* as a possible causative agent, especially in the elderly or where there is a history of recent antibiotic use. Other common infective causes include *Campylobacter* and *Salmonella*. Inflammatory causes of diarrhoea include ulcerative colitis, Crohn's disease, ischaemic colitis and radiotherapy-induced colitis. Diarrhoea can be present in numerous other gastrointestinal conditions such as appendicitis and diverticulitis.

Table 1 **Causes of vomiting other than gastroenteritis with key diagnostic clues**

Age group	Condition	Diagnostic clues
Any age	Raised intracranial pressure or other intracranial pathology	No diarrhoea, persistent vomiting, associated headache
Infants less than 3 months, most commonly at around 3 weeks	Pyloric stenosis	Projectile vomiting, failure to thrive (low weight and length for age), palpable mass in epigastrium with feeding
Any age but generally under 18 months	Intussusception	No diarrhoea, bile-stained vomit, episodic abdominal pain, blood-stained stools
Female of childbearing age	Pregnancy	No diarrhoea, amenorrhoea
Any age	Diabetic ketoacidosis	No diarrhoea, dehydrated, unwell
Any age	Uraemia secondary to renal failure	A very high blood urea (greater than 40 mmol/L) is very emetogenic and the patient may vomit profusely
More common in the elderly but any age	Bowel obstruction	No diarrhoea, other symptoms or signs of obstructed bowel – distended abdomen, absolute constipation (for faeces and flatus), colicky abdominal pain. Incarcerated hernia at any site (always check for a groin hernia in patients of any age who present with vomiting)
Commonly elderly females but either sex	Acute closed angle glaucoma	No diarrhoea, painful red eye

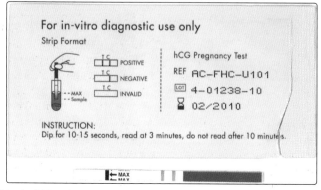

Fig. 1 **Positive bedside urine pregnancy test** in a young woman who presented with vomiting.

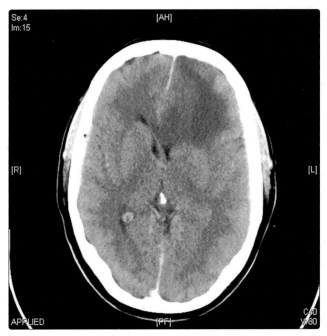

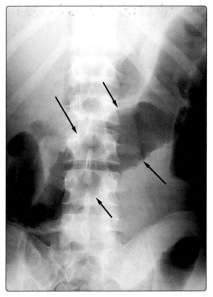

Fig. 3 **Abdominal x-ray showing toxic megacolon** (arrows).

Fig. 2 **Contrast-enhanced CT scan of the head** showing a left frontal tumour with mass effect. This middle-aged man presented to the emergency department with vomiting and mild headache.

History

There may be a history of ingestion of a suspicious meal or other family members affected suggesting an infective cause. It is essential to ask about both the nature of the stool (colour, consistency) and the frequency of passing stool. Bloody diarrhoea may be infective (especially *Campylobacter*) or inflammatory (especially ulcerative colitis). It is important to gain an idea of the quantity of blood and also the appearance, fresh, altered, mixed or separate. Recent antibiotic usage and taking a proton pump inhibitor are both risks for *Clostridium difficile* infection.

Examination

Any marked abdominal tenderness or signs of peritoneal irritation will require investigation and admission for observation.

Investigations

Check serum amylase or lipase if any associated abdominal pain, to rule out pancreatitis. Renal function needs to be assessed if the diarrhoea is profuse or the patient is clinically dehydrated. A stool culture ought to be sent although this often takes at least 48 hours for a result. If the patient is discharged, follow-up of the result is essential; 'food poisoning' of any cause is a notifiable disease and in the UK the Health Protection Agency must be informed. In patients with known or possible ulcerative colitis who are

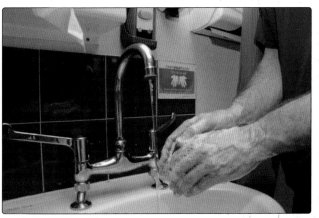

Fig. 4 **Hand washing with soap** is essential before and after any contact with patients with diarrhoeal illness.

systemically unwell with pyrexia, tachycardia and abdominal pain, toxic megacolon needs to be considered. With toxic megacolon a plain abdominal x-ray will show a dilated colon, greater than 5.5 cm in diameter (Fig. 3).

Emergency management

Rehydration is the key to initial management. In adults intravenous rehydration with 0.9% saline is the preferred fluid. Potassium chloride may be added if the initial potassium is low or low normal. The maximum rate that potassium chloride can be administered is 20 mmol per hour. If an inflammatory cause is suspected then visualization of the mucosa (sigmoidoscopy, rigid or flexible) will be required. If the patient is well this may be possible on an outpatient basis but commonly with this group of

patients the diarrhoea is so profuse that they require admission. Meticulous infection control measures are paramount in patients with diarrhoea. Cleaning hands with alcohol preparations is not sufficient; hands must be properly washed with soap before and after any patient contact (Fig. 4).

Key points

- Be very cautious about making the diagnosis of gastroenteritis if there is vomiting but no diarrhoea.

- Always check for femoral hernia in any age.

- Consider *Clostridium difficile* in patients with diarrhoea who have been taking antibiotics or are on a proton pump inhibitor. The patient will need to be barrier nursed.

Acute renal failure

Acute renal failure is the sudden loss of the ability of the kidneys to excrete waste products and concentrate urine without losing electrolytes. In the emergency department the key is to identify the presence of acute renal failure, diagnose the underlying cause and rapidly institute emergency management. Identification is based principally on the history but may be suspected from examination and confirmed on blood testing. The immediate emergency management largely involves the treatment of hyperkalaemia. High serum potassium excites the myocardium and is the commonest electrolyte abnormality leading to cardiac arrhythmias and cardiac arrest. It is essential to treat hyperkalaemia promptly and effectively. The other key step in the emergency department management is to identify patients that require urgent dialysis and facilitate this in association with either a renal physician or intensive care team. Causes of renal failure are best considered as pre-renal, renal or post-renal in origin (Fig. 1).

History

Two components to the history are important, firstly to identify the existence of renal failure and secondly to identify possible causes. The existence of renal failure may be suspected in patients with known renal impairment who present with symptoms to suggest deterioration. Symptoms of renal failure may be very non-specific. A high serum urea causes lethargy and also nausea and vomiting. There may be a reduction in the production of urine or complete anuria. Anuria suggests a post-renal cause such as bladder outlet obstruction and acute retention of urine from an enlarged prostate. A history of recent illness such as a streptococcal illness or Henoch–Schönlein purpura and a comprehensive history of recent medications taken may give valuable clues to the underlying aetiology.

Examination

Uraemia may cause a pericardial or pleural effusion. Pericardial effusion may be detected by distended neck veins and muffled heart sounds, and the ECG shows electrical alternans, alternating large and small QRS complexes due to movement of fluid in the pericardial sac altering the conduction of the electrical activity. Pleural effusions may be detected by reduced breath sounds and stony dullness to percussion. Abdominal examination may reveal a large bladder suggestive of bladder outflow obstruction.

Investigations

Urine testing: urinalysis and urgent microscopy (Fig. 2, Table 1). Infection is suggested by presence of leucocytes and nitrites on urinalysis and leucocytes and possibly organisms seen on microscopy. Proteinuria on urinalysis and red cell casts with microscopy suggest acute glomerular nephritis. Granular casts suggest acute tubular necrosis.

Blood tests: the serum creatinine and urea will enable you to quantify the degree of renal impairment. The potassium is the most important

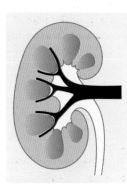

Pre-renal

- **Hypovolaemia from any cause**
  - Blood loss
  - Excessive fluid loss from diarrhoea and vomiting
  - Excessive loss from an ileostomy
- **Hypotension from any cause such as**
  - Septic shock
  - Cardiogenic shock
  - Addison's disease

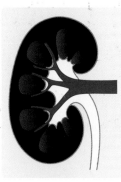

Renal

- **Acute tubular necrosis**
  - Following episode of renal ischaemia
  - Due to direct toxins such as myoglobin (with rhabdomyolysis), aminoglycosides and radiology contrast medium
- **Acute glomerular nephritis**
  - Post infectious most commonly following Group A, betahaemolytic streptococcal infection
  - Complicating systemic illness such as Henoch–Schönlein purpura
  - Due to intrinsic renal disease
- **Acute interstitial nephritis**
  - Most commonly due to drugs such as NSAIDs

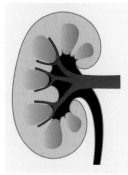

Post-renal

- **Bladder outflow obstruction**
- **Bilateral ureteric obstruction**
- **Bilateral renal calculi**

Fig. 1 **Important emergency department causes of renal failure.**

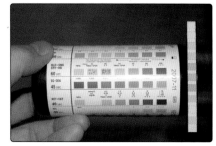

Fig. 2 **Dipstick urine testing.**

Table 1 **Parameters assessed by dipstick urinalysis**
Glucose
Bilirubin
Ketones
Specific gravity
Blood
pH
Protein
Urobilinogen
Nitrates
Leucocytes

Table 2 Treatment of hyperkalaemia (potassium >6.5 mmol/L)

1. Calcium chloride 10% or calcium gluconate 10%; 10 mL intravenously (rule of 10s). Calcium is a membrane stabilizer for myocardial cells. It will not lower the serum potassium but stabilizes the myocardial cell membrane. Repeat doses may be required if the hyperkalaemia persists with ECG changes for longer than 30 minutes.
2. Salbutamol nebulizer 10–20 mg in an adult.
3. Insulin-dextrose. A mix of 50 mL 50% dextrose plus 10 units of a short-acting insulin (Actrapid) given over 20 minutes. This will help to reduce the serum potassium by driving the ions intracellularly. Monitoring of the blood glucose is essential.

Table 3 Main indications for consideration for emergency filtration or dialysis

- Acidosis: serum bicarbonate <12 mmol/L, arterial pH <7.15
- Pulmonary oedema: it is important to remember that conventional treatments for a patient with pulmonary oedema are unlikely to be successful in patients with severe renal impairment and volume overload
- Hyperkalaemia: serum potassium >7.0 mmol/L

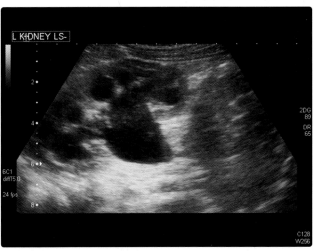

Fig. 3 **Ultrasound image showing distended renal calyces** in a left kidney with hydronephrosis in a patient with acute renal failure.

electrolyte to assess and act on in the emergency department. If elevated, emergency treatment is required (Table 2).

ECG: important to look for any signs of hyperkalaemia, peaked T waves or broadening of the QRS complex.

Ultrasound: an ultrasound scan may identify an abnormality with the kidneys such as an obstructive uropathy with hydronephrosis (Fig. 3).

Emergency management

It is essential that a patient with hyperkalaemia has cardiac monitoring in a closely monitored environment and is treated urgently. Dehydrated patients with pre-renal failure should be rehydrated with intravenous crystalloid.

Insertion of a urinary catheter allows close monitoring of urine production and will also relieve the obstruction if the cause of the acute renal failure is bladder outflow obstruction.

Involve renal physicians early if there is evidence of renal inflammation associated with acute renal failure or if the patient requires urgent haemodialysis (Table 3). If the patient is very unwell then haemofiltration in the intensive care unit may be required.

Key points

- Hyperkalaemia requires prompt identification and urgent treatment.
- Early ultrasound and sending a urine for microscopy (particularly looking for casts) is helpful in identifying the aetiology of the renal failure.
- Always consider the need for dialysis, especially if the patient has pulmonary oedema.

Urinary tract problems

Haematuria

Haematuria, blood in the urine, may be either visible to the human eye (macroscopic) or detected only on urine dipstick testing (microscopic). Common causes of microscopic haematuria include infection, trauma and occult malignancy.

Causes of macroscopic haematuria

- Ureteric calculi: the patient will have experienced pain, commonly loin, but sometimes lower abdomen or groin pain. The pain is typically colicky and can be excruciating.
- Infection: haemorrhagic cystitis, a severe inflammatory infection of the bladder, can cause haematuria.
- Trauma: in the context of blunt abdominal trauma, if macroscopic haematuria is present, then imaging with contrast-enhanced CT is indicated. In major trauma it is possible to have a significant renal injury with no haematuria. If only microscopic haematuria is present, the mechanism of injury was not significant, and if there is no associated abdominal tenderness, then it is reasonable to adopt an expectant policy. The urine needs to be rechecked in approximately one week to ensure that the haematuria has resolved. Persistent microscopic haematuria always requires investigation and referral to a urologist.

Ureteric colic

Be wary of making the diagnosis of renal colic in patients over 50 years of age; always consider the possibility of pain from a leaking aortic aneurysm. Also, consider non-urological causes for microscopic haematuria: appendicitis and leaking aortic aneurysms may both cause microscopic haematuria. If there is abdominal tenderness (as opposed to loin tenderness) renal colic is less likely. Urinalysis shows microscopic haematuria in over 95% of cases of ureteric colic. Be very cautious about diagnosing renal colic in someone who has no microscopic haematuria, as this is very unusual. Check the renal function (urea/creatinine and

electrolytes), FBC and CRP. If a microcytic (low mean cell volume, MCV) and hypochromic (low mean cell haemoglobin, MCH) anaemia is detected, this picture of iron deficiency anaemia suggests a chronic blood loss. The white cell count and CRP may be elevated in infection. Sepsis in a patient with an obstructed kidney from a calculus is a urological emergency; if the obstruction is not removed or the kidney drained (with a urostomy) the kidney may be irreversibly damaged. In suspected ureteric colic there are several possible imaging modalities that can be utilized (Table 1). An abdominal CT without contrast is the gold standard. Plain abdominal films are generally unhelpful as stones are difficult to identify with any accuracy and it is not possible to assess ureteric dilatation. Renal tract ultrasound lacks sensitivity but may show an obstructive uropathy in the setting of ureteric colic (Fig. 1); it is the initial investigation of choice in pregnant patients. A CT will identify the presence of calculi with accuracy (Fig. 2), identify the presence of complications of calculi such as ureteric obstruction and may also identify a possible alternative diagnosis for the patient's symptoms (such as a leaking aortic aneurysm, appendicitis, diverticulitis or other renal tract pathology).

Table 1 **Accuracy of imaging modalities for ureteric colic**			
Imaging technique	Positive predictive value (%)	Negative predictive value (%)	Accuracy (%)
Helical CT	97	100	98
Plain radiography	90	51	70
Intravenous urography	93	31	60
Ultrasound	100	30	46

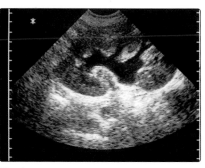

Fig. 1 **Renal ultrasound showing dilatation of pelvicalyceal system.**

Emergency management

Adequate analgesia is essential in ureteric colic. Non-steroidal anti-inflammatory drugs (NSAIDs) have been shown to be as effective as opiates in treating pain from ureteric calculi. Some patients will require both an NSAID and an opiate. Ensure adequate hydration with intravenous fluids and, if the patient has nausea or has vomited, an anti-emetic is indicated. If the diagnosis is clear, the renal function is normal, the patient does not have a known abnormal renal tract (such as a solitary kidney), there is no suggestion of infection, and the pain settles, then an outpatient approach to management is reasonable. A plain CT abdomen and appropriate follow-up can be arranged on an outpatient basis. Persistent microscopic haematuria requires investigation to rule out an occult malignancy.

Urinary tract infections

Lower urinary tract infections (UTIs) involve the bladder and urethra, whereas pyelonephritis involves the kidneys and is more serious. A UTI is defined as a culture of pure growth of 10^5 organisms. Clearly this definition is not of much help in patients presenting to the emergency department since culture results commonly takes 48 hours. Local symptoms of UTI include dysuria, frequency and incontinence and systemic symptoms are fever, rigors, vomiting (in children) and confusion (in the elderly). At the extremes of age, local symptoms are often absent with non-specific systemic symptoms predominating. Examination may show signs of infection such as fever and tachycardia or there may be suprapubic tenderness. Often there will be very little to find on examination. Renal angle tenderness suggests pyelonephritis and is more worrying. Urinalysis is a point of care test that involves a dipstick of a urine sample. Ideally the urine ought to be midstream. Urinalysis tests for the presence of leucocytes, nitrites, blood and protein. All of these parameters may test positive with a urinary tract infection but the presence of leucocytes and nitrites is more specific.

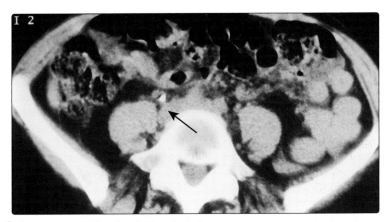

Fig. 2 **Non-contrast CT showing right ureteric stone.**

The leucocytes test depends upon detection of the enzyme leucocyte esterase. The nitrite test relies on the fact that most organisms causing UTIs will convert urinary nitrates to nitrites. The sensitivity and specificity of the presence of leucocytes or nitrites is less than 100% and the figures quoted for their presence predicting a UTI are very variable. Urgent urine microscopy may be helpful although this is time-consuming. The urine is examined for the presence of leucocytes and bacteria. Greater than five leucocytes per high powered field suggest a UTI. The presence of bacteria on Gram staining is very specific for UTI but not sensitive. In patients with suspected UTI it is helpful to send the urine for culture but a system needs to be in place for the follow-up of positive results. Antibiotic treatment of suspected UTIs depends on local sensitivities. The commonest organism causing UTI is *E. coli*. Other common pathogens are *Enterococcus, Klebsiella, Pseudomonas* and *Proteus*. *E. coli* is increasingly resistant to traditional antibiotics such as amoxicillin, oral cephalosporins and trimethoprim. Quinolones (e.g. norfloxacin), which have a much greater sensitivity, are now the antibiotics of choice for uncomplicated UTI. Systemically well patients are normally treated as outpatients but those with complicated UTIs (extremes of age, solitary kidney, systemic symptoms, immunocompromised patients, structural abnormality of renal tract) will require admission. Patients with suspected pyelonephritis generally require admission to ensure adequate hydration and response to treatment.

Retention of urine

Acute retention of urine is an inability to pass urine from the bladder and should not be confused clinically with anuria. In males, the commonest cause is bladder outflow obstruction, which in turn is most commonly caused by benign prostatic hypertrophy. Other causes include urethral strictures, blood clots and malignancy. The patient, generally a middle-aged or elderly man, will not be able to pass urine, although there may be overflow dribbling. There may be abdominal discomfort in the suprapubic region and on examination there will be tenderness and stony dullness to percussion. Always consider a neuropathic cause for retention especially in patient groups where retention is uncommon (e.g. women). Neurological conditions causing acute retention include multiple sclerosis and cauda equina syndrome (see 'Back pain' chapter). Medications such as anticholinergics can cause acute retention, and a careful drug history is important. Treatment involves passing a Foley catheter; in adult males this is normally a size 16F. This allows the bladder to be drained. Occasionally a Foley catheter cannot be passed, and suprapubic catheterization will be required.

Key points

- Never assume a diagnosis of ureteric colic in patients over 50 years.
- Ureteric colic is less likely in the absence of haematuria.
- Macroscopic haematuria in trauma is an indication for CT scanning.
- Always check for persistent haematuria.
- Urinary tract infections are a common cause of sepsis, and of confusion in the elderly.

Male genital problems

A spectrum of conditions affecting the male genital tract may present to the emergency department. The patient is commonly embarrassed and a sympathetic approach is important.

Testicular torsion

Testicular torsion must be considered in anyone complaining of groin or testicular pain. Torsion generally occurs in a bimodal age distribution, either in infants or in adolescents. Do not be deceived by a history of trauma; patients sometimes relate their testicular pain back to an irrelevant trivial injury. Also, traumatic testicular torsion is well described. There is an overlap in the presentation of torsion and infection (epididymitis and orchitis); distinction can be difficult. With torsion, the pain is often more sudden in onset compared with infection, where the pain is more gradual in onset. Always have a chaperone with you when examining the genitalia. Palpate both testes, feeling for the body of the testicle and the epididymis. The position of both testicles is important to note. In torsion, the testicle is tender and tends to lie higher and in a more horizontal position (Fig. 1). Check the cremasteric reflex; this involves stroking the inside of the thigh and watching for contraction of the ipsilateral cremaster muscle and elevation of the testicle.

This reflex may be quite subtle but is often lost in testicular torsion. Testicular ultrasound may be helpful in distinguishing between torsion and infection, particularly if Doppler ultrasound is used to demonstrate blood flow in the testicular artery. Clinical suspicion should predominate since a normal ultrasound does not always rule out torsion. If torsion is strongly suspected then referral for surgical exploration and not unnecessary investigation and delay is required. If torsion is a possibility then a urology review is always indicated.

The hydatid of Morgagni is an appendage of the testicle that may undergo torsion. The pain is localized to the appendage on the upper pole of the testis and the 'blue dot' sign if present is indicative. The 'blue dot' sign is where the ischaemic appendage is visible through the skin (Fig. 2). If the diagnosis is certain then a conservative approach is reasonable; if there is doubt it is safest to treat as a possible testicular torsion.

Epididymitis and orchitis

Infective causes of male genital pain are epididymitis and orchitis; there is overlap between the two conditions. Infection tends to affect men over 35 years and is very uncommon in men under 20 years of age. In more elderly men it is commonly associated with a

lower urinary tract infection caused by Gram-negative bacteria. In younger men it may be a manifestation of a sexually transmitted disease such as chlamydial infection. Treatment involves antibiotics, analgesics and advice to wear underwear that supports the scrotum. Urinalysis may show some indication of infection but blood tests are generally not helpful. Mumps can cause an orchitis, but in this case the symptoms are bilateral and other features of mumps will be present.

Fournier's gangrene

Fournier's gangrene is a necrotizing fasciitis of the scrotum. It is rare but life-threatening if not identified early and treated aggressively. Early on the appearance is of a cellulitis affecting the external genitalia. This progresses, occasionally rapidly, over hours to necrosis and gangrene. Treatment is with aggressive resuscitation, antibiotics and surgical debridement.

Torn frenulum

A torn frenulum is seen in adolescents after sexual activity. Occasionally the frenulum will require suturing for haemostasis but if the bleeding has stopped a conservative approach and a period of abstinence from sexual activity is all that is required.

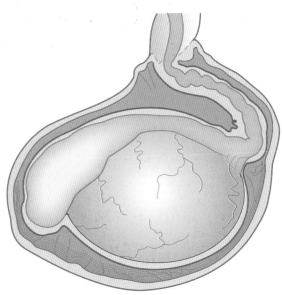

Fig. 1 **Bell-clapper (horizontal) testis.**

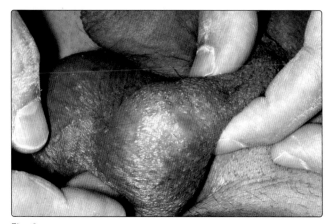

Fig. 2 **'Blue dot' sign indicative of torsion of hydatid of Morgagni.**

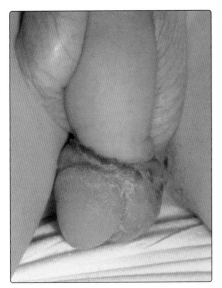

Fig. 3 **Paraphimosis;** note swelling of the glans.

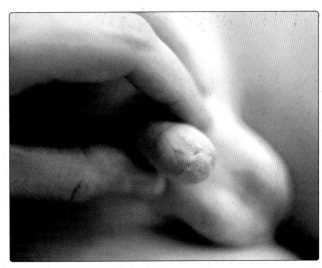

Fig. 4 **Phimosis;** the foreskin cannot be retracted.

Paraphimosis and phimosis

A paraphimosis is where the foreskin is retracted over the prepuce and cannot be reduced (Fig. 3). The band around the prepuce can be very tight and the situation exacerbated by local oedema. Ensure the patient has plenty of analgesia; a penile block may help. Local anaesthetic is infiltrated around the base of the penis; ensure that plain local anaesthetic is used without the addition of adrenaline (epinephrine). Adrenaline causes vasoconstriction and could cause penile ischaemia. The paraphimosis can normally be reduced by longitudinal traction of the penis. If this fails surgical intervention may be required.

A true phimosis develops over years. The foreskin becomes non-retractile and the aperture progressively stenoses (Fig. 4). The patient presents with difficulty passing urine; there may be retention of urine and even an obstructive uropathy.

Trauma

With genital trauma consider the possibility of sexual assault. Most haematomas will resolve without intervention, patients often require reassurance since the appearance of bruised genitalia is often quite alarming.

Priapism

Priapism is the presence of an involuntary persistent painful erection. Its occurrence is unrelated to sexual stimulation and is an emergency. A key factor in the examination is that the glans is not swollen. It can be caused by medications such as sildenafil, by haematological conditions such as sickle cell anaemia and by spinal cord injury. Ischaemic priapism is an emergency and requires aspiration of blood from the corpus. Involve the urology team at an early stage.

Paediatric considerations

- Boys may not volunteer that their genitalia are painful and may present with lower abdominal pain.
- Torsion can occur at any age, including newborns.
- Infective causes of testicular pain are very rare in children. Be very wary of making the diagnosis of epididymitis in an adolescent; torsion is much more likely.

Key points

- In anyone presenting with testicular pain consider the possibility of torsion.
- If torsion is possible then referral for surgical exploration is mandatory.
- Features of cellulitis in the male genital region may be an early manifestation of Fournier's gangrene.

Headache

Introduction

Headache is very common; it is the main symptom in up to 5% of all patients who attend the emergency department. Although most headaches have a benign underlying aetiology, the emergency physician must differentiate which headache represents a life-threatening disorder.

Headaches can be classified into primary headaches (with no underlying pathology) and secondary headaches. Primary headache syndromes such as migraine, tension headache or cluster headaches usually presently slowly or are recurrent. In contrast, most secondary headaches (such as subarachnoid haemorrhage, meningitis and low CSF pressure headache) tend to be single events developing over a period of seconds to weeks.

Key diagnostic points

A clear history is the most important tool when assessing patients with headache (Table 1). Details of all medications should be noted since the commonest cause of a chronic headache is medication-overuse resulting from frequent intake of analgesic medication (NSAIDs, paracetamol or opiate-based analgesics).

Table 1	**Key points in history**
Onset	Seconds to minutes (SAH)
	Hours to days (meningitis)
	Days to months (raised ICP)
Character	Sudden, severe 'like being hit by a bat' (SAH)
	Pulsating (migraine)
	Boring (cluster headache)
	Tenderness (giant cell arteritis)
Location	Unilateral (migraine, cluster headache)
	Bilateral
	Occipital (SAH)
Triggers	Trauma (SAH, haematoma, carotid dissection)
	Oversleeping, hunger, alcohol (within hours) and change in temperature (migraine)
	Alcohol, glyceryl trinitrate (cluster headache)
	Lying down, crouching, coughing and straining, nausea and vomiting (raised ICP)
Associated symptoms	Flashing lights (migraine)
	Nausea (migraine)
	Infective symptoms such as fever (meningitis)

Examination is often normal in the patient presenting with headache. In addition to a full neurological examination, key signs to look for are:

- fever, rash, neck stiffness and photophobia (meningitis)
- temporal artery and scalp tenderness (giant cell arteritis)
- loss of venous pulsations with or without papilloedema seen by fundoscopy (raised ICP).

Investigations

Other than an ESR in the case of giant cell arteritis, blood tests do not inform the cause of headache. A head CT scan is important in the diagnosis of suspected subarachnoid haemorrhage, raised intracranial pressure, haematomas or tumours and some cases of meningitis. All first or worst headaches presenting to an emergency department warrant a head CT scan as do patients with focal signs or reduced conscious level. Further investigations such as lumbar puncture or MRI may be indicated.

Red flags in the history and examination, suggesting a serious cause for the headache are:

- new onset headache
- history of recent trauma
- fever or rash (meningitis)
- focal neurological signs or altered consciousness
- symptoms and signs of raised intracranial pressure
- scalp tenderness or jaw claudication (giant cell arteritis).

Causes

Secondary headaches
Subarachnoid haemorrhage
This usually presents with a sudden onset headache. Patients classically describe the headache 'like being hit at the back of the head'. There may be associated signs of meningism (neck stiffness and photophobia) and occasionally focal neurological signs. Mortality is high, with 25% of patients dying within 24 hours and another 25% dying in hospital. CT scan of the head within 24 hours is over 90% sensitive for detecting subarachnoid blood (Fig. 1). If the CT is normal, a lumbar puncture should be performed looking for xanthochromia (a yellow discoloration of CSF caused by bilirubin resulting from the breakdown of haemoglobin) (Fig. 2). This may not be detectable within the first 12 hours of headache onset. Management is aimed at preventing secondary complications, such as vasospasm, with adequate intravenous hydration, analgesia and calcium channel blockers such as nimodipine. Eighty per cent of non-traumatic subarachnoid haemorrhages are caused by ruptured saccular arterial aneurysms. Untreated, there is a 3% risk per year of aneurysmal rebleeding. Definitive management therefore includes obliterating the detected aneurysm either by an intravascular procedure or by open surgery.

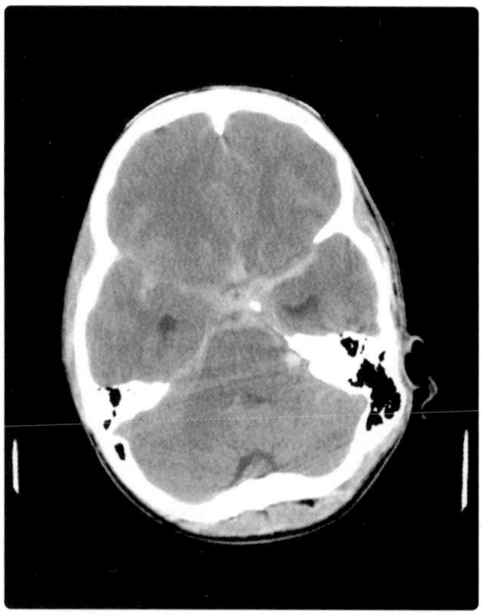

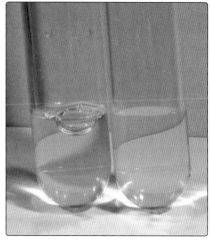

Fig. 1 **CT scan showing subarachnoid blood.**

Fig. 2 **Xanthochromia CSF compared to normal CSF.**

Subdural haematoma

This can present with headache, particularly if chronic. A history of preceding trauma is often not forthcoming or deemed trivial in nature. Associated alteration in consciousness and focal neurological signs can accompany a rapidly enlarging haematoma, although can be absent in the chronic form. A low threshold for head CT imaging is needed to avoid missing this diagnosis, especially in elderly patients or patients with alcohol dependence.

Cerebral venous thrombosis (dural sinus thrombosis)

This may present as a non-specific headache, with features of raised intracranial pressure (headache worse on lying flat or coughing and straining, nausea, and sixth nerve palsy) and focal signs or evidence of encephalopathy. Diagnosis is confirmed by specific radiological investigations such as CT venogram or MRI.

Giant cell arteritis

Always consider in any headache patient over the age of 50. Failure to recognize this disorder can lead to irreversible blindness secondary to anterior ischaemic optic neuropathy. Typical features are temporal artery tenderness with scalp pain, jaw claudication and episodes of amaurosis fugax. The erythrocyte sedimentation rate (ESR) is usually greater than 50 mm/hour. A temporal artery biopsy may confirm the diagnosis, although a negative biopsy does not exclude giant cell arteritis since parts of the artery may be normal (so-called 'skip-lesions'). If the diagnosis is suspected clinically, treatment with high dose steroids must be started immediately.

Meningitis

Meningitis is an important differential for acute or subacute headache and is discussed in the 'Meningitis and encephalitis' chapter.

Acute closed angle glaucoma

This is an ophthalmological emergency. This diagnosis must always be considered in the patient presenting to the emergency department with a headache accompanied by a painful red eye.

Primary headaches

Tension-type headache

The commonest form of headache, it is often described as a tight band around the patient's head. The cause is unknown although stress is often associated. Analgesia is often ineffective and reassurance and relaxation exercises can be helpful.

Migraine

Characterized by episodic, recurrent moderate to severe headaches lasting 4–72 hours which are pulsating in character and can be unilateral, these headaches may be associated with photophobia (fear of light), phonophobia (fear of sounds), osmophobia (fear of smells) and nausea. A minority of patients will describe a preceding aura lasting 5–60 minutes. This aura may be visual (positive features such as flickering lights/fortification spectra or negative features such as visual field defects), somatosensory (positive features such as paraesthesia or negative in the form of numbness) or manifest as dysphasic speech disturbance. Treatment consists of acute relief medication such as a 5-HT1 agonist (sumatriptan) or a combination of paracetamol, a non-steroidal anti-inflammatory drug and an anti-emetic. If headaches are frequent, then prophylactic medication can be considered, such as a beta-blocker, tricyclic antidepressant or certain anti-epileptic drugs.

Cluster headache

This belongs to a rare group of specific headaches characterized by strictly unilateral head pain associated with autonomic symptoms and signs. Once seen, cluster headache is never forgotten and female patients will often state that the pain of cluster headache is more severe than labour pains. The headache itself is usually located around the eye and temple. There may be unilateral photophobia, in contrast to migraine which is usually bilateral. Autonomic features include lacrimation, conjunctival injection, ptosis, miosis, nasal blockage or rhinorrhoea, forehead sweating and ipsilateral eyelid oedema. In contrast to migraine, the patient is often restless. The attacks last between 15 and 180 minutes. Many patients will experience 'cluster periods' lasting weeks to months separated by periods of remission. Management consists of acute relief medication, high flow oxygen and subcutaneous 5-HT1 agonist (sumatriptan).

Emergency management

A detailed history is the key to risk stratifying patients presenting to the emergency department with a headache. All 'first or worst' sudden headaches should be considered as possible subarachnoid haemorrhages and investigated. CT and lumbar puncture should be considered together. For other headaches, MRI is the investigation of choice if CT is unremarkable. Primary headache syndromes may be relieved with specific treatments. Most patients benefit from simple analgesia and rehydration. Escalation up the analgesia ladder often has little short-term benefit and can lead to a medication-overuse headache. Discussion with a neurologist is usually indicated to discuss which patients should be followed up in clinic.

Key points

- History is important in diagnosing headache causes.
- Very rarely does examination identify the cause of headache.
- It is helpful to divide headaches into primary and secondary causes.
- CT and lumbar puncture should be considered together as investigation for suspected subarachnoid haemorrhage.

Seizures

Up to 10% of the population will have a seizure during their lifetime. A single seizure in a patient presenting to an emergency department (ED) may be part of an epilepsy disorder, an isolated seizure ('first fit') or the result of a specific underlying disorder (provoked seizure). Epilepsy is defined as a tendency to recurrent seizures, each seizure being an abnormal neurological episode caused by an abnormal discharge of neurons.

Diagnosis and classification

In the ED, it is important to differentiate seizures from a syncopal episode (see 'Blackouts and syncope' chapter). The diagnosis of epilepsy is clinical, based on the history from the patient and witnesses, and aided by investigations such as EEG and CT scan. Examination is usually normal unless there is an underlying disorder causing a provoked seizure. Examine for evidence of structural brain disease, especially if the seizure is of a focal type.

Epilepsy can be classified according to the seizure type (Fig. 1) and according to the epilepsy syndrome. Patients may have more than one type of seizure within their epilepsy syndrome. The old terms 'petit mal' and 'grand mal' are now rarely used. Three main types of epilepsy syndrome exist:

- generalized: associated with diffuse, generalized discharge of neurons
- focal: neurons discharge from a specific area of the brain that may remain localized or become generalized.
- provoked: secondary to acute abnormalities.

Investigations

All patients presenting with a seizure should have their blood glucose checked. In patients with known epilepsy who have recovered completely after a seizure, blood tests will be of little value, although anticonvulsant drug blood levels can be measured to assess compliance. Epileptic patients who have an atypical seizure or who remain obtunded should be considered for full biochemical tests and head CT scan.

An EEG is helpful in characterizing the epilepsy syndrome but a normal EEG does not exclude epilepsy. Only in rare circumstance, e.g. non-convulsive status or suspected encephalitis, is an EEG useful in the ED. All patients with suspected meningitis (neck stiffness, photophobia, fever) or a focal brain lesion should have a head CT scan.

Single seizure

Many patients present to ED with a first ever generalized convulsion or a blackout that resembles a seizure. Assessment is aimed at identifying any underlying or treatable cause (Table 1).

During the post-ictal period patients often have loss of airway reflexes and are best nursed in the recovery position (Fig. 2).

Table 1 **Acute cause of seizures**
Hypoxia
Hypoglycaemia
Head trauma
Meningitis and encephalitis
Metabolic disorders, including hyponatraemia, hypocalcaemia, eclampsia
Drug overdose, including alcohol, tricyclics, anticonvulsants, cocaine
Drug withdrawal, including alcohol, benzodiazepines, anticonvulsants
Cerebral tumour or stroke
Fever (in children)

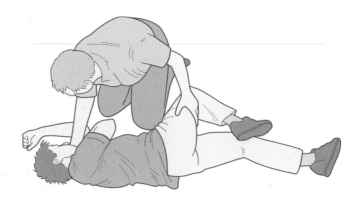

Fig. 1 **Seizure types.**

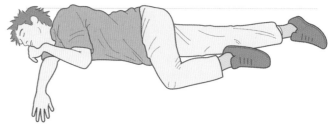

Fig. 2 **Recovery position.**

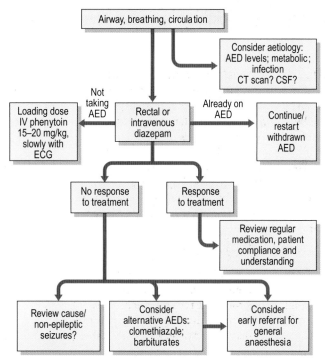

Fig. 3 **Management of convulsive status epilepticus.** AED, anti-epilepsy drug.

If fully recovered, a patient with a first seizure may be discharged home with follow-up in a neurology clinic. A diagnosis of epilepsy is not made after a single seizure and no anticonvulsants are commenced. Patients should be advised not to drive or operate complex machinery before their neurology review.

Emergency management

Status epilepticus is defined as a seizure or seizures occurring for 30 minutes, either continuously or intermittently but without full recovery. The seizures may be generalized or focal or rarely there may be a non-convulsive status with a confusional state with or without abnormal motor activity. Status epilepticus may be the first presentation of epilepsy. The longer the seizure activity continues the more refractory to treatment it becomes.

Resuscitation is aimed at stabilization of ABC, termination of the seizures and treating any underlying cause (Fig. 3). After checking the blood glucose, first line treatment is administration of an intravenous benzodiazepine (diazepam, midazolam or lorazepam). This may be followed by a loading dose of phenytoin (Table 2). If the seizure continues, the patient will need to be given a general anaesthetic (using thiopental).

Table 2 **Drugs for status epilepticus**

Drug	Dose IV	Alternative routes
Lorazepam	0.1 mg/kg	
Diazepam	0.2–0.3 mg/kg	0.3–0.5 mg/kg rectally
Midazolam	0.1 mg/kg	0.2 mg/kg intranasal or buccal
Phenytoin	15–20 mg/kg loading dose	
Thiopental	2–4 mg/kg for anaesthesia	

Key points

- Look for an underlying cause for seizures as many of these conditions are serious and/or treatable.
- Do not overlook alcohol withdrawal or encephalitis as a possible underlying cause.
- Status epilepticus is a medical emergency.
- Advise on driving restrictions and document clearly.

Vertigo and giddiness

Introduction

The terms 'giddiness', 'dizziness', 'vertigo', 'muzzy head' and 'off balance' are often used by patients to convey a number of symptoms. Direct questioning is usually needed to elicit the exact nature of the patient's complaint.

Vertigo is an illusion of rotation due to an asymmetric disorder of the peripheral labyrinths of the inner ear, or the central connections including the vestibular nerve, nuclei and the cerebellum. The patient feels as if either they, or the environment, is rotating or, less commonly, tilting. It is associated with nausea, vomiting and unsteadiness. It is always temporary, always made worse by movement of the head and almost never causes loss of consciousness unless this is secondary to a fall or other complication.

Key diagnostic points

Most causes of vertigo can be identified by a thorough history and examination (Table 1). Only rarely are further tests required. Of key importance is the need to distinguish peripheral vestibular lesions from central vestibular connections.

Specific examination tests

- *Head impulse test* (Fig. 1). The patient sits upright with gaze fixed on a target roughly 3 metres away and is instructed to keep looking at the target whilst the examiner turns their head. Starting with the head slightly turned to one side, turn the head rapidly in a horizontal direction to the other side to about 20°. Watch the eyes for corrective eye movements (saccades). Corrective saccades after a head thrust in one direction indicate that there is a peripheral vestibular lesion affecting that side.
- *Positional test (Dix–Hallpike test)*: With the patient sitting upright on the bed turn the head 45° to one side, then lay the patient back quickly with the head turned until their head is extended over the end of the bed with one ear downwards; examine for nystagmus. If present, note the latency (time taken for the nystagmus to start after the manoeuvre), the direction of nystagmus in relation to

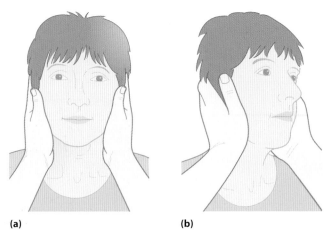

(a) **(b)**

Fig. 1 **Head impulse test.** Patient sits upright with gaze fixed on a target roughly 3 m away and they are instructed to keep looking at the target whilst the examiner turns their head rapidly in a horizontal direction to about 20°. Watch the eyes for corrective eye movements (saccades).

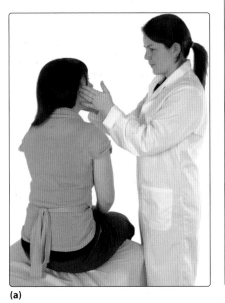
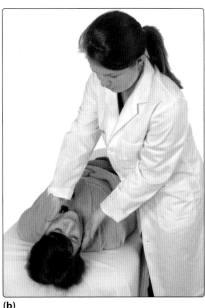

(a) **(b)**

Fig. 2 **Positional (Dix–Hallpike) test. (a)** With the patient sitting upright on the bed turn the head 45° to one side. **(b)** Then lay the patient back quickly with the head turned until their head is extended over the end of the bed with one ear downwards; examine for nystagmus. The classic result of the Hallpike test, seen in benign paroxysmal positional nystagmus (BPPV), is nystagmus after a latency of 2–6 seconds which is mixed rotatory and horizontal (seen as down towards the lower ear), associated with vertigo and nausea which wane as the nystagmus reduces over the subsequent 30 seconds.

the downward ear, and whether the nystagmus fatigues over time (wait for 60 seconds). The classic result of the Hallpike test, seen in benign paroxysmal positional vertigo (BPPV), is nystagmus after a latency of 2–6 seconds which is mixed rotatory and horizontal (seen as down towards the lower ear), associated with vertigo and nausea, which wane as the nystagmus reduces over the subsequent 30 seconds (Fig. 2).

Table 1 **Key points in history and examination**	
Vertigo	Acute or gradual onset; intermittent or sustained
Auditory dysfunction	Hearing loss or tinnitus; ear discharge or pain
Associated neurology	Diplopia; ataxia or dysarthria; sensory or motor dysfunction
Medication	Anticonvulsant toxicity; aminoglycosides
Eye movements	Nystagmus (rotatory, horizontal, vertical or mixed)
Gait and balance	Ability to stand and walk unaided; Romberg's test

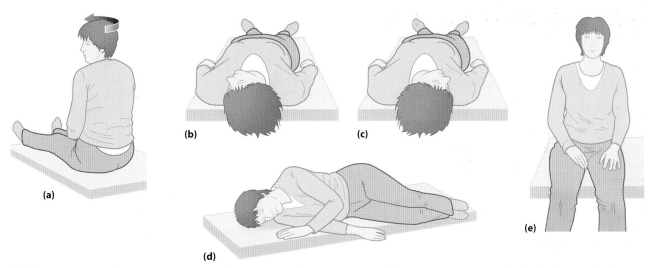

Fig. 3 **Epley's manoeuvre: each position is held for 30–60 seconds (a–e).** Starting with the patient sitting up, turn their head 45° to one side, then follow the sequence through **b** to **d**, holding each position for 30–60 seconds; then sit the patient up again.

■ *Blocking visual fixation of nystagmus*: An ophthalmoscope can be used to block visual fixation and allow easier detection of a spontaneous nystagmus. The patient is asked to cover one eye with their hand while the fundus of the other eye is viewed with the ophthalmoscope. A common result is for initially unapparent nystagmus to become obvious or for known nystagmus to increase in amplitude. This is associated with a peripheral vestibular lesion. It is important to note that because the optic nerve head is behind the centre of rotation of the eye the nystagmus is in the opposite direction to what is observed normally.

Investigations

MRI of the brain, caloric testing or auditory evoked potentials may be indicated in investigating central causes of vertigo. A CT scan only rarely identifies a cause.

Causes

■ Benign paroxysmal positional vertigo (BPPV): this is the commonest cause of vertigo, causing an intermittent, positional vertigo. It is generally thought to be caused by the movement of otolith particles within the semicircular canals of the inner ear; it may follow viral infection or head injury. Diagnosis is via the Hallpike positional test, which gives the classical findings outlined above.
■ Vestibular neuronitis: also called labyrinthitis and vestibular neuritis. It often follows viral infection and

can occur in epidemics. The head impulse test is invariably positive but the rest of the neurological examination is normal.
■ Ménière's disease: this presents with spontaneous, well-defined, prolonged episodes of vertigo that can last from 20 minutes to 24 hours. It is often associated with deafness and tinnitus, which can take a few days to resolve after the vertigo settles.
■ Vertebrobasilar circulation infarct and haemorrhage: tends to cause sudden, severe vertigo with vomiting and instability such that the patient struggles to stand unaided, even with eyes open. There may also be other neurological symptoms such as headache, visual disturbance, diplopia, dysarthria, weakness or numbness.
■ Brainstem lesions such as infarction, tumours (especially acoustic nerve tumours) or multiple sclerosis may cause sustained vertigo.

Emergency management

Suspicion of a central cause depends on recognizing when the signs and symptoms presented by the patient do not match the features of any of the peripheral disorders with reasonable accuracy. Although readily available, CT scans have a low diagnostic yield, being unable to detect many posterior fossa lesions as well as demyelination. The investigation of choice for a central cause is an MRI or, if vertebrobasilar insufficiency or vertebral artery dissection is suspected, MR angiography. If MRI is unavailable it may be safe to observe the patient if there is only mild concern, as in those

with a peripheral cause the nystagmus will improve significantly over 48 hours.

Vestibular sedatives can be used in the acute phase when symptoms are most pronounced. Drugs used include antihistamines e.g. cinnarizine or betahistine, dopaminergic antagonists e.g. prochlorperazine, or anticholinergic agents e.g. hyoscine. Vestibular sedatives may delay compensation of vestibular function and should only be used for a short time. Patients can be taught graded exercises to encourage retraining of central mechanisms.

Epley's manoeuvre (Fig. 3) can be used to reposition and remove debris in the semicircular canals and so treat BPPV. This manoeuvre can be performed in the emergency department although it sometimes needs to be repeated several times over the course of days.

Key points

■ It is important to establish the presenting complaint truly is vertigo.

■ A number of bedside tests can be easily learned.

■ Associated neurological symptoms, lack of auditory symptoms, severe imbalance and persistent, severe vertigo are historical features suggestive of a central cause.

■ Any neurological signs, nystagmus of a central type or not reduced by fixation, an abnormal response to the Hallpike test, a negative head impulse test or an inability to stand up even with eyes open are suggestive of a central cause.

■ MR imaging is the modality of choice for suspected central causes.

Weakness and sensory loss

Introduction

Weakness and sensory symptoms are common and can arise from lesions at every level of the nervous system. Not all limb weakness is secondary to a stroke (CVA). Sensory symptoms can occur in isolation or in conjunction with motor weakness. They do not occur in diseases that solely affect muscle or the neuromuscular junction, such as motor neuron disease. The commonest sensory symptoms are numbness, tingling, pins and needles or pain. It may be difficult for the patient to describe the exact nature of their sensory disturbance or to localize the area of sensory change.

Key diagnostic points

Determine the time course of the symptoms and the exact nature of the complaint. Patients may complain of weakness when they mean fatigue or poor coordination. Loss of joint position sense may be described as clumsiness. Numbness, tingling and pins and needles can mean different things to different patients.

The history should establish whether there are other symptoms such as difficulty swallowing, any abnormality of speech, vision or urination, any recent head trauma and relevant past medical history (especially hypertension, diabetes, previous strokes).

Examination for weakness should assess for wasting, fasciculation, posture, power, tone and reflexes. Assessing tone and reflexes requires the patient to be relaxed or distracted by conversation. Tone may be decreased, i.e. 'flaccidity', or increased, i.e. 'spasticity'. In an acute upper motor neuron (UMN) lesion, e.g. with a stroke, tone may be temporarily flaccid before becoming increased. A reliable assessment of power cannot be undertaken if the patient is confused, has pain-limiting movements (such as arthritis) or has significant coordination problems.

The distribution of weakness is important in helping identify the site of neurological lesion, e.g. paraplegia, hemiplegia or ascending weakness. Reflexes are increased in UMN lesions and decreased in lesions of the lower

motor neurons (LMN) or muscles. Reflexes may be absent in the early stages of an UMN lesion. The plantar reflex is typically upgoing in UMN lesions, but can be inconsistent (Fig. 1). Assess gait if possible; this may demonstrate a hemiplegic, waddling (myopathic) or steppage (LMN) gait.

Examination of sensation involves assessment of all five modalities: light touch, pin-prick, joint position sense, vibration sense and temperature. The different modalities are mainly carried in two tracts (dorsal column and spinothalamic tract) within the spinal cord; a preliminary sensory examination can focus on just light touch and joint position.

Like weakness, the distribution of sensory changes is important. Hemisection of the spinal cord will lead to contralateral loss of light touch, pin prick and temperature with ipsilateral loss of vibration and joint position sense below the level of the lesion. A dorsal column lesion will

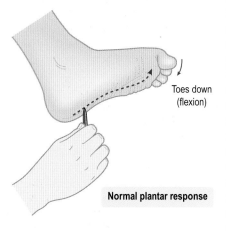

Normal plantar response

Toes down (flexion)

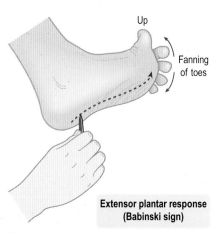

Up

Fanning of toes

Extensor plantar response (Babinski sign)

Fig. 1 **The plantar reflex.**

lead to loss of vibration and joint position sense below the lesion level with preservation of other modalities. A brainstem lesion, such as a stroke or tumour, will typically lead to complete contralateral body sensory loss with ipsilateral sensory loss in the face. Localized spinal cord lesions like a disc prolapse will lead to sensory loss in a dermatomal distribution.

Important emergency investigations to consider are head CT scan to diagnose strokes (bleed or infarct), subdural bleeds or tumours, and spine MRI to diagnose cord compression. Spinal cord compression requires emergency surgery, while some very recent strokes can be treated with thrombolysis (within 3 hours of presentation).

Investigations for suspected lower motor neuron weakness are rarely performed in an emergency department.

Causes

Upper motor neuron weakness
Lesions of the brain, brainstem and spinal cord cause upper motor neuron signs and the weakness has a pyramidal pattern, particularly affecting extensor muscles in the legs, and flexors in the arms. Brain hemisphere (cortex) or brainstem lesions will cause contralateral weakness affecting the face, arm or leg opposite to the side of the lesion. There may be associated cranial nerve or sensory signs. The commonest cause of acute upper motor neuron weakness is stroke, a brain injury of a vascular origin (Table 1). This may be cerebral

Table 1 **Causes of weakness**
Stroke
Multiple sclerosis
Tumour
Subdural haematoma
Spondylosis
Spinal abscess/inflammation
Motor neuron disease
Polio
Neuropathies:
Guillain–Barré
Diabetes
Nutritional deficiencies
Myasthenia gravis
Myopathies:
Muscular dystrophy
Polymyositis
Functional weakness

infarction (80%), cerebral haemorrhage (15%) or subarachnoid haemorrhage (5%). Strokes are the third most common cause of death in the western world, and even if survived, many patients are left dependent on long-term care. Most cerebral infarctions are due to thromboembolic disease, which is more likely in patients with hypertension, diabetes or a smoking history.

The clinical features of a stroke depend on the area of brain affected, which in turn depends on the cerebral vessel affected. Anterior circulation strokes occur with thromboembolic disease affecting branches of the middle and anterior cerebral arteries. Total occlusion of the middle cerebral artery (MCA) leads to contralateral hemiplegia, hemisensory loss, homonymous hemianopia and deviation of the eyes toward the side of the lesion. Branch occlusions lead to incomplete syndromes. Left-sided MCA lesions lead to dysphasia, either expressive or receptive, or even global aphasia. Posterior circulation strokes occur with disease of the vertebral, basilar or posterior cerebral arteries or their branches. Thromboembolus of these vessels can give combinations of contralateral homonymous hemianopia, contralateral hemisensory loss or disturbance of higher function such as memory, speech or cortical blindness. Posterior circulation strokes can also give cerebellar signs.

A transient ischaemic attack (TIA) is defined as a brief episode of neurological dysfunction caused by focal brain or retinal ischaemia, with clinical symptoms typically lasting less than one hour, and without evidence of acute infarction on imaging. They are mainly caused by emboli and can occur in the anterior or posterior circulation giving temporary symptoms and signs similar to strokes. A particularly common TIA of the anterior circulation is transient monocular blindness or 'amaurosis fugax'. The aim of management of TIAs is to prevent a future stroke.

Urgent investigations should be aimed at looking for an underlying cause such as carotid stenosis (listen for bruits) or cardiac emboli (ECG for atrial fibrillation). Long-term aspirin, carotid endarterectomy or anticoagulation (if patient has atrial fibrillation) all reduce the risk of ischaemic stroke or recurrent TIA. Risk stratification for admission or discharge from the emergency department is important. The ABCD[2] risk stratification tool can be used to help predict the level of risk for early stroke (Table 2).

Lower motor neuron weakness

Lesions of the lower motor neuron, anterior horn cell or peripheral nerves produce LMN weakness. Neuropathies usually produce a distal weakness, although this can be generalized. Guillain–Barré syndrome is an acute demyelinating neuropathy. It usually presents with mild peripheral weakness, often with sensory symptoms, but can progress rapidly to a severe proximal weakness with involvement of cranial nerves and autonomic nerves. Management is supportive, often with ventilatory support as well as specific treatments such as plasma exchange and immunoglobulin injections.

Neuromuscular junction weakness

This is much less common, and usually due to myasthenia gravis. This autoimmune disease classically causes a variable, fatiguable weakness with no sensory loss. Antibodies against the acetylcholine receptor compete with released acetylcholine, interfering with the neuromuscular transmission. The more the muscle is used, the weaker it becomes. The muscles most commonly affected are: face, eyelids, proximal arm and respiratory. Patients often present insidiously with ptosis or diplopia and can develop a myasthenic crisis with life-threatening respiratory compromise.

Muscle weakness

Unlike lower motor neuron, reflexes are preserved in muscle weakness (sensation is also normal). It normally occurs in a proximal limb distribution. These myopathies are often inherited such as muscular dystrophy. Acquired myopathies are often metabolic, for example with renal or liver failure, but can also be inflammatory as with polymyosis.

Sensory loss

Sensory disturbance can be transient or persistent. The cause may originate in the brain (tumour, demyelination, TIAs and CVAs or epilepsy), the spinal cord (demyelination, cervical spondylosis), nerve roots (radiculopathy) or peripheral nerves (diabetic neuropathy). Sensory disturbances can also be unexplained or psychogenic in origin.

Table 2 **The ABCD[2] score for identification of individuals at high early risk of stroke after a TIA**	
Clinical feature	**Score**
A (Age)	1 point if ≥60 years
B (Blood pressure)	1 point if ≥140/90 mmHg
C (Clinical features)	2 points for unilateral weakness, 1 point for speech disturbance without weakness
D (Duration of symptoms)	1 point for 10–59 minutes, 2 points for ≥60 minutes
D (Diabetes)	1 point

Total score	Stroke risk	Action
Scores 0–3	Low risk	Outpatient investigation
Scores 4–5	Moderate risk	Urgent investigation
Scores 6–7	High risk	Admission and urgent investigation

Key points

- Strokes are a major cause of mortality and morbidity in the UK.
- Examination will suggest the site of neurological lesion.
- All TIAs must be risk stratified (ABCD[2]).
- Thrombolysis may be an option for strokes presenting within 3 hours.

Confusion

Introduction

Confusion is a common presentation to the emergency department (ED), especially in elderly patients, and has many causes (Table 1). The presentation of 'confusion' lies along a spectrum of altered conscious level with normal consciousness at one end and coma at the other (see 'Coma' chapter). Many alternative labels are used to describe acute confusion: delirium, acute organic brain disorder, acute confusional state or organic psychosis. Patients with dementia, aphasia (receptive or expressive) or psychosis can mistakenly be diagnosed as acutely confused (Table 2).

Key diagnostic points

History

The history is of vital importance. Confusion typically presents over the course of hours or days and is usually fluctuating in nature. Confused patients typically have reduced arousal, with poor short-term memory, reduced attention spans and poorly organized thinking. Demented patients usually have normal arousal but a progressive decline in cognitive function over years.

Taking a useful history from a confused patient can be very difficult; most are slow to answer and can be emotionally labile often with agitation.

A corroborated history from a spouse or career is helpful and will give information on the patient's premorbid mental function and whether there are any other medical problems that increase the risk of confusion, e.g. diabetes, Parkinson's disease, cardiovascular disease or alcohol problems. A recent history of a fall raises the possibility of a head injury with a subdural bleed causing confusion (Fig. 1).

The patient may present to the ED alone; access to the patient's medical notes and information from the GP or carers (residential home staff, day centre staff, even neighbours) is vital in making an accurate assessment.

Examination

Apart from assessment of the patient's higher cerebral function, neurological examination may show signs of meningitis, hydrocephalus, a recent seizure or a cerebrovascular event. Focal signs are unusual and would suggest an intracranial lesion such as subdural haematoma. The Glasgow Coma Score (GCS) is a standard way of recording the level of consciousness. Higher mental function testing will show disorientation (in time, place or person) and abnormal attention. Scoring systems such as the Abbreviated Mental Test Score are used in an ED setting to assess higher mental function (Table 3). General examination is important to look for signs of infection, metabolic

Table 2 **Differences between dementia and acute confusion (delirium)**

	Dementia	**Delirium**
Onset and course	Slow onset over months or years	Sudden onset over hours or days
Speech	Normal	Slurred
Attention	Normal	Inattentive, easily distracted
Memory	Gradual memory loss	More forgetful than usual
Hallucinations	Possible	Common
Mood	Normal or depressed	Anxious, fearful, suspicious, indifferent
General health	Usual	Sign of illness or drug side effects

Table 1 **Causes of acute confusion**

Systemic	Metabolic
	Hyper- or hyponatraemia
	Hypercalcaemia
	Hypoglycaemia
	Hepatic failure
	Hypothyroidism
	Toxic
	Drugs, especially antiparkinsonian medications and illicit drugs
	Toxins – alcohol or alcohol withdrawal
	Infections
	Septicaemia, urinary tract infections, pneumonia
Intrinsic	Infectious
	Meningitis, encephalitis, malaria
	Paroxysmal
	Epilepsy, ictal or post-ictal
	Immunological
	Lupus
Vascular	Post-stroke
	Subarachnoid haemorrhage
Extrinsic	Subdural haemorrhage
	Post-traumatic
	Hydrocephalus

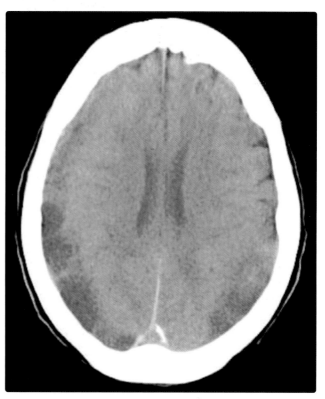

Fig. 1 **CT head scan showing bilateral subdural haematomas.**

Table 3 **The Abbreviated Mental Test Score is a useful screen in patients with suspected cognitive impairment; the maximum score is 10 and a score below 7 suggests cognitive impairment**

Question	Requirement for positive score
Age	Score for exact age only
Date of birth	Score for correct date and month
Year	Score for current year only
Time of day	Score if correct to the nearest hour
Place	Score if exact address or name of hospital given ('in hospital' is insufficient)
Monarch (or head of state)	Score for current monarch only
Year of First World War	Score for year of start or finish
Counting backwards from 20 to 1	Score if no mistakes or subject corrects himself or herself spontaneously
Recognition of two people	Score if roles of two people correctly recognized – e.g. doctor and nurse
Recall of three point address such as 42 West Street	Score if registered correctly near beginning of test and on recall at end of test

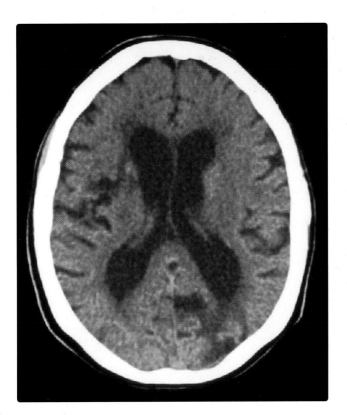

Fig. 2 **CT scan of hydrocephalus.**

disturbance (liver failure, renal failure) or endocrine dysfunction (hypothyroidism, diabetes).

ED management

All confused patients in the ED should have the following blood tests: U&Es, glucose, LFTs, calcium and FBC. In the elderly, urinary and respiratory infections are common causes of confusion. Urinalysis and chest x-ray are useful investigations; other tests may include thyroid function tests, drug screen, blood cultures and blood gases. Many patients warrant head CT scan to exclude a focal brain lesion, subarachnoid haemorrhage, hydrocephalus (Fig. 2) or prior to lumbar puncture in suspected meningitis. Acutely confused patients need to be admitted to hospital for further investigations and nursing care.

Key points

- Many terms are used to denote confusion.
- Confusion should be distinguished from dementia, aphasia or schizophrenia.
- An accurate history is the most important part of assessment.

Meningitis and encephalitis

Infections of the central nervous system are relatively rare. Bacterial meningitis, viral meningitis and encephalitis often have similar overlapping clinical features and can be considered together as meningoencephalitides. Since the introduction of the *Haemophilus influenzae* type B (HiB) vaccine, bacterial meningitis has changed from being primarily a disease of young children (median age 15 months) to mainly a disease of young adults (median age 25 years). The commonest organisms in adults are *Streptococcus pneumoniae*, *Neisseria meningitides* and *Listeria monocytogenes*. Epidemics of bacterial meningitis occur with *N. meningitides*, especially in young adults.

Bacterial meningitis has a mortality rate of around 10%, with up to 20% of patients having some sequelae, most commonly hearing loss, epilepsy, higher function deficits or extremity amputations.

The main differential diagnoses for bacterial meningitis are other types of meningoencephalitides or subarachnoid haemorrhage (see 'Headache' chapter). Aseptic meningitis describes clinical meningitis of non-bacterial aetiology, including viral meningitis, tubercular meningoencephalitis and inflammatory meningitis caused by sarcoid or malignancy.

Key diagnostic points

The classic features of meningitis are fever, headache and neck stiffness. This triad is present in approximately two-thirds of patients with bacterial meningitis. Fever is the most common complaint, present in up to 97% adults, while neck stiffness occurs in roughly 90%. Other features include:

- vomiting
- photophobia
- Kernig's sign; extending the knee while the hip is flexed causes back pain
- altered mental state
- seizures
- focal signs
- petechial or purpuric rash, often associated with meningococcal meningitis or septicaemia (Fig. 1)

- septic shock – may be the main presentation with few signs of meningism; more common at the extremes of age.

The clinical presentation may be atypical in patients with impaired immunity, diabetes, alcohol abuse or previous neurosurgery. In these patient groups a high level of suspicion is required. Appropriate investigations are discussed below with emergency treatment.

Viral meningitis is usually less severe than bacterial with an absence of petechial rash and more mild headache and neck stiffness. In many cases, it is not possible to differentiate viral from bacterial and analysis of cerebrospinal fluid (CSF) is required. Tuberculous meningitis is a more chronic process with a longer history of malaise, fever and headache. It may present more subtly with multiple cranial nerve palsies. Cerebrospinal fluid analysis is not specific, although very low CSF glucose levels are suggestive.

Encephalitis can present as an acute meningitis-type illness but may feature

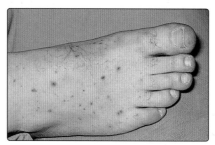

Fig. 1 **Typical meningococcal rash.**

primarily altered behaviour, confusion or seizures. Viral encephalitis may be caused by herpes simplex (HSV), Epstein–Barr virus, adenovirus or rarely rabies. It can occur in epidemics. HSV encephalitis typically affects the temporal lobes with behavioural and speech changes, hemiplegia and seizures frequently leading to short-term memory problems even after recovery.

Emergency management

Investigations

Bacterial meningitis is a medical emergency and treatment should not be delayed pending investigations. All suspected cases should have blood cultures taken and antibiotics administered. Lumbar puncture with laboratory examination of the CSF is important in diagnosis (Fig. 2). Lumbar puncture should be deferred until after a head CT scan (or MRI) if the patient has any focal neurology, signs of raised intracranial pressure, altered mental state or seizures. Interpretation of CSF analysis can be challenging with the immediate CSF Gram stain only being diagnostic in up to two-thirds of patients with bacterial meningitis (Table 1). Culture of the CSF improves the sensitivity but this can take up to 48 hours; ambiguous analysis can present a challenge. If the patient has had antibiotics prior to lumbar puncture (perhaps only by a few hours) then caution is required when interpreting CSF analysis.

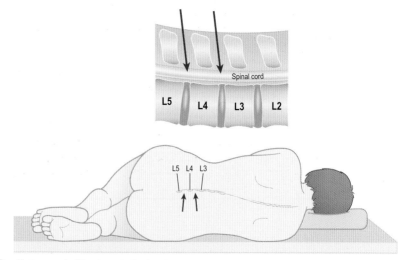

Fig. 2 **Anatomical landmarks for lumbar puncture.**

Table 1 Typical changes in cerebrospinal fluid in different types of meningitis

	Cell count	Differential	CSF protein	CSF glucose
Bacterial	>200/µL	Polymorphs	>1.5 g/L	<40%
Viral	50–200/µL	Lymphocytes	<1.0 g/L	Normal
Tuberculous	50–500/µL	Lymphocytes	>1.0 g/L	<40%
Partially treated bacterial	50–500/µL	Mainly lymphocytes	Variable	Normal or reduced
Normal	<5/µL	Lymphocytes	< 0.45 g/L	>60% of blood glucose

Detection of bacterial antigen in CSF before culture is available can be undertaken either by latex particle agglutination or more commonly polymerase chain reaction (PCR). PCR is particularly useful in detecting viral pathogens and is much more sensitive than viral culture. For herpes simplex type 1 virus, PCR has a sensitivity of >95% and a specificity of 100%. PCR is also helpful in suspected tuberculous meningitis as culture of *Mycobacterium tuberculosis* can take up to 6 weeks.

Newer CT scans often reveal signs of meningeal inflammation in bacterial meningitis (Fig. 3). In viral encephalitis, MRI can show diagnostic temporal lobe changes while EEG may show a suggestive pattern (Fig. 4).

Treatment

Early administration of intravenous antibiotics is imperative. A 30 minute door to antibiotic time should be aspired to. Initially the causative organism is unknown and an empirical regime is required. International guidelines recommend ceftriaxone (or another third generation cephalosporin) with or without vancomycin. Antibiotic resistance varies widely and local protocols are important. In neonates and the elderly the incidence of *Listeria monocytogenes* and enterococci is much higher and warrants the addition of ampicillin. Antibiotic regimes may need to be altered for immunocompromised patients. Adjunctive treatment of meningitis with corticosteroids is controversial, although there is evidence that a dose of dexamethasone at the time of first antibiotic reduces neurological sequelae.

Viral meningitis can be treated conservatively, usually with analgesia and fluid rehydration. If the diagnosis is in doubt, especially in possible cases of partially treated bacterial meningitis, antibiotics should be continued. Tuberculous meningitis requires triple therapy with isoniazid, ethambutol and rifampicin (plus pyrazinamide) for 9 months.

In patients with clinical or CSF features of herpes encephalitis, empirical treatment with aciclovir should be initiated. Without treatment HSV encephalitis has a mortality of 80%, falling to 30% with aciclovir.

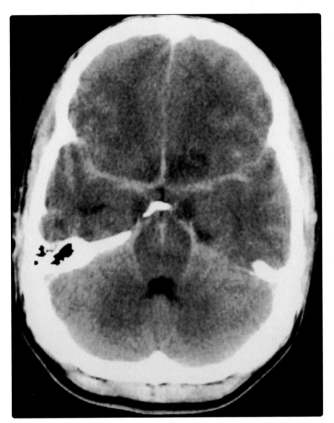

Fig. 3 **CT scan showing the extensive inflammation sometimes seen in tuberculous meningitis.**

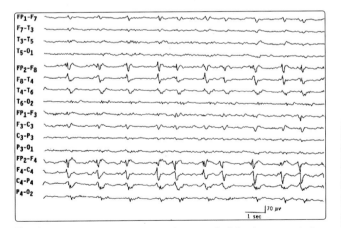

Fig. 4 **EEG in a case of herpes simplex encephalitis,** showing periodic epileptiform discharges occurring over the right temporal region every 1 to 2 seconds.

Key points

- Bacterial meningitis is an emergency and antibiotics should be started before cultures are available.
- The classic signs of bacterial meningitis are: fever, headache and neck stiffness.
- Meningitis and encephalitis may overlap in their presentations.
- Analysis of CSF is essential in making a specific diagnosis.
- Herpes simplex encephalitis is frequently fatal if left untreated.

The patient with disturbed behaviour

Patients may present to the emergency department voluntarily seeking help for a mental disorder or they may be brought by carers, relatives or even the police, usually following a display of disturbed behaviour. A disturbed patient may be suffering from a psychiatric illness, an organic brain lesion, a personality disorder or an emotional upset.

Differential diagnosis

Acute confusional state

Delirium or acute confusion may be the cause of disturbed behaviour, or may coexist with mental illness (see 'Confusion' chapter). Be aware that patients with abnormal behaviour initially labelled as psychiatric often have a final diagnosis of a medical condition. Acute onset confusion with disorientation, hallucinations, delusions, clouding of consciousness and impaired memory may well result in disturbed or violent behaviour, especially in the elderly. Features which increase the likelihood of a medical cause for disturbed behaviour are: first presentation, disorientation, fluctuating conscious level, visual hallucinations, use of drugs and neurological signs or symptoms.

Life-threatening medical conditions that can cause sudden onset of disturbed behaviour include:

- meningoencephalitis
- hypoglycaemia
- hypoxia
- hypertensive encephalopathy
- intracranial haemorrhage
- poisoning
- seizures
- acute organ failure.

Antipsychotic medication can result in acute confusion. Sedation may be required to allow adequate assessment of the patient.

Psychoses

Psychoses are mental illnesses characterized by loss of insight and abnormal behaviour. Schizophrenia and mania are important causes of acutely disturbed behaviour presenting to the emergency department. Schizophrenia is characterized by thought disorder, delusion and typically auditory hallucinations. A

patient with previously well-controlled psychosis may present acutely to the emergency department due to omitting drug therapy, loss of support network or an external pressure.

Drug-induced psychosis can occur with prescribed drugs such as central nervous system depressants, beta-blockers or digoxin or with recreational drugs such as cocaine, amphetamines or LSD.

Alcohol related

Alcohol withdrawal may occur acutely, within 6–12 hours of abstinence. The patient can present with agitation, tremor and sweating. Delirium tremens occurs after 24–72 hours of abstinence; in addition to tremor, agitation, fever and tachycardia it features an acute confusional psychosis with visual hallucinations. Patients with alcohol withdrawal require admission for intravenous multivitamins (Pabrinex) as well as sedation with a benzodiazepine (chlordiazepoxide or diazepam). Alcohol withdrawal can also present to the emergency department as seizures and, rarely, as acute alcohol hallucinosis.

Chronic alcohol abuse can lead to inadequate B vitamin levels in the brain resulting in Wernicke's encephalopathy (ophthalmoplegia, ataxia and peripheral neuropathy) or Korsakoff's psychosis (loss of short-term memory with confabulation). At-risk patients (chronic alcohol abuse with any intercurrent illness) should be given intravenous vitamins.

Depression and self-harm

Depressed mood can be a feature of psychosis but more commonly exists as a neurotic depression. Patients with low mood often have sleep disturbance (classically difficult getting to sleep in neurotic depression and early morning wakening in severe or psychotic depression), loss of appetite, and difficulties with relationships and work. It is essential to ask about suicidal thoughts; questioning is not associated with any increase in suicide attempts. Patients often present after a 'loss' event such as bereavement, separation from partner or loss of employment. Figure 1 shows the main features of severe depression.

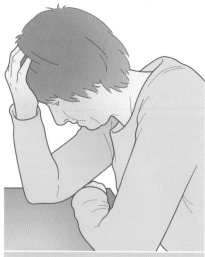

- Significant change in weight
- Insomnia
- Extreme tiredness
- Diminished ability to think/concentrate
- Feelings of worthlessness and guilt
- Continuing thoughts of death or suicide

Fig. 1 **Symptoms of severe depression.**

If a patient appears to be severely depressed or expresses suicidal ideation they should be referred for a full psychiatric assessment. It is not appropriate to start antidepressants in the emergency department and this should be deferred to the patient's psychiatrist or GP.

Self-harm accounts for 1–2% of UK emergency department attendances. Self-harm may present as either poisoning or self-inflicted injury. Self-harm carries a significant mortality; 1% of patients who harm themselves will successfully commit suicide within the subsequent 12 months. All patients who present with self-harm should undergo a full psychiatric assessment including a suicide risk assessment. Scoring systems such as the SAD PERSONS system can be useful (Table 1). A score <6 suggests low risk and is very predictive for safe hospital discharge with no mortality at 6 months.

Key diagnostic points

History

Disturbed patients should be managed in a non-confrontational, non-judgemental manner. Care needs to be taken to ensure the safety of staff.

Table 1 **SAD PERSONS scoring system**	
Variable	**Score**
Sex: male	1
Age: <19 or >45	1
Depression: hopelessness	2
Psychiatric care: previous self-harm or psychiatric illness	1
Excessive drug use	1
Rational thinking loss: severe depression with psychotic feature	2
Single, separated, divorced, widowed	1
Organized attempt	2
No life supports: social isolation	1
States future intent: continued suicidal ideation	2

Table 2 **The mental state assessment**
General description: appearance, behaviour, attitudes
Cognition: consciousness, orientation, memory, intelligence
Thought processes: content and form
Perception
Speech
Mood and affect
Insight and judgement

Potentially aggressive patients are best interviewed in a designated room with two doors and easy communications to call for assistance.

A full psychiatric history includes asking the patient to list their complaints, with history of any previous psychiatric problems. Obtain a drug history (medicines, recreational drugs and alcohol) and the contact details of any agencies the patient is involved with. Carers may suggest stressors in the patient's recent past which could precipitate or exacerbate disturbed behaviour. Common presentations include: an episode of self-harm, an acute emotional upset, an exacerbation of a known psychiatric illness with the patient requesting help or admission, and acutely disturbed or bizarre behaviour in a patient lacking insight into their problems.

The patient and carers should be questioned for neurological symptoms, including headaches, loss of consciousness or speech impairment. Episodes of confusion or syncope are very suggestive of an organic brain disorder. Evidence of recent infections, trauma (especially head injury), dyspnoea or risk factors for HIV infection should be sought.

Alcohol is commonly associated with disturbed or violent behaviour and is a significant risk factor for attempted or actual suicide. Screening questions can be used such as the CAGE questionnaire.

Examination

Physical examination is directed towards identifying an organic cause for the disturbed behaviour and should include neurological examination as well as temperature, blood glucose, examination for signs of head injury and signs of infection. A mental state examination (MSE) should follow a standardized format (Table 2).

Following an MSE, it is usually possible to identify the most likely underlying problem, the degree of patient insight and probability of cooperation, and whether the patient will be better managed as an inpatient. Mental state examinations should occur in a private, quiet room where the patient feels secure. Medical and nursing staff should be aware of risk factors for patient violence and consider the need to be accompanied by security guards or police.

About 20% of psychiatric patients have a medical condition requiring treatment and often contributing to the acute behaviour disturbance. Investigations to be considered include urine drug screen, septic screen, head CT scan, EEG and lumbar puncture.

Emergency management

Non-pharmacological techniques are the mainstay of managing acutely disturbed patients. Treat any organic cause of confusion such as hypoglycaemia, hypoxia or metabolic derangement. Drugs are required for patients who are extremely agitated or aggressive who cannot be managed by counselling. Haloperidol is usually the first choice, it rarely cause respiratory depression but is associated with extrapyramidal side effects. Benzodiazepines (lorazepam, midazolam) can be used for short-term sedation; these are best avoided in delirium since they can cause increased confusion.

Physical restraint should be limited to an absolute minimum to prevent the patient from causing injury to themselves or others. Communication with the disturbed patient, constant explanation and reassurance are always preferred, and commonly the most effective, option.

Key points

- It is important to differentiate psychiatric illness from organic disease as a cause of disturbed behaviour.

- A mental state examination is essential.

- Always consider alcohol intoxication or withdrawal as a potential cause of disturbed behaviour.

- Drugs and physical restraint should be reserved for patients who are extremely agitated.

The poisoned patient and toxidromes (1)

Exposure to any substance in sufficient quantity can be harmful. Substances that cause harm after exposure to small quantities are described as having high toxicity. Ricin, a highly potent toxin derived from the castor bean, can be lethal following exposure to less than 3 µg/kg. Other substances, such as water, become toxic only when consumed in large quantities. All drugs, including recreational drugs, have a therapeutic dose range beyond which the harmful effects outweigh the potential benefits. With such a large number of potential toxins, clinicians are often initially unable to identify the substance involved in poisoning, especially if the patient is unconscious. Instead clinicians rely on the identification of constellations of signs and symptoms. Many common toxins can often be grouped together into families, each producing a syndrome with characteristic signs and symptoms. These toxic syndromes are known as toxidromes (Fig. 1).

Poisoning causes over three thousand deaths per year in the UK, one-third of which are accidental. Paediatric poisoning and opiate poisoning account for the majority of accidental poisonings. Approximately half a million poisoned patients are admitted to hospital each year in the UK. Paracetamol poisoning alone accounts for 70 000 admissions per year. UK legislation limiting availability of paracetamol in 1998 has resulted in a decrease in case fatality.

Clinical features of toxidromes

Anticholinergic (e.g. tricyclic antidepressants, antipsychotics)

Tachycardia, hypertension and peripheral vasodilatation with hyperpyrexia. Pupils are dilated, with dry mucous membranes, urinary retention and reduced gut motility. Confusion, coma or seizures are frequently seen.

Opiate (e.g. heroin, morphine)

Bradycardia, hypotension and hypothermia. Pupils are constricted. Respiratory depression and coma are frequent features. Reduced gut motility and hyporeflexia can occur. External signs such as needle tracks may be seen.

Sedatives (e.g. benzodiazepines)

Respiratory depression and reduced level of consciousness. Pupils are not usually affected. Slurred speech, ataxia and blurred vision may occur.

Sympathomimetic (e.g. cocaine, amphetamine)

Like anticholinergic toxidromes, features include tachycardia, hypertension and hyperpyrexia. However, pupils are dilated and mucous membranes are wet with increased perspiration and increased gut motility. Confusion and seizures can occur along with increased muscle activity and hyperreflexia.

Cholinergic (e.g. organophosphate pesticides)

Diarrhoea, urinary frequency, constricted pupils, bradycardia and bronchospasm. Vomiting, lacrimation and salivation are also common features of this toxidrome.

Emergency management

Strong odours, evidence of chemical burns and multiple casualties with unexplained symptoms should alert the clinician and special precautions may need to be taken before proceeding further. Consider the need for decontamination and avoid contamination of the emergency department (see the 'Hazardous material and CBRN incidents' chapter). Initially utilize the standard ABCDE approach. Poisoned patients frequently present with a limited history. Specific laboratory investigations will be directed by the history of substance exposure, the timing of this exposure, the presence of toxidromes and/or the suspicion of exposure to a particular substance that is amenable to quantitative laboratory analysis.

Patients with signs of circulatory collapse will require intravenous fluid resuscitation. Initiate cardiac monitoring, and obtain a 12-lead ECG. If urine can be obtained, perform a urine toxicology screen.

Assess the Glasgow Coma Scale score and perform a mini neurological examination, including pupil size/reactivity and examination for lateralizing signs. Assess for and treat seizure activity or hypoglycaemia. Undress the patient and examine thoroughly, looking in particular for local signs such as needle track marks or signs of a specific toxidrome, for example dry mucous membranes.

History

The initial focused history is aimed at determining the likelihood of exposure to a toxic substance. Ambulance staff should be questioned before they leave. Was a suicide note found? Were there any empty medication bottles or blister packs? Was there evidence of alcohol consumption? Friends and family may be able to provide important information. When was the patient last known to be well? What

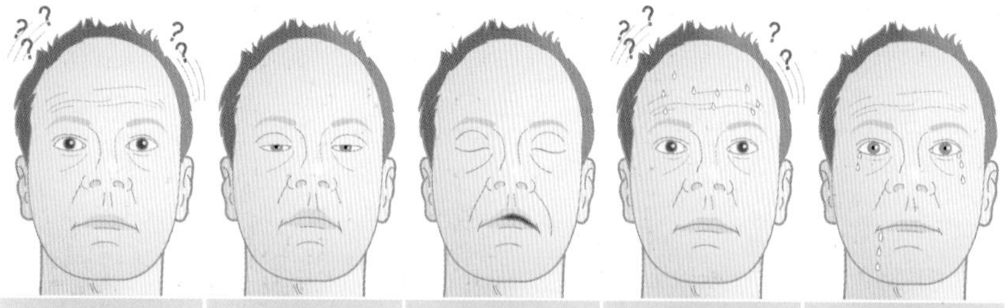

Anticholinergic	Opiate	Sedative	Sympathomimetic	Cholinergic
Confusion	Coma	Blurred vision	Confusion	Wheeze
Seizure	Hypotension	Slurred speech	Seizure	Bradycardia
Hypertension	Brachycardia	Hypoventilation	Hypertension	Diarrhoea
Tachycardia	Hypoventilation		Tachycardia	Urinary frequency
Hyperpyrexia	Constipation		Hyperreflexia	
Constipation	Hyporeflexia		Diarrhoea	
Urinary retention	Needle tracks			

Fig. 1 **Toxidromes.**

Table 1 Sources of information

British National Formulary (www.bnf.org)
Guy's and St Thomas' Medical Toxicology Unit
  (http://www.medtox.org/info)
National Poisons Information Service
Toxbase (www.toxbase.org)
Tel: 0870 600 6266

Table 2 Common antidotes

Substance	Antidote
Opiates	Naloxone
Tricyclic antidepressants	Bicarbonate
Calcium channel blockers	Calcium
Beta-blockers	Glucagon
Organophosphates	Atropine
Cyanide	Sodium nitrite or dicobalt edetate
Hydrofluoric acid	Calcium gluconate
Iron	Desferrioxamine
Digoxin	Digoxin-specific antibody fragments
Paracetamol	N-acetylcysteine, methionine
Anticoagulants	Phytomenadione (vitamin K)

medications were available in the household? What potentially toxic substances could the child have come into contact with? Conscious patients will often be able to give accurate information on the nature of the substance or combination of substances consumed. Where details of the substance are known there are several national sources of information available which can provide general information on the management of all potential poisons as well as specialist advice (Table 1).

Examination

The initial focused examination includes information gathered in the ABCDE assessment. Examine for specific signs suggestive of the common toxidromes. For example, signs of reduced level of consciousness, respiratory depression, hyporeflexia and miosis would suggest an opiate toxidrome. This is a condition with a specific antidote (naloxone), the use of which can have dramatic results. Consider symptoms and signs in unison and assess whether in combination they fit the pattern of a particular toxidrome.

Antidotes and activated charcoal

Specific antidotes to consider at an early stage include naloxone, bicarbonate, calcium, glucagon, atropine and sodium nitrite (Table 2).

However, the vast majority of poisons have no specific antidote and treatment is largely supportive.

Activated charcoal is highly effective at gastric decontamination if given within one hour of ingestion. Charcoal binds to toxins and prevents absorption. It can be administered after one hour in delayed presentations where anticholinergic (reduced gut motility) or modified release drugs have been consumed.

Further assessment, decontamination and enhanced elimination

Once resuscitative measures have been undertaken and the patient is stable a detailed assessment can be made, including psychiatric assessment if possible. A full system and external examination is required to exclude associated problems such as aspiration pneumonitis, rhabdomyolysis and injury.

Further methods of decontamination may be appropriate in exceptional circumstances including gastric lavage and whole bowel irrigation. Gastric lavage is only effective if performed within one hour of exposure and requires a protected airway. Whole bowel irrigation is considered in iron and lithium poisoning (not inactivated by charcoal) and some modified release drugs.

Enhanced elimination techniques include repeated doses of activated charcoal, haemodialysis or urine alkalinization. These techniques can be used to enhance elimination of certain drugs after they have been absorbed, for example repeated activated charcoal in carbamazepine poisoning.

Disposition

The majority of poisoned patients are admitted to hospital for observation and supportive treatment. Patients requiring airway protection or ventilatory support are managed in a critical care area. Patients with conduction defects and arrhythmias are managed in a cardiac monitoring area.

Common drugs causing poisoning

Paracetamol poisoning

Paracetamol (acetaminophen) is available without prescription on its own or combined with other drugs such as codeine, ibuprofen, caffeine and pseudo-ephedrine.

The toxicity of paracetamol in overdose is the result of a toxic metabolite (N-acetyl-p-benzoquinone imine, or NAPQI) that is formed (via cytochrome p-450 action) and that accumulates in unusually large amounts once the non-toxic preferential routes of metabolism are saturated.

NAPQI is normally metabolized with glutathione to an inactive compound, but when produced in large amounts the availability of glutathione is soon depleted and hepatotoxicity results.

Clinical features

The toxic dose of paracetamol is 150 mg/kg body weight. For those who are at high risk (alcoholics, malnourished, those taking enzyme-inducing drugs) the amount required to cause hepatotoxicity is lower.

In the first few hours following ingestion of a large dose of paracetamol the main features are abdominal pain, nausea and vomiting. If untreated, hepatoxicity develops causing right upper quadrant pain and tenderness. Over the course of the next 48 hours symptoms of acute hepatic failure develop such as jaundice, hypoglycaemia, hepatic encephalopathy and bleeding. Symptoms of associated renal failure may also be seen.

Treatment

N-acetylcysteine (NAC) should be administered in those patients who are at risk of developing hepatotoxicity as determined by their paracetamol blood level taken at 4 hours post ingestion (Fig. 2). Treatment should be commenced by 8 hours post ingestion to minimize the risk of hepatotoxicity.

Oral methionine is an alternative but tends to be less effective than intravenous NAC as the patient may vomit and not fully absorb the appropriate dose.

Patients presenting post 8 hours from ingestion and who have taken >150 mg/kg should have NAC started immediately, prior to the paracetamol level becoming available. If the level comes back below the treatment line and the patient is asymptomatic then the NAC can be stopped.

In very late presentations there is some evidence that NAC may still be helpful even after 24 hours post ingestion in those who have taken a significant overdose.

The poisoned patient and toxidromes (2)

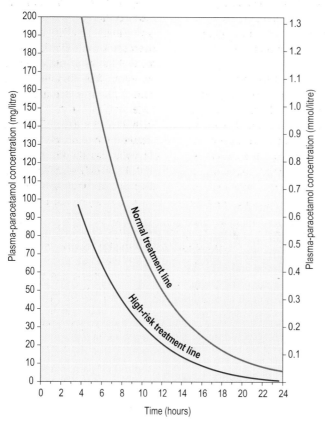

Fig. 2 **Graph for treatment of paracetamol poisoning.**

In those that do suffer a degree of liver damage the first parameter to change is the prothrombin time/INR and this is used to monitor the progress of such patients. Liver function tests (AST and ALT) may reach very high levels (>10 000 U/L) after 24 hours.

Salicylate poisoning

Salicylates (acetylsalicylic acid, ASA, aspirin) remain widely available over the counter. Aspirin levels usually peak within 2 hours of therapeutic dosing but may be delayed for up to 6 hours if enteric coated formulations have been taken. Salicylates impair cellular respiration by uncoupling oxidative phosphorylation. They stimulate respiratory centres in the medulla, producing a primary respiratory alkalosis. Salicylates simultaneously and independently produce a primary metabolic acidosis. Eventually metabolic acidosis becomes the primary acid–base abnormality as salicylates enter cells and poison mitochondria.

Clinical presentation

The degree of clinical toxicity can be predicted from the dose ingested; however the most useful features in assessing the patient are the clinical signs and symptoms, acid–base status and serum salicylate concentrations.

Common clinical features include nausea, vomiting and tinnitus. Severe poisoning may produce confusion, agitation, coma and convulsions. CNS features are less common in adults than in children.

Metabolic and acid–base differences

Adults and children over the age of 4 years present with a mixed respiratory alkalosis and metabolic acidosis, with normal or high arterial pH.

Children aged 4 years or less often have a dominant metabolic acidosis with low arterial pH.

Initial management

Serum salicylate concentration should be taken at least 2 hours (in symptomatic patients) or 4 hours after ingestion, since it may take several

hours for peak plasma concentrations to occur. Repeat levels should be taken after a further 2 hours because of the possibility of continuing absorption.

Emergency treatment includes oral activated charcoal in patients who present within one hour of ingestion. A second dose of charcoal is indicated if the plasma salicylate concentrations are increasing, suggesting delayed gastric emptying.

Further treatment depends on the severity of poisoning.

Patients with **mild poisoning** (children with plasma salicylate <350 mg/L and adults with <500 mg/L) usually need only increased oral fluids.

In **moderate poisoning** (salicylate >350 mg/L in children and >500 mg/L in adults) intravenous fluids should be commenced to ensure an adequate urine output. Elimination of salicylate may be increased by alkalinization of urine by administration of intravenous sodium bicarbonate. The optimum urine pH is 7.5–8.5 and should be measured hourly.

Haemodialysis is the treatment of choice for **severe poisoning** (salicylate level >900 mg/L (6.4 mmol/L)). Haemodialysis is also indicated in patients who have a severe metabolic acidosis (pH <7.2) or persistently high salicylate concentration unresponsive to urinary alkalinization.

Tricyclic poisoning

Tricyclic antidepressants (TCAs) such as amitriptyline, dothiepin and imipramine are antidepressants and pain modulators that are frequently taken in overdose, often in combination with analgesics, benzodiazepines and alcohol. They are particularly toxic and may cause serious illness and death even with the ingestion of as little as 20 mg/kg.

TCA metabolites are renally excreted. They are highly protein bound with a high volume of distribution and so have a prolonged half-life (up to 48 hours). The main pharmacological effects of TCAs include:

1. anticholinergic action
2. myocardial membrane effect
3. alpha-adrenergic blockade
4. inhibition of noradrenaline reuptake.

The appearance of symptoms and signs of toxicity can develop rapidly (Table 3).

Cardiovascular and CNS features are most serious. Patients may have an acidosis on blood gas measurement. Acidosis can be either respiratory, metabolic or a mixed picture. In the presence of an acidosis the cardiovascular effects become more pronounced and potentially fatal arrhythmias can occur. QRS widening on the ECG is the best predictor of toxicity (Fig. 3). Symptoms/signs of serious toxicity almost always present within 6–9 hours of ingestion, but may then persist for 48–72 hours.

Management
Initial assessment should follow the ABCDE approach.

All patients should be fully monitored and receive oxygen, IV access, blood gas analysis, 12 lead ECG and baseline biochemistry (including 4 hour paracetamol and salicylate levels).

Any patient who has signs of cardiovascular or neurological instability, or if there is QRS widening on the ECG, should receive an immediate intravenous bolus of sodium bicarbonate (1 mmol/kg) regardless of the blood pH.

Prevention of absorption
There is some evidence to suggest that absorption can be decreased by the administration of activated charcoal. Gastric lavage may be helpful if the overdose is large and the patient is within 1 hour of ingestion. Both methods may require the patient to have formal airway protection in the presence of a reduced level of consciousness.

Supportive treatment and further monitoring
Any patient who has taken a TCA overdose should be closely monitored for 6–9 hours or until they are symptom free. Comatose patients should be intubated and ventilated in order to avoid further complications such as aspiration. Seizures should be treated with benzodiazepines. Arrhythmias should be treated initially with intravenous sodium bicarbonate. Hypotension may be treated with intravenous glucagon.

Table 3 **Clinical effects of TCAs**

Anticholinergic effects	CNS effects	Cardiovascular effects
Blurred vision, dry mouth	Agitation	Tachycardia
Urinary retention	Anxiety	Prolongation of PR interval
Dilated pupils	Confusion	Heart blocks
Tachycardia	Coma	Prolongation of QRS interval and QT segment
Impaired sweating	Seizures	Ventricular tachyarrhythmias
Thermoregulation disruption	Ophthalmoplegia	Cardiac arrest – asystole
Various GI effects	Rigidity	Hypotension

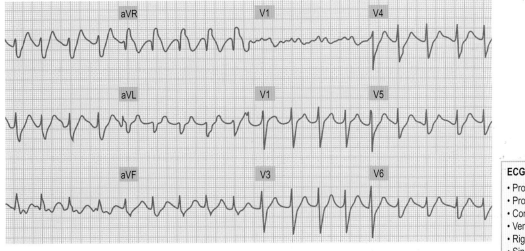

ECG signs in TCA poisoning
- Prolonged QRS
- Prolonged QT interval
- Conduction abnormalities
- Ventricular dysrhythmias
- Right axis deviation
- Sinus tachycardia

Fig. 3 **Electrocardiogram with signs of tricyclic toxicity.**

Key points

In a potentially poisoned patient:

- Consider the need for decontamination.
- Actively look for the presence of a toxidrome.
- Consider specific antidotes.
- Consider the need for activated charcoal (reduce absorption).
- Consider the need for enhanced elimination.

Paracetamol

- Blood paracetamol levels should be taken at 4 hours post ingestion.

- Paracetamol levels are unreliable in staggered overdoses or when the ingestion is more than 12 hours ago.
- If in doubt, treat with NAC and ensure it is started within 8 hours.

Salicylates

- Diagnosis is clinical.
- Confirm by measuring serum salicylate levels.
- Treatment is with activated charcoal and alkaline diuresis, or haemodialysis.
- Repeat the salicylate levels if raised.

Tricyclics

- Patients require close monitoring for 6–9 hours or until they are symptom free.
- Treatment with intravenous bicarbonate may be life-saving.
- Full supportive care with intubation and ventilation is often required.

Hazardous material and CBRN incidents

Release of chemical, biological, radiological and nuclear (CBRN) materials can occur without warning as a result of a wide range of events including industrial accidents, terrorism and natural outbreaks of communicable diseases. This might involve chemical fires, chemical contamination of the environment, or the deliberate release of chemicals or poisons. A CBRN event might involve old tyres being ignited and releasing clouds of toxic smoke, an acid leak out of a tanker creating noxious gas or an explosion that rips through an industrial plant. The key to the management of CBRN incidents is preparedness. In the UK the Health Protection Agency (HPA) coordinates the national response (http://www.hpa.org.uk/).

Patients with CBRN contamination require meticulous decontamination prior to being allowed in to the emergency department (ED). Mass casualty decontamination is the responsibility of the fire and rescue service. Admission of contaminated patients into the ED can be disastrous. If the ED is contaminated it will be rendered unusable and this will present a far greater risk to the community as a whole. Decontamination involves removal of all clothing and thorough washing of the entire body with plain soap and plenty of water. These simple decontamination measures will be sufficient for the vast majority of chemical exposures. Further specific advice can be sought from the HPA, regional poisons centres or TOXBASE (Fig. 1).

Chemical hazards

Nerve agents are toxic chemical warfare agents, chemically related to organophosphorus insecticides. They include sarin, which was used in the 1995 terrorist attack on the Tokyo underground system. These agents inhibit acetylcholinesterase, producing parasympathetic effects, copious secretions, bronchospasm, bradycardia, abdominal cramps, diarrhoea, constricted pupils, muscle fasciculation, weakness, respiratory paralysis,

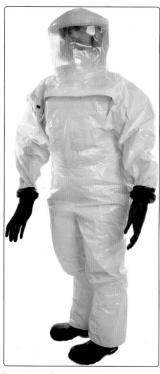

Fig. 1 **Healthcare worker in personal protective clothing.**

tachycardia, hypertension, confusion, convulsions and coma. Death is caused by respiratory arrest. Three types of antidote are used in treatment of nerve agent poisoning and have a synergistic effect: atropine antagonizes the effects of acetylcholine at muscarinic receptors, particularly effective in decreasing secretions and treating bradycardia; pralidoxine reactivates inhibited enzyme, thereby decreasing the amount of excess acetylcholine; and diazepam for CNS protection.

Every major ED should be able to respond to a chemical incident by instigating the following measures:

- Avoid contamination of hospital facilities by isolating and streaming contaminated patients.
- Use appropriate facilities and equipment for their chemical decontamination.
- Instigate immediate appropriate treatment according to chemical exposure.
- Involve the appropriate agencies such as the HPA.

Biological hazards and infectious diseases

Examples of such incidents that have resulted in serious disruption to EDs include anthrax, SARS and avian flu (see 'Tropical diseases and fever in the returning traveller' chapter).

Anthrax is an acute disease of herbivorous mammals, caused by the bacterium *Bacillus anthracis*, and is highly lethal. It can form long-lived spores. Humans acquire it through contact with infected animals or contaminated products by inhalation, ingestion or direct wound contact. Anthrax spores can be grown outside the body and used as a biological weapon but cannot spread directly from human to human. The 2001 US anthrax attacks occurred when letters containing the anthrax spores were mailed to several news media offices and two US Senators, killing five people and infecting 17 others. Several buildings needed isolation or decontamination at enormous cost.

Radiological/Nuclear

Nuclear accidents have occurred quite frequently over the last half century resulting in human exposure to radioactive substances. Meticulous decontamination is paramount. Geiger-Muller instruments may be required to detect exposure. Management is supportive.

Key points

- Emergencies, outbreaks of disease, and chemical incidents have the potential to cause disruption for communities on a large scale.

- Disease outbreaks and chemical incidents can develop very rapidly – so preparation and emergency planning are essential components in minimizing the impact on the public (Fig. 2).

- Be alert to the unusual, the unexpected, and the case that 'just doesn't fit'.

IF ANY OF THE FOLLOWING UNUSUAL CLINICAL PRESENTATIONS OCCUR – CONSIDER DELIBERATE RELEASE

- Usually large numbers of patients present over a period of time
- Cases linked by epidemiological features
  - Similar features/similar geographical area
  - **STEP 1-2-3** (see Box)
- Signs/symptoms unusual or unusually severe
- Known cause but unusual in UK or where acquired
- Known cause but not responding to standard therapy
- Unknown aetiology

CBRN INCIDENTS
hpa.org.uk/emergency/CBRN.htm

CBRN incidents: clinical management and health protection

Consider the risk of transmission or contamination to staff and/or other patients

*Isolate patient
*Use standard personal protective equipment (PPE) – wear gloves, gown and mask (add eye protection if patient coughing or vomiting)

STEP 1-2-3

The following precautions should be taken before continuing with the assessment

First actions:

ONE Casualty
  Treat as **normal**

TWO Casualties
  Have a low index of suspicion but otherwise treat as normal

THREE Casualties or More
  Initial assessment should be outside the department, use **PPE**, ask for **Specialist Help**

ACUTE
- Over minutes to hours
- Occur in circumscribed geographical area
- Occur in people who may have shared a known common exposure

DELAYED
- Over hours to days or days to weeks
- May or may not occur in geographical clusters
- May or may not occur in people who have shared a known common exposure
- Detected by surveillance

Most likely: **CHEMICAL**

Other possibilities: **Biological toxins**
Radiological

Most likely: **INFECTIOUS AGENT**

Other possibilities: **Radiological**
Chemicals (latent period)
(Psychological)

- **STAFF PROTECTION (PPE), HOSPITAL PROTECTION (air conditioning, isolation)**
- **INITIAL CLINICAL ASSESSMENT, HISTORY AND LIFE SAVING MANAGEMENT**

In a chemical incident prompt decontamination may be life saving. In a radiological incident triage and treat life threatening injury before decontamination; if the patient's clinical condition permits, decontaminate first and then treat. Initiate local/regional contingency plans.

DECONTAMINATION

Rinse-Wipe-Rinse

Step 1

Gently wash affected areas with soapy water (0.9% saline for open wounds and eyes):
- this dilutes the contaminant and removes particles and water based chemicals

Step 2

Wipe affected areas gently but thoroughly with sponge or soft brush or washcloth:
- this removes organic chemicals and petrochemicals

Step 3

Gently rinse affected areas

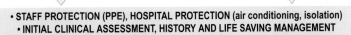

1. Seek expert advice locally*

2. Ensure safety of self, other staff and patients

3. Detailed clinical assessment – use standard PPE
- Nature and time course of symptoms
- Detailed clinical history
- Identify possible recent risk factors:
  - Where has the patient been?
  - What has the patient been doing?
  - With whom or what has the patient had contact

***Inform local HPU IMMEDIATELY**
http://www.hpa.org.uk/larshpus.htm

SEEK EXPERT ADVICE

4. Management as per best available advice
- Take samples for laboratory investigations
- Treatment or Prophylaxis as indicated

5. Record information and communicate with
- Senior clinician
- Hospital management
- Infection control
- Local medical microbiologist and chemical pathologist
- Laboratory
- Local HPU
- Chemical Hazards and Poisons Division/ National Poisons Information Service
- Local Radiation Protection Advisor

Fig. 2 **Suspected CBRN emergency clinical situation algorithm.**

Plant and animal toxins

Plants

Although serious poisoning rarely occurs, some plants are very poisonous.

Small amounts of foxglove (Fig. 1) or wild arum can cause nausea, vomiting and stomach cramps, large amounts are potentially fatal. Rhubarb leaves contain the same harmful chemicals, glycosides. Other poisonous plants include laburnum, poppies and deadly nightshade.

Serious poisoning as a result of eating mushrooms is rare. Mushrooms found in the garden may cause nausea, vomiting and occasionally, hallucinations. Early development of such symptoms (in the first two hours) is generally associated with a good prognosis. The Amanita family (Fig. 2), which includes the death cap fungus (*Amanita phalloides*) and destroying angel (*Amanita virosa*), can cause severe symptoms and death. After several hours, there is sudden abdominal pain, persistent vomiting and watery diarrhoea. There may be an apparent recovery, but then, after a couple of days, hepatic, renal and cardiac failure develops.

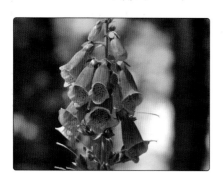

Fig. 1 **The flower of the foxglove plant.**

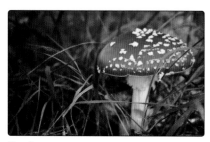

Fig. 2 **A poisonous mushroom from the Amanita family.**

Treatment

Treatment of plant poisoning includes identification of the plant, prevention of absorption by activated charcoal, and symptomatic treatment.

Cholinergic features ('SLUDGE': salivation, lacrimation, urinary incontinence, diarrhoea, GI upset and hypermotility, emesis) can be treated with atropine. Always consult a local toxicology centre (Toxbase/National Poisons Information Service).

Animal toxins – marine poisoning

Various species of fish and shellfish contain poisonous toxins. Ciguatera toxin can be present in various fish species, including barracuda, sea bass, and many tropical reef fish. Ingestion of the toxin causes nausea, vomiting, watery diarrhoea, numbness and tingling. Treatment is symptomatic.

Tetrodotoxin poisoning can follow ingestion of puffer fish. Symptoms include numbness of lips, tongue, face and extremities, sensations of lightness or floating, dizziness, extensive muscle weakness as well as gastrointestinal symptoms.

Scromboid poisoning occurs after eating fish that contain high levels of histamine. Symptoms and signs resemble an allergic reaction. Treatment is supportive and includes intravenous antihistamine.

Marine envenomation

Most serious envenomations occur in the warm waters of the Indo-Pacific region.

Surface stings

This common mechanism of envenomation involves a system of glands able to discharge venom through a tube into the skin.

They are found in the:

- *Physalia* (Portuguese man of war/bluebottles)
- fire corals/corals
- anemones
- jellyfish.

Effects range from severe burning pain with localized skin erythema, through mild systemic upset, to severe systemic reactions involving vomiting, chest pain, convulsions and respiratory failure.

Extremely toxic species are found in tropical waters:

- box jellyfish (*Chironex fleckeri*) and
- Irukandji syndrome (*Carulia barnesi*).

Treatment involves supportive care and administration of antivenom. Vinegar should be applied for 30 minutes or until the pain subsides, followed by removal of the nematocysts. Local application of ice packs or hot-water immersion provides analgesia.

Stings/skin puncture

Several species of marine animals cause a 'sting' by deeply puncturing the victim's skin and introducing venom.

This group includes:

- sea urchins
- cone shells
- starfish
- stingrays
- catfish
- weever fish (Europe)
- Scorpaenidae: lionfish (Fig. 3), scorpion fish, and the lethal stonefish.

Envenomation produces severe localized pain, swelling and often tissue necrosis. Systemic symptoms may be mild or severe with cardiorespiratory collapse in the case of the stonefish.

Treatment is supportive and includes antivenom where available (stonefish), rinsing with fresh water, removal of

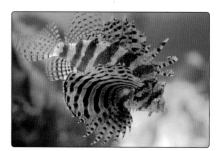

Fig. 3 **A lionfish.**

any foreign body, adequate haemostasis and then immersion in hot water. Typically, spines and stingers are radio-opaque, so x-rays or ultrasound may be used to locate any remaining pieces.

Bites

Species that envenomate by biting include octopi and sea snakes. The blue-ringed octopus has caused several fatalities.

Sea snakes' envenomation can lead to severe systemic symptoms including cardiovascular or neurological system failure. There is no specific antivenom, but symptoms may respond to multivalent snake antivenom.

Non-marine envenomation

Snake bites

Only one-tenth of the 3000 species of snake in the UK worldwide are dangerous to humans.

There is only one indigenous poisonous snake in the UK, the adder (Fig. 4), but other species of snakes may be found in zoos or private collections. The three families of snakes are the Elapidae (land snakes like cobras, mambas and kraits), the Viperidae (adder, common viper) and the Hydrophiladae (sea snakes).

Major symptoms of envenomation include:

- coagulopathy
- neurotoxicity
- myopathy
- cardiac effects such as hypotension, arrhythmia.

First aid involves transportation of the victim to hospital, lying still, with a pressure immobilization bandage in situ. Only bring the snake if safe to do so!

In the emergency department do not remove pressure bandages. Initial management involves an ABCDE assessment with resuscitation as appropriate.

Look for signs of ptosis, ophthalmoplegia and muscle weakness; bleeding from gums or IV sites; and tender lymphadenopathy. Only then inspect the bite site, cutting the bandage away at the site of the bite only.

In addition to urinalysis and standard blood tests, swab the bite and collect urine for Venom Detection Kit (VDK). Observe the patient for 24 hours; if signs of systemic envenomation develop, process the VDK, ask an expert to identify the snake and administer the appropriate antivenom.

Dangerous insects and spiders

Insects and spiders can inflict injury in the form of bites, stings and allergic reactions.

Few spiders, arthropods and insects are capable of causing death. In most spider or insect bites, rest and elevation, local application of ice packs or local heat, simple analgesics and antihistamines are all that is required. Venomous species, where treatment with antivenom may be required, include:

- black widow (Fig. 5)
- brown recluse spider
- redback spider
- funnel web spider
- tarantula (non-fatal).

Other venomous insects (Hymenoptera) include ants, wasps and bees. As well as painful local reactions, toxic reactions may result from multiple stings. Symptoms include gastrointestinal dysfunction, fainting, muscle spasms and convulsions. In some patients, life-threatening anaphylactic reactions may occur.

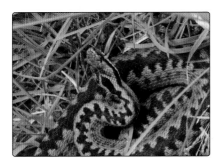

Fig. 4 **The adder, or common viper,** is the only poisonous snake indigenous to the UK.

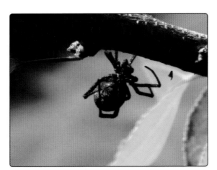

Fig. 5 **The black widow spider.**

Key points

- Most bites and stings cause localized reactions.
- Application of local heat or immersion in hot water will help relieve the pain of many localized reactions.
- Be aware of the possibility of systemic reactions and the need for rapid treatment.
- For up-to-date management of animal poisoning and envenomation consult a local toxicology centre (Toxbase/NPIS).

Heat and cold emergencies

Heat emergencies

Sunburn

Sunburn is an acute inflammatory reaction of the skin following exposure to the sun's ultraviolet radiation. The skin is warm, erythematous, oedematous and may blister. In extreme cases the patient may require fluid resuscitation and the burns require appropriate management as for burns in general (see 'Burns' chapter). In most cases symptomatic treatment is all that is required.

Thermoregulatory failure

Heat exhaustion and heat stroke represent a spectrum of disease where normal thermoregulatory mechanisms are impaired after exposure to heat. This may be further classified as either exertional (e.g. marathon runners in hot conditions) or non-exertional (e.g. the elderly during a summer heat wave). In exertional heat illness the situation is exacerbated by dehydration and loss of salt. The hallmark of heat illness is loss of normal thermoregulatory mechanisms with an elevated core body temperature. There is a blurring of the margin between heat exhaustion and heat stroke but in heat stroke the core body temperature will be markedly elevated (greater than 40°C) and there will be central nervous system impairment; either confusion or decreased GCS score.

History

The ambient atmospheric temperature will be raised; there may be a history of exercise. Symptoms initially are non-specific such as fatigue, lethargy, headache and myalgia.

Examination

The patient will be pyrexial. Progression to heat stroke with rapid elevation of the body temperature and CNS deterioration may be rapid. The patient may be clinically dehydrated (dry mucous membranes) but this is not a prerequisite.

Emergency management

The key is to aggressively manage the hyperpyrexia. This is most effectively achieved by stripping the patient, and spraying them with a fine mist of water using hand-held sprays (Fig. 1) and fanning the patient, ideally with an electric fan. Ice packs may be placed in the groin and axillae but care needs to be taken to limit the skin exposure to the ice to avoid skin damage. Rehydrate either orally or intravenously and correct any electrolyte abnormalities.

Cold injury

Cold injury can either cause local injury, for example with frostbite, or systemic illness as with hypothermia.

Frostbite

Frostbite is caused by freezing of the tissues with the development of ice crystals. It affects body extremities, commonly digits and the nose. The affected body part is painful and there is often some sensory disturbance such as numbness. The pain may be throbbing or burning in nature. There will be skin changes ranging from erythema and blistering through to frank tissue necrosis and gangrene. The key to management is adequate analgesia and rapid, moist rewarming. Moist rewarming involves submerging

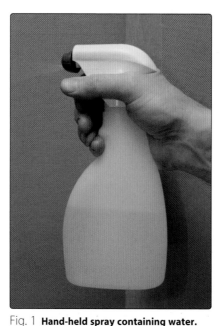

Fig. 1 **Hand-held spray containing water.**
When used in conjunction with an electric fan is an effective method for cooling patients with exertional heat stroke.

the affected body part in a water bath maintained at 40°C. Dry heat is to be avoided. Surgical intervention is deferred as long as possible until clear demarcation has occurred; this commonly takes weeks or months. There is no role for early surgical debridement and no pharmacological agents have been shown to be of any benefit.

Hypothermia

Hypothermia is classified as mild (32–35°C), moderate (30–32°C) and severe (<30°C). Once identified, rewarm the patient either passively or actively.

History

Hypothermia tends to affect specific groups. The commonest group encountered are elderly patients who are found on the floor of their home after a period of time. In the elderly always consider what has caused the patient to be in a position to become hypothermic as well as treating the hypothermic state. There are many possible underlying aetiologies; important ones to consider are injuries from a fall (such as a fractured neck of femur), sepsis (such as a urinary tract infection) and endocrine illness, particularly hypothyroidism. Hypothermia may be the first presentation of hypothyroidism.

In other groups there will normally be a history of cold exposure; in young adults this is commonly associated with intoxication of some description. Hypothermia is common in individuals who have been submerged in water.

Examination

Measurement of the core body temperature is best achieved using a low reading rectal thermometer (Fig. 2). A general examination should be carried out to help identify a possible cause for the hypothermia.

Investigations

In the elderly, investigations are geared towards identifying an underlying cause and are dictated by the clinical situation encountered, for example x-ray of hip, urinalysis or checking thyroid function. ECG may show J waves (Fig. 3).

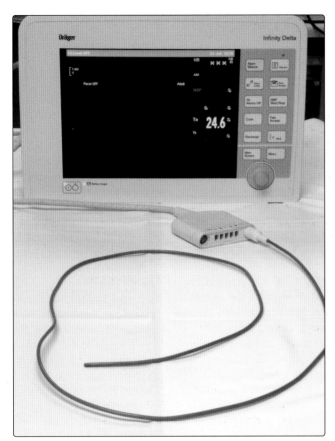

Fig. 2 **Low temperature rectal probe** used to measure and monitor core temperature (in this case reading 24.6°C).

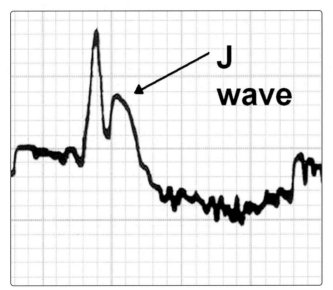

Fig. 3 **Lead III of an electrocardiogram** of an elderly woman who was found on the floor in her house with a fractured hip and a core temperature of 29°C. J wave is clearly demonstrated.

Table 1 **Methods of rewarming the hypothermic patient**
Passive external
Removal of wet clothes
Warm blankets
Warm environment
Active external
Heated forced air warmers (such as a Bair Hugger®)
Warmed humidified oxygen
Active internal
Extracorporeal rewarming methods
Cardiopulmonary bypass
Haemofiltration
Haemodialysis
Heated irrigation by infusing warm fluid into:
Thoracic cavity using chest drains
Peritoneal cavity using peritoneal dialysis catheter
Bladder using urinary catheter
Warmed intravenous fluids (minimal effect)

Movement of hypothermic patients should be undertaken carefully as it may precipitate an arrhythmia. In cardiac arrest the hypothermic myocardium is resistant to defibrillation and the circulation time is much slower. Efforts are concentrated on rewarming. No adrenaline is given until the core temperature is greater than 30°C. With defibrillation, when the temperature is less than 30°C a single shock is delivered but not repeated again until the core temperature is greater than 30°C.

Obviously dead people are cold and so the decision to actively rewarm someone in cardiac arrest needs to be carefully considered and is most appropriate where there has been a rapid cooling.

Paediatric considerations

Infants have a high surface to body ratio and so become hypothermic more quickly.

Key points

Heat emergencies

- Heat exhaustion and heat stroke represent a spectrum of illness where there is loss of normal thermoregulation, and pyrexia.

- With heat stroke the body temperature is >40°C and there is CNS impairment.

- Treatment is by cooling and rehydrating the patient.

Cold injury

- Treatment of frostbite is analgesia and moist rewarming.

- With hypothermic patients consider what may have caused them to become hypothermic.

Emergency management

Rewarm the patient. There are three classes of rewarming techniques: passive external, active external and active internal (Table 1). With passive external rewarming no external heat is added; the patient's own metabolic processes generate heat. This is the simplest and slowest rewarming method. In general, with mild and moderate hypothermia and in the elderly where the hypothermia has developed over many hours, external techniques are sufficient. In younger individuals, in severe hypothermia, and where there has been a more rapid cooling (for example if caught in an avalanche) then an active internal approach is more appropriate.

Electrical and water induced injury

Electrical injury and lightning injury

Although there are some similarities between electrical and lightning injuries, important differences exist.

Electrical injury can be divided into high and low voltage injury (greater or less than 1000 volts). Electrical injury broadly causes four types of injury:

- burns
- deep tissue injury to muscles, nerves and vessels
- cardiac injury
- blast type injury, for example fractures and cervical spine injury.

Consider the possibility of all four types of injury in anyone presenting having sustained an electrical injury. With an electrical injury, current passes through the tissues and dissipates heat. It is the dissipation of heat that is responsible for damage to deep structures. Different body structures offer a different resistance to the current; muscle offers a high resistance whilst nerves (which are used to conducting current) and vessels (filled with fluid, a good conductor) offer less resistance. When electricity passes through structures with a higher resistance, such as muscle, more heat is generated leading to greater damage.

With lightning injury, deep tissue injury and burns are very unusual. Lightning consists of a current of millions of volts which lasts a fraction of a second (Fig. 1). This may strike the individual directly, arc from an adjacent structure (such as a tree) or cause a stride voltage (current spreads out across the ground for a variable distance from the strike). Instead of passing through an individual there is the phenomenon of flashover where the lightning is conducted over the surface of the skin rather than through the body.

With electrical injury it is imperative to establish the voltage of the supply. Mains supply in Europe is 220–240 volts alternating current (AC) and electrical shocks are relatively common. High voltage shocks are usually sustained by accidentally cutting through a high voltage line, often an underground line which has been struck with an implement such as a spade. Electrical injuries are particularly dangerous in pregnancy; all pregnant patients who sustain an electrical injury require a period of observation and fetal monitoring.

Examination

Check for signs of deep injury such as muscle tenderness, vascular or nerve injury. Check for entry and exit wounds. Consider possibility of a compartment syndrome resulting from muscle injury (see 'Compartment syndrome' chapter) or of a cardiac injury. Check for any associated blast type injury that may have resulted from the individual being thrown a distance.

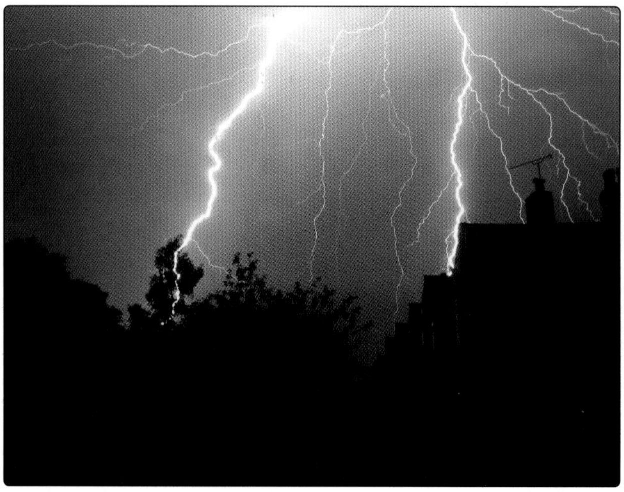

Investigations

An ECG is mandatory in all electrical injuries. If there is any suggestion of muscle injury with rhabdomyolysis, then measurement of creatine kinase is indicated.

Emergency management

If a low voltage (240 volts) shock has been sustained, the ECG is normal and there is no evidence of deep tissue injury (such as muscle tenderness) then reassurance is all that is required. Most burns are flash burns and are managed as for burns in general (see 'Burns' chapter).

If muscle injury is suspected, consider firstly the possibility of a compartment syndrome and secondarily rhabdomyolysis. Rhabdomyolysis is the breakdown of muscle and leads to myoglobin release into the circulation. Myoglobin deposits in the renal tubules causing acute tubular necrosis and acute renal failure. The urine often develops a dark colour, which is similar in appearance to tea (Fig. 2). Treatment involves close monitoring of urine production and ensuring that there is an adequate diuresis by keeping the patient well hydrated with intravenous fluids.

In general if someone survives the initial lightning strike then they are likely to survive. Lightning can cause injury to all body systems, particularly the central nervous and cardiovascular systems. The diagnosis is normally clear with a thunderstorm having been in the vicinity. Blast type injury and perforated tympanic membranes are common following a lightning strike.

Water induced injury – drowning and near drowning

Drowning is defined as death from submersion in fluid, usually water. Near drowning is survival for longer than 24 hours after a submersion episode. Traditionally drowning is subdivided into wet and dry drowning. Wet drowning is more common and involves aspiration of fluid. Dry drowning is where laryngospasm

Fig. 1 **Lightning** – millions of volts for a fraction of a second.

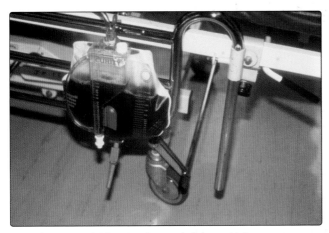

Fig. 2 **Urine containing myoglobin secondary to rhabdomyolysis.**

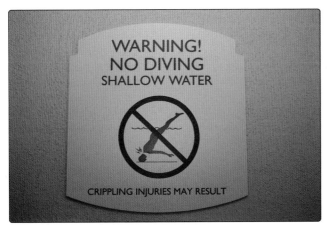

Fig. 3 **Beware of associated injuries** in drowning and near drowning patients.

occurs with subsequent cerebral hypoxia, but with little, if any, direct pulmonary injury. There is a bimodal age presentation with one peak in preschool children and the other in teenagers and people in their early twenties. Alcohol consumption is commonly a contributory factor in the latter group. In warm climates such as Australia, where there are a high number of swimming pools, drowning is the second commonest cause of death in children after road trauma.

History
The diagnosis is not in doubt; there will be a history of submersion.

Patients who are not in cardiac arrest may have respiratory symptoms such as cough or shortness of breath, or if there has been a period of cerebral hypoxia there may be neurological impairment which may manifest as either a depressed GCS, agitation, or less commonly, focal neurology. If there is a history of diving into shallow water consider cervical spine injury (Fig. 3).

Examination
Perform an ABCDE assessment, with a careful respiratory examination. Always consider the possibility of hypothermia.

Investigations
Chest x-ray may show pulmonary oedema, but this may be delayed in its presentation. Image the cervical spine if there is a history of diving into shallow water.

Emergency management
Provide respiratory support as appropriate; this may involve intubation to maintain oxygenation. Treat hypothermia. Exclude associated injuries (such as cervical spine injury).

If the patient is in cardiac arrest post submersion and is hypothermic, the decision needs to be made as to whether to commence rewarming before terminating attempts at resuscitation. While hypothermia provides a degree of neuroprotection, the more prolonged the resuscitation the higher the incidence of significant neurological impairment if the resuscitation attempts are successful (see 'Cardiac arrest' chapter).

Key points

Electrical injury and lightning injury

- Patterns of injury with high voltage electrical shock and lightning injury are different – muscle injury is common following high voltage electrical injury but rare following lightning strike.

- Non-pregnant patients with a normal ECG and having sustained a mains voltage shock generally require reassurance only.

- All pregnant patients who have sustained an electrical shock, no matter what the voltage, require a period of observation and monitoring.

- Consider the possibility of associated blast type injury.

Water induced injury

- Pulmonary complications may be delayed; consider the need for observation in seemingly well patients.

- Assess for hypothermia.

- Consider the possibility of associated injury, especially cervical spine injury if there is a history of diving.

The painful joint

A single acutely painful swollen joint (monoarthritis) can be caused by a variety of pathologies. The first priority is to exclude septic arthritis, as prompt aggressive treatment will lead to a better outcome.

Causes of acute monoarthritis

Crystal arthropathy, trauma and infection are the most common causes of an acutely painful joint. It is useful to categorize acute monoarthritis into three broad categories:

- inflammatory – infection, crystal arthropathy, rheumatological conditions
- traumatic
- non-inflammatory – degenerative disease, avascular necrosis.

History

Determine the speed of onset. An acute monoarthritis usually develops over a few days (less than 2 weeks). A rapid onset, over hours to days, suggests bacterial infection or crystal arthropathy. Fungal and mycobacterial infections are generally rare and have a slower onset, but can mimic an acute bacterial arthritis. Is this an acute exacerbation of longstanding joint pain, pre-existing osteoarthritis?

Pain and swelling commonly follow trauma: a knee that swells immediately following trauma suggests a haemarthrosis and cruciate ligament injury; a twisting injury and gradual swelling over 24 hours suggests a meniscal injury. Ask directly about penetrating injuries to the joint. Thorn injuries may cause synovitis several months after the original injury.

A flitting polyarthritis may be caused by rheumatic fever or gonococcal arthritis. Obtain a sexual history and ask about any intravenous drug usage. Take a travel history, noting the possibility of tick bites; rickettsiae may cause joint pain (Lyme disease). The patient's age is important; pseudogout tends to affect the elderly; disseminated gonococcal infection, reactive arthritis and ankylosing spondylitis generally affect young adults.

Examination

Check vital signs for evidence of sepsis/infection. Is the patient unwell or toxic, or is this purely a localized problem? Be aware that in immunocompromised or immunosuppressed patients signs and symptoms may be masked or milder. Examine the affected joint systematically (look, feel, move). Ensure that the pain is coming from the joint in question, as pain may be referred. Pain from the hip can be referred to the knee, especially in children. Pain may also be due to pathology of associated soft tissues such as a bursa. Hip pain may be caused by trochanteric bursitis rather than true joint pathology. True hip joint pain is usually felt in the groin. Signs of infection such as erythema, swelling and tenderness may be absent in deep joints such as the hips.

Perform a thorough general examination looking for a generalized rash or pustules (gonococcal infection), subcutaneous tophi (gout), conjunctivitis (Reiter's syndrome/reactive arthritis), or a cardiac murmur and splinter haemorrhages (endocarditis).

Special investigations

Synovial fluid

Aspirate the joint if infection is a possibility. Send the synovial fluid for urgent Gram stain, culture and microscopy, looking for bacteria, crystals, white cell count and differential. Aspiration of frank blood indicates a haemarthrosis, usually following trauma. Fat globules suggest an underlying fracture which may not be visible on the x-ray (an occult fracture). Overlying cellulitis is a relative contraindication to aspiration of a joint. Aspirate the joint fully until it is dry; it is therapeutic for a septic arthritis and will improve the patient's symptoms. Normal synovial fluid is transparent and essentially colourless; inflammatory synovial fluid is turbid and non-transparent. A synovial fluid WCC of $>50\,000 \times 10^9$ with relative neutrophilia is very suggestive of infection. Microscopy may reveal crystals: Calcium pyrophosphate dihydrate crystals of pseudogout (CPPD) are rhomboid in shape and weakly positively birefringent. Monosodium urate crystals (gout) are needle shaped and strongly negatively birefringent (Fig. 1). Do not be totally reliant on the synovial fluid WCC and be aware that septic arthritis may coexist with a crystal arthropathy.

Blood tests

No blood test is highly sensitive or specific for the diagnosis of monoarthritis. Obtain FBC, ESR, CRP, blood cultures, and uric acid. Although commonly raised, the white cell count **may** be normal in septic arthritis. The ESR and CRP are usually elevated, but may also be elevated in a non-infectious inflammatory arthritis. The serum uric acid levels may be normal in acute gout. Similarly a raised uric acid does not confirm gout. Blood cultures are positive in around half of the cases of septic arthritis. Antibody tests for HIV and Lyme disease should be considered if appropriate. In the

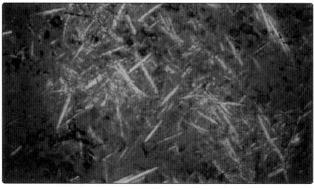

Fig. 1 **Needle-shaped negatively birefringent monosodium urate crystals of gout.**

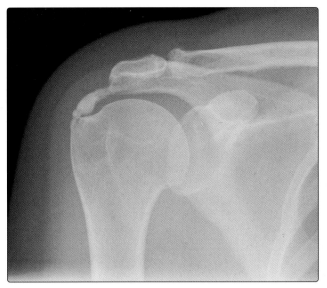

Fig. 2 **AP radiograph of the shoulder showing acute calcific tendonitis;** note calcification in supraspinatus tendon in subacromial space.

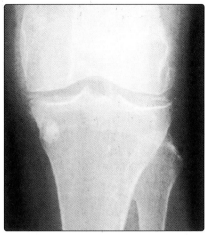

Fig. 3 **AP radiograph of the knee showing chondrocalcinosis of the menisci.**

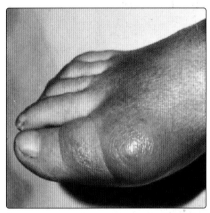

Fig. 4 **Acute gout affecting MTP joint of big toe.**

emergency setting, tests like rheumatoid factor, antinuclear factor and HLA B27 are not indicated.

Radiology

Plain x-rays are indicated if the patient gives a history of trauma, and also to rule out underlying bony abnormalities as a cause for the pain.

X-rays may show:

- soft tissue swelling
- acute bony problems like slipper upper femoral epiphysis (SUFE) of hip in adolescents
- chronic degenerate changes of the joint or bone, e.g. osteoarthritis, rheumatoid arthritis or avascular necrosis
- calcification – chondrocalcinosis of knee menisci, acute calcific tendonitis of the rotator cuff (Figs 2 and 3)
- periosteal reaction of osteomyelitis (after 10 to 14 days of symptoms).

Radionuclide scanning is useful to detect infection in deep-seated joints. Ultrasound is very useful to detect effusions, and will aid aspiration of deeps joints. MRI is the gold standard; it provides information on the joint, effusion, the bone and the associated soft tissues.

Surgery

An arthroscopy and biopsy can be diagnostic and therapeutic.

Septic arthritis

Staphylococcus aureus is the commonest pathogen in septic arthritis. Other organisms include streptococci and Gram-negative bacteria. Anaerobic and Gram-negative infections occur in immunocompromised patients; gonococcal arthritis is the commonest type of non-traumatic acute monoarthritis in young, sexually active individuals.

Crystal arthropathy

An important clue in the diagnosis of crystal-induced arthritis is a history of an acute onset of monoarthritis that resolves spontaneously.

Gout tends to affect peripheral cooler joints such as the big toe, foot, ankle, knee, wrist, finger and elbow. It typically affects the MTP joint of the big toe, with a rapid onset that may wake the patient. Acute gout may be difficult to distinguish from infection; in gout the patient may have a low grade fever and an acutely painful, erythematous inflamed joint (Fig. 4). Gout usually resolves spontaneously over 1–2 weeks. Treatment of the acute attack is directed at reducing pain and inflammation, usually with an NSAID. If a patient cannot tolerate an NSAID, an alternative is colchicine. This is an effective treatment but may cause diarrhoea and vomiting. Allopurinol is used to prevent further episodes if the patient has frequent episodes. Allopurinol is contraindicated during an acute attack and may precipitate an attack when commenced. Pseudogout or calcium pyrophosphate disease (CPPD) is caused by the deposition of calcium pyrophosphate dihydrate crystals and predominantly affects the knees and wrists. Radiographs may demonstrate chondrocalcinosis (meniscal calcification) (Fig. 3). Treatment is symptomatic with analgesia, particularly NSAIDs.

Non-inflammatory

Acute exacerbations of osteoarthritis may occur spontaneously or follow increased activity. There is usually a history to suggest chronicity. X-rays will demonstrate longstanding arthritic changes. Osteonecrosis or avascular necrosis (AVN) may give symptoms of a monoarthritis with pain on weight bearing, limping and reduced range of movement. X-rays may be normal; a bone scan or MRI will demonstrate early changes of AVN.

> ### Key points
>
> - There are several causes for a monoarthritis but always exclude septic arthritis.
>
> - Ensure the pain represents a true monoarthritis and is not referred pain from another joint or from the tissues adjacent to the joint.
>
> - Do not blindly start antibiotics in suspected septic arthritis; obtain all specimens first, including blood cultures and synovial fluid aspirate.

Non-traumatic musculoskeletal emergencies

Most musculoskeletal disorders can and should be managed in the primary care setting, allowing continuity of follow-up. However, some musculoskeletal disorders present more acutely, resulting in an emergency department attendance. Some musculoskeletal emergencies, such as infection, affect all parts of the body (upper limb, lower limb and spine), whereas some are particular to a certain anatomical region, such as acute calcific tendonitis of the shoulder.

History

Define the main complaint; this is commonly pain. Was there any precipitating event such as increased or unusual activity? Always enquire about trauma. Was the onset acute, or is this an acute exacerbation of an underlying chronic disorder? Enquire about alleviating and aggravating factors, and what treatment has been tried so far? Take a general medical history noting any predisposition to infection, history of malignancy and previous surgery.

Examination

Follow the simple LOOK, FEEL, MOVE approach. Expose the affected area, maintaining the patient's dignity; always examine the joint above and the joint below.

LOOK – for any swelling, scars, sinuses, erythema, how the patient holds the limb or walks.
FEEL – for temperature of a joint, for effusions, to localize areas of tenderness.
MOVE – active, passive and special movements/tests.

Consider the overall general condition of the patient including vital signs and temperature; is the patient toxic, or are there any systemic features of disease such as pitting of the nails in psoriasis?

General emergencies

- Infection
- Sickle cell crisis
- Oncological
- Rheumatological

- Compartment syndrome, this may occur in the absence of trauma (see 'Compartment syndrome' chapter)
- Crystal arthropathy (see 'The painful joint' chapter).

Infection

Musculoskeletal infection is common and may present as infection of the skin (cellulitis), joint (septic arthritis) or bone (osteomyelitis). A variant of cellulitis is necrotizing fasciitis and this is a true emergency (see 'Common rashes in adults' chapter). Always consider and actively exclude infection whenever a patient presents with a painful joint or bone. In up to half of cases of osteomyelitis there will be a history of preceding trauma. (See 'The painful joint' and 'The limping child' chapters.)

Perform a thorough local and systemic examination; look for signs of sepsis including pyrexia, tachycardia and hypotension. Special investigations include FBC (be aware that a normal white cell count (WCC) does not exclude infection), inflammatory markers ESR and CRP (again the sensitivity for both of these in ruling out sepsis is not 100%), radiographs (signs of osteomyelitis may take 10–14 days to develop). Obtain blood cultures at presentation. They will not help in the emergency department but may become positive a few days later. For presumed bone or joint infection it is often best not to blindly start antibiotics unless the patient is systemically toxic; obtain specimens first. For possibly infected joints, aspiration of the joint with urgent microscopy of the aspirate is indicated. Generally it is advisable not to aspirate an artificial joint (hip or knee) in the emergency department. Involve the orthopaedic team early in suspected infected joint replacements; most total knee replacements remain painful, bruised and swollen for many weeks following the surgery and may look infected.

Sickle cell crisis

Musculoskeletal manifestations of sickle cell disease include vaso-occlusion, and superimposed infection (see 'Anaemia and bleeding disorders' chapter). Vaso-occlusive crises present with severe localized pain, local tenderness, swelling and erythema. Pyrexia and a raised WCC are common and create difficulties in excluding concomitant infection.

Patients with sickle cell disease are more susceptible to osteomyelitis, Salmonella being the classically described causative organism. However, osteomyelitis in patients with sickle cell disease may also be caused by common organisms including Staphylococcus aureus. The signs and symptoms of osteomyelitis are very similar to those of a vaso-occlusive crisis. If infection is suspected, obtain the usual bloods including blood cultures and obtain a senior opinion.

Oncological musculoskeletal emergencies

Primary musculoskeletal tumours are rare. Metastatic tumours to bone are relatively common. Metastases to bone may weaken it, leading to a pathological fracture. If a patient with known cancer presents with bone pain obtain a radiograph, and, if a lytic lesion is present, refer to the orthopaedic team for consideration of prophylactic fixation (Fig. 1). If the radiograph is normal, further investigation, such as a bone scan, may be required. Always consider the possibility of spinal cord compression in patients who have malignant disease and present with back pain. Oncology patients may be neutropenic, predisposing them to bone and joint infection; the presentation may also be a little atypical (see 'Oncology emergencies' chapter).

Musculoskeletal emergencies associated with rheumatoid arthritis

Rheumatoid arthritis is generally a chronic disease, but complications may arise acutely. An acute exacerbation of joint pain may be due to the disease process; however, always be vigilant to the possibility of superimposed infection (see 'The painful joint' chapter). Acute synovitis may lead to nerve compression syndromes, for example median nerve (acute carpal tunnel syndrome) and posterior interosseous nerve (wrist drop). Chronic synovitis and attrition of

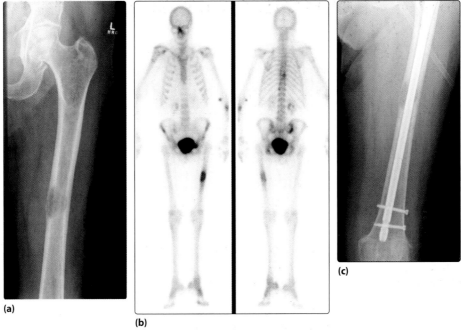

(a)

(b)

(c)

Fig. 1 **Patient with known lung cancer presented with thigh pain. (a)** Radiograph showing lytic lesion involving >50% width of left femoral shaft. **(b)** Nuclear medicine bone scan of same patient; note intense increased uptake in left femur and a few hot spots around the left elbow. **(c)** Postoperative radiograph following prophylactic femoral nailing.

tendons may lead to an acute closed tendon rupture (commonly to the little finger) or synovial cyst rupture (may present similar to a DVT).

Upper limb

Painful shoulder
Tendonitis of the shoulder is common and is often self-limiting. The pain may be severe and unrelenting, often worse at night. Exclude infection based on history, physical examination, blood tests and occasionally joint aspiration. If severe, obtain a radiograph looking for acute calcific tendonitis (most commonly the supraspinatous tendon). Adhesive capsulitis (frozen shoulder) also starts with acute severe pain and may begin spontaneously or following minor trauma. It is associated with diabetes and in diabetics is more resistant to treatment. Treat symptomatically with analgesics (NSAIDs) and consider a steroid injection. For calcific tendonitis, needle barbotage (breakdown of the calcific deposit) under local anaesthetic and ultrasound guidance may help.

Hand infections
Hand infections are common. Prompt aggressive treatment is required to limit morbidity and maximize function:

- felon – infection of the pulp space
- paronychia – infection around the nail fold
- web space infections – infections in the web space may track and point

dorsally resulting in a 'collar button' abscess
- midpalmar, thenar and hypothenar space infection – these are all potential spaces in the hand that may become infected
- acute flexor tenosynovitis of the hand – may be inflammatory or infective in nature. Kanaval's signs of an infected flexor tendon sheath include:
- finger held in slight flexion
- fusiform swelling
- flexor tendon sheath tenderness
- pain on passive finger extension.

Lower limb

The differential diagnosis of lower leg pain is wide.

Potential causes of leg pain
- Musculoskeletal – cramps, strain, stress fractures, compartment syndrome (acute, chronic)
- Vascular – venous (acute DVT, chronic venous insufficiency), arterial (chronic peripheral vascular disease, acute ischaemia either thrombosis or embolism)
- Metabolic – hypokalaemia, gout, diabetes mellitus (peripheral neuropathy)
- Infection – cellulitis, septic arthritis, osteomyelitis
- Neoplastic – primary bone tumours are rare, metastatic bone disease is more common
- Referred pain – sciatica, degenerative disc disease, spinal infection, spinal stenosis, nerve entrapment.

History
The history should give clues on the nature of the disorder: age is an important discriminator, acuity of onset, risk factors for DVT or arterial disease, history of malignancy, associated symptoms, back pain, neurological symptoms.

Examination
LOOK – is the leg swollen, red or pale, evidence of chronic venous insufficiency (hyperpigmentation)?
FEEL – palpate for areas of tenderness (calf tenderness), check capillary refill, palpate pulses (femoral, popliteal, dorsalis pedis, posterior tibial), examine the back and abdomen
MOVE – move all the joints, check motor power, sensation and reflexes.

Special tests
- Radiographs may be necessary to exclude underlying bony pathology.
- Ankle-brachial pressure index (ABPI) – the pulse may be palpable in peripheral vascular disease; the ABPI should not be less than 1.0.
- D-dimer blood test and ultrasound – see 'Thromboembolic disease' chapter.

> **Key points**
>
> - Take a thorough history; examine systematically – LOOK, FEEL, MOVE.
> - Actively exclude serious diagnoses such as joint infection, DVT and malignant disease.
> - Consider referred pain as the cause of the pain.

Back pain

Back pain is very common. Most people will experience back pain at some time in their lives and generally this will improve within one month. It is important to decide if the back pain is simple mechanical back pain, or part of a more sinister process.

Serious causes of back pain to consider and exclude are:

- malignancy – either primary or secondary deposits
- infection – discitis, epidural abscess, osteomyelitis
- trauma
- referred pain such as with a leaking abdominal aortic aneurysm
- cord compression resulting in neurological deficit (cauda equina syndrome).

Take a thorough history, paying particular attention to the red flags which may suggest a sinister feature to the back pain (Table 1).

Examine for vertebral deformity (kyphosis or scoliosis), local inflammation or tenderness, range of movement and straight leg raising.

A general examination should include:

- vital signs including temperature
- look for evidence of possible malignancy:
  - breast
  - thyroid
  - renal
  - lung
  - prostate (rectal examination for prostate and also check sphincter tone and test peri-anal sensation)
- examine the abdomen – always exclude abdominal aortic aneurysm (by bedside ultrasound or CT if over 60 years)

- perform a thorough neurological examination, including checking dermatomes and myotomes (Fig. 1) including rectal examination.

If the onset is acute, there are no red flags, and neurological and general examination is normal, then no further special investigations are required. Otherwise, depending on the clinical scenario, obtain an FBC, ESR and CRP (infection, myeloma), PSA (prostatic carcinoma), serum protein electrophoresis (myeloma), bone chemistry (tumour/metastasis) and consider imaging.

Imaging. Plain radiographs are indicated if there is a history of trauma and bony tenderness. Plain radiographs are neither sensitive nor specific enough to rule out infection or malignancy. If infection or malignancy is strongly suspected, then an MRI scan is the modality of choice, with radionucleotide scan (bone scan) being an alternative.

Once sinister causes for back pain have been considered and excluded, identify the mechanical cause of the back pain:

- leg pain, sciatica (suggests either disc herniation or spinal stenosis)
- spinal claudication (spinal stenosis)
- segmental instability (spondylolysis/listhesis)
- low back pain (simple mechanical back pain).

Malignancy

Metastatic spinal disease is 25 times more common than primary tumours of the spine. The most common metastatic neoplasms are breast, lung, prostate, kidney tumours, lymphoma and multiple myeloma (Fig. 2). Night pain and pain at rest suggest a possible spinal malignancy. Epidural compression and onset of myelopathy secondary to spinal metastasis is a true neurological emergency; refer immediately to a spinal surgeon and oncologist. Radiotherapy or urgent surgery is often required. Surgery is indicated if:

- the diagnosis is in doubt (tissue required for diagnosis)
- there is mechanical instability of the spine
- there is severe, rapid or progressive neurological deterioration.

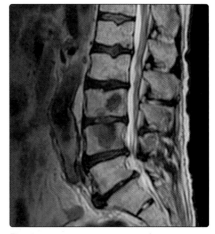

Fig. 2 **MRI lumbar spine (sagittal T2 with fat suppression)** showing metastatic tumour deposits in the lower lumbar vertebral bodies.

Table 1 **Red flags with back pain**
■ Age: less than 20 years and over 55 years
■ Recent significant trauma, or milder trauma, age >50 years
■ Night pain
■ Thoracic pain
■ Previous medical history – carcinoma, immunosuppression steroids, HIV
■ Systemic symptoms – unexplained fever, unexplained weight loss
■ Neurological symptoms or signs
■ Structural deformity
■ Intravenous (IV) drug use
■ Duration greater than 6 weeks

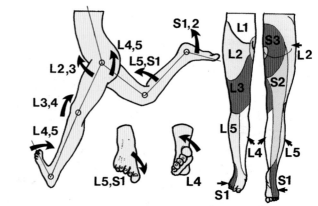

Fig. 1 **Dermatomes and myotomes** in the lower limb.

Infection

Spinal infections may be acute (bacterial infections) or chronic (e.g. fungal or mycobacterial infections). Suspect spinal infection in any patient who has recently had a spinal procedure and has focal severe pain, not relieved by rest. Patients with an epidural abscess may not present with the classic triad of fever, spine pain and neurological deficit. Have a high index of suspicion in elderly patients. Obtain a white cell count, CRP and ESR in patients who have red flags for infection. MRI is the investigation of choice. Tuberculosis has a predilection for the spine and may cause vertebral collapse and a sharply angulated deformity (Pott's disease).

Disc herniation and cauda equina syndrome

Patients with disc herniation usually present with the acute onset of low back pain that radiates into the buttocks and thighs and down one leg (sciatica) (Fig. 3). Neurological symptoms and signs depend on the level and severity. The straight leg raise test is sensitive but non-specific. With large herniations, the cauda equina may become involved causing bilateral motor weakness of the lower extremities, and bladder and bowel symptoms. The patient may experience urinary symptoms (incontinence, frequency or retention of urine), bowel symptoms (incontinence) or paraesthesia in the saddle area. If cauda equina syndrome is suspected obtain an emergency MRI and refer immediately to a spinal surgeon. Cervical disc herniation presents with neck and upper limb pain, paraesthesia with or without weakness in the

distribution of the affected nerve root (Fig. 4). Thoracic disc herniation is rare, but because there is relatively less space available for the cord in the thoracic spine, cord injury and paralysis below the waist is possible.

Spinal stenosis

Spinal stenosis is a degenerative condition with narrowing of the spinal canal. Patients present with neurogenic claudication. This is leg pain that is brought on by walking and is relieved by sitting or flexing forward. Spinal stenosis may also be associated with cauda equina syndrome.

Spondylolysis and spondylolisthesis

Spondylolysis may be congenital or acquired. It is characterized by a defect

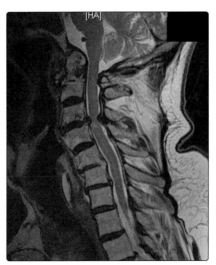

Fig. 4 **MRI cervical spine (sagittal T2 with fat suppression)** showing cord compression anteriorly from a broad-based disc and posteriorly from ligament hypertrophy. Note the subtle signal change in the cord.

or stress fracture in the pars interarticularis. Patients present with low back pain and stiffness, and the pain increases when they bend backwards.

Spondylolisthesis is where one vertebra slips forward on the vertebra below. This may be due to a spondylolysis or be degenerative in origin. Patients present with back stiffness and pain, occasionally sharp shooting pain into the buttocks and leg. Some patients will describe a 'slipping sensation' when standing up.

Low back pain

The most common form of back pain is simple mechanical back pain. Degenerative disc disease and facet joint arthritis place increased stress on the intervertebral ligaments. Most simple mechanical back pain will resolve with symptomatic treatment within one month. It is important to remember 'backs that move do better than backs that don't'. Prolonged absolute bed rest and inactivity is not good for mechanical back pain. Suggest relative rest, avoiding strenuous activity but remain as mobile as possible.

Paediatric considerations

- Significant back pain in prepubertal children is usually due to serious pathology and needs to be taken seriously and investigated.
- Back pain in adolescents may have a benign cause (overuse, sport or backpacks) which should improve with rest and symptomatic treatment.
- Approach as for adult back pain; red flags, history and physical examination and investigate as appropriate.

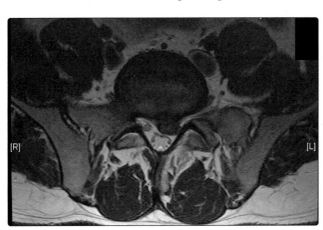

Fig. 3 **MRI lumbar spine (axial T2 with fat suppression)** showing large left posterior disc protrusion at L5/S1 compressing the L5 nerve root.

Key points

- Actively exclude sinister causes of back pain based on history (red flags) and examination.
- Always actively exclude a cauda equina syndrome and be vigilant for possible infective causes especially in the elderly.
- MRI is usually the imaging modality of choice in the absence of trauma.
- Always consider and exclude abdominal aortic aneurysm in older patients.

Sepsis

Often sepsis goes either undetected or undertreated. The body responds to infection by mounting an inflammatory response. The presence and severity of this response can be assessed by identifying the systemic inflammatory response syndrome (SIRS; Table 1). In the emergency department the presence of SIRS plus a presumed bacterial infection defines sepsis. Early identification of sepsis and aggressive early treatment has been shown to reduce mortality.

The commonest sources for sepsis are respiratory and urinary tract infections with other important sites being the central nervous system (meningitis), skin (cellulitis, necrotizing fasciitis (Fig. 1)), abdomen (appendicitis, diverticulitis) and facial infections (dental infections, ENT infections).

History

It is important to identify both the presence of sepsis and also the site of the infection. Often the patient presents with symptoms suggestive of a particular infection, and SIRS is diagnosed indicating a more serious manifestation of this particular infection. Occasionally the presentation is not so clear and a patient presents with sepsis with no specific symptoms or easily identifiable source. A careful history is essential to help identify both the presence of sepsis and a possible source. This latter presentation is particularly common at the extremes of age, in infants and in the elderly, especially where there is cognitive impairment with dementia.

Table 1 **Systemic inflammatory response syndrome (SIRS) in adults is defined as the presence of two or more of the following four features:**

1. Temperature <36°C or >38°C
2. Respiratory rate >20 breaths per minute
3. Heart rate >90 beats per minute
4. White blood cell count <4 × 10⁹ cells/L or > 12 × 10⁹ cells/L

Examination

An initial primary survey should determine the cardiorespiratory status of the patient. A thorough systemic examination can help to identify a possible source for the sepsis. Ensure that the patient is fully exposed. In children, search carefully for a non-blanching rash suggestive of meningococcal disease and check for signs of meningeal irritation (neck stiffness, photophobia). In the elderly a careful check for cutaneous infections is needed, particularly the lower legs and feet as this is a site that is often overlooked.

Investigations

These are guided to a certain degree by the history and examination. Check the urine; in the extremes of age symptoms and signs of a urinary tract infection are often absent. A chest x-ray (Fig. 2) is necessary if there are any respiratory symptoms, any abnormality of respiratory examination or if no source for sepsis is clearly identified. Blood tests include an urgent full blood count (white cell count will help to diagnose SIRS), blood cultures (before antibiotics wherever possible), serum lactate (very important in quantifying the degree of sepsis) and other blood tests to help identify end organ injury (renal function, liver function and coagulation). If tissue is not well perfused, lactate, a byproduct of anaerobic metabolism, will accumulate leading to a lactic acidosis. A serum lactate > 4 mmol/L suggests significant tissue hypoperfusion. Serum lactate can often be measured using a point of care test (POCT).

Emergency management

Once sepsis has been identified, urgent aggressive management is imperative. If SIRS is identified the sepsis resuscitation bundle must be initiated (Table 2). Some components of the bundle can be initiated easily (such as measuring lactate, taking blood cultures, giving antibiotics, oxygen and fluids) whilst other require more

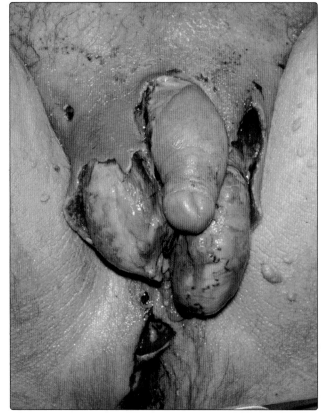

Fig. 1 **Fournier's gangrene (necrotizing fasciitis of the male perineum)** after surgical debridement.

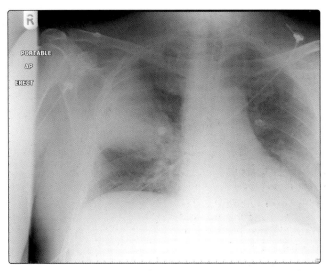

Fig. 2 **Chest x-ray showing pneumonia** (right middle lobe); a common source of sepsis.

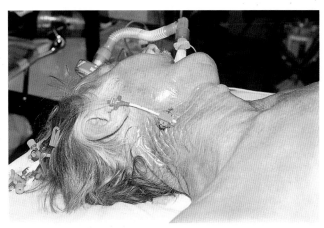

Fig. 3 **An internal jugular central venous catheter in situ.**

Table 2 **Targets for sepsis management in adults (sepsis resuscitation bundle)**
1. Measure serum lactate
2. Obtain blood cultures before giving antibiotics
3. Give broad spectrum antibiotics
4. Treat hypotension or raised lactate (or both) with fluids
5. Give vasopressors for ongoing hypotension (maintain mean arterial pressure (MAP) >65 mmHg)
6. Maintain adequate central venous pressure (8–12 mmHg)
7. Maintain adequate central venous oxygen saturations (>70%)
8. Maintain urine output >0.5 mL/kg/h

expertise (such as the use of vasopressors and measurement of central venous pressure and central venous oxygen saturations). Measurement of central venous pressure and central venous oxygen saturations requires the presence of a central venous line (Fig. 3) (see 'Central venous catheterization' chapter). It is essential that simple yet important first steps are initiated early whilst senior help is sought for the technically more difficult components of the sepsis bundle. Patients with established SIRS often require ongoing care in an intensive care setting.

For further information see http://www.survivingsepsis.org/.

Paediatric considerations

Always check for a non-blanching rash and signs of meningism (photophobia, neck stiffness, irritability).

Key points

- Sepsis is often undertreated or not recognized early.

- Sepsis is SIRS associated with an infection, proven or suspected.

- Severe sepsis is sepsis associated with organ dysfunction.

- Septic shock is sepsis associated with hypotension despite adequate volume resuscitation.

- Initiate the sepsis bundle early.

- Central venous access is best obtained under ultrasound guidance.

Human immunodeficiency virus (HIV), blood-borne and sexually transmitted infections

Human immunodeficiency virus (HIV) and AIDS

Acquired immunodeficiency syndrome (AIDS) is a set of symptoms and infections resulting from the damage to the human immune system caused by the human immunodeficiency virus (HIV).

HIV impacts on emergency medicine in several ways:

- Patients with known HIV present with illness.
- Patients present with possible transmission of HIV having sustained either a needlestick injury or an exposure to body fluids.
- New presentation of HIV; this is relatively unusual but it is important to have a high index of suspicion in high risk groups (Table 1).

Patients with known HIV

Acute complications affecting patients with known HIV are generally related to either infection or to a complication of drug therapy. Infections can affect any body system and are much more likely when the CD4 count falls to below 50 cells/µL (Fig. 1). Combination therapy from the three groups of antiretroviral agents has been found to be most effective and is known as highly active anti-retroviral therapy (HAART). Generally HAART is considered when the CD4 count falls to below 350 cells/µL. Anti-retroviral therapy can cause significant side effects including bone marrow suppression, rashes, gastrointestinal symptoms and jaundice. Reaction to a constituent of HAART should be considered as a possible cause of symptoms in a patient with known HIV.

Needlestick injuries and exposure to body fluids

Needlestick injuries can be sustained in either a healthcare setting, for example whilst taking blood, or alternatively in the community, for example a child pricking themselves on a discarded needle in a playground. All hospitals will have a designated protocol for the management of needlestick injuries and for exposure to body fluids. Types of high risk injury include penetration with a hollow needle, injury with an obviously contaminated needle and injury from a needle that had previously been inserted into a vessel. Other possible means of transmission include spills onto broken skin, body fluid contact with mucous membranes, human bites and sexual assault. Diseases that may be transmitted are HIV, hepatitis B (HBV) and hepatitis C (HCV). The risk of seroconversion if you sustain a hollow needle injury from an infected individual with HIV is approximately 0.3% and for HCV is 0.85%. If the HIV and hepatitis status of the donor is unknown, it is very useful to obtain consent and send a serum sample for urgent HIV and hepatitis screen. Specific immediate treatments exist for reducing the risk of transmission of HBV and HIV, but none exists for HCV. For HBV an accelerated course of immunization is advised, with the first dose being given in the emergency department. For HIV, consider the need for post-exposure prophylaxis (PEP). This is a considered decision and is largely based upon the two factors outlined above, namely the status of the patient and the type of injury sustained. If doubt exists consult an infectious disease specialist prior to beginning PEP, which can be stopped if the donor is found to be HIV negative on testing. In the case of possible transmission of HCV, blood is taken and stored so that if transmission does occur evidence exists for any compensation claim.

Sexually transmitted infections (STIs)

The most important STIs, excluding HIV, are chlamydia, gonorrhoea, genital herpes, *Trichomonas* infection,

Table 1 **High risk groups for HIV infection**
■ Unprotected sexual intercourse
■ Men who have sex with men
■ Intravenous drug users
■ Recipient of blood transfusion before 1985
■ Maternal HIV infection

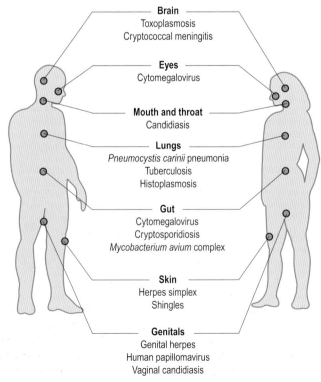

Brain
Toxoplasmosis
Cryptococcal meningitis

Eyes
Cytomegalovirus

Mouth and throat
Candidiasis

Lungs
Pneumocystis carinii pneumonia
Tuberculosis
Histoplasmosis

Gut
Cytomegalovirus
Cryptosporidiosis
Mycobacterium avium complex

Skin
Herpes simplex
Shingles

Genitals
Genital herpes
Human papillomavirus
Vaginal candidiasis

Fig. 1 **Opportunistic infections in HIV infection.**

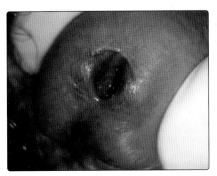

Fig. 2 **Mucoid discharge due to chlamydial urethritis.**

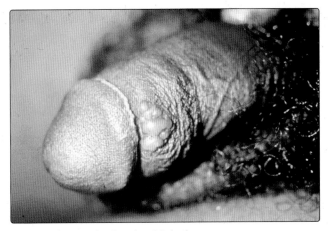

Fig. 3 **Vesicles due to herpes simplex virus 2 infection.**

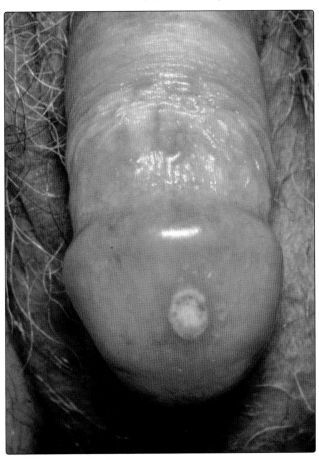

Fig. 4 **Genital ulcer on glans penis, primary chancre of syphilis.**

human papillomavirus (HPV) and syphilis. Contact tracing, microbiology swab taking and initiation of treatment are all important components of the management. Confidentiality and sympathy are essential since people commonly feel embarrassed. Take a thorough sexual history including number of partners, use of barrier methods (condoms) and previous STIs. A urethral discharge in a man may be due to chlamydial infection or gonorrhoea. In chlamydial urethritis there is dysuria and the discharge is mucoid (Fig. 2), whilst in gonorrhoea the discharge is characteristically purulent and profuse. In women, *Trichomonas* may cause a green frothy vaginal discharge, but with vaginal discharges, consider non-sexually transmitted causes such as bacterial vaginosis and candidiasis (white curd-like discharge). Genital ulcers are most commonly caused by herpes simplex virus (HSV) (Fig. 3) but also consider syphilis (Fig. 4). Many hospitals provide excellent clinics where patients can self-present if they suspect an STI. Such clinics may provide a more efficient and private service than a busy emergency department and if possible patients should be redirected there.

Key points

- Always consider the possibility of HIV infection in high risk patients.
- Carefully risk assess the likelihood of viral transmission with needlestick injuries.
- Genitourinary medicine clinics provide the optimal environment for assessment of patients with suspected sexually transmitted infection.

Tropical diseases and fever in the returning traveller

Tropical diseases are infectious diseases that are more widespread in the tropics and subtropical regions and tend to disproportionately affect poor or remote populations in developing regions of the Americas, Asia and Africa.

Many air travellers visit these regions and are exposed to these diseases, most notably malaria and hepatitis. While tropical disease must always be considered in the febrile unwell returning traveller, more common non-tropical conditions such as viral illnesses and other sources of sepsis must not be overlooked (Table 1).

Malaria

Fever in a traveller within 3 months of departure from a malaria-endemic area should be investigated thoroughly. Malaria is the major cause of sickness and death in many developing countries (Fig. 1). It is an infective disease caused by four species of the genus *Plasmodium*:

- *P. falciparum*
- *P. ovale*
- *P. vivax*
- *P. malariae*.

The infection is spread by female *Anopheles* mosquitoes.

Clinical features

P. falciparum malaria is the most severe, being characterized by paroxysms of chills, sweats and haemolysis. Cerebral malaria is a potentially fatal complication.

The incubation period is generally 7 to 14 days but may be up to a year, if the patient is semi-immune or has taken prophylaxis.

There is a prodrome of flu-like symptoms with headache, malaise, myalgia and anorexia. Following the prodrome the patient develops paroxysms lasting 8 to 12 hours with sudden coldness followed by a severe rigor for up to an hour, then a high temperature, vomiting, flushing and sweating. Paroxysms are generally daily but may be irregular.

On examination the patient may be anaemic, jaundiced and have hepatosplenomegaly without lymphadenopathy or a rash.

Diagnosis

A diagnosis is achieved by repeated microscopy of thick and thin blood films. Thick films are more sensitive at identifying infection with parasites whilst the thin films help to identify the particular species of *Plasmodium* involved. In partially treated patients, if blood smears are negative, bone marrow smears may be required. Antigen detection tests are available for

use in areas where microscopy is not available, or where laboratory staff are not experienced at malaria diagnosis. Malaria antibody detection tests are performed using the indirect fluorescent antibody (IFA) test. The IFA procedure can be used to determine if a patient has been infected with *Plasmodium*. Because of the time required for development of antibody and also the persistence of antibodies, serological testing is not practical for routine diagnosis of acute malaria. However, antibody detection may be useful for testing a patient with a febrile illness who is suspected of having malaria and from whom repeated blood smears are negative. Always seek expert help and/or consult local protocols.

Treatment

This is dependent on the organism and resistance.

Chloroquine is the standard treatment for *P. vivax* and *P. ovale* malaria. Relapse may occur due to persistent hepatic forms, hypnozoites. Treatment with antimalarials should be followed with a course of primaquine for 21 days.

Active malaria infection with *P. falciparum* is a medical emergency requiring admission to hospital. Severe infection should be treated with intravenous quinine, especially in the light of considerable worldwide chloroquine resistance. Exchange transfusion may be indicated where

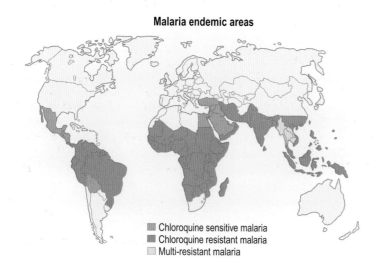

Malaria endemic areas

■ Chloroquine sensitive malaria
■ Chloroquine resistant malaria
□ Multi-resistant malaria

Fig. 1 **Malaria endemic areas.**

Table 1 **Tropical diseases and causes of fever**	
Tropical diseases	**Most common causes of fever after travel to the tropics**
Malaria	Respiratory infection
Dengue fever	UTI
African trypanosomiasis	Pharyngitis
Leishmaniasis	Diarrhoeal illness
Schistosomiasis	Malaria
Cholera	Meningitis
Yellow fever	Hepatitis
Tuberculosis	Dengue fever
Chagas disease	Enteric fever (typhoid)
Leprosy	Epstein–Barr virus
Lymphatic filariasis	Rickettsia
Onchocerciasis	Amoebic liver abscess
Ebola haemorrhagic fever	Tuberculosis
Lassa fever	Acute HIV

there is a very high parasitaemia. Blood glucose should be monitored regularly and corrected where necessary. In cerebral malaria ventilation is common and consideration should be given to treatment with intravenous mannitol for cerebral oedema. After treatment, a single dose of Fansidar should be considered.

The most important factors determining survival in falciparum malaria are early diagnosis and prompt initiation of appropriate treatment.

Traveller's diarrhoea

Antimotility agents, such as loperamide, are safe and efficacious for mild to moderate cases of traveller's diarrhoea in adults; most acute cases of this diarrhoea respond to a single dose or 3-day course of antimicrobial therapy (e.g. ciprofloxacin).

Persistent diarrhoea in returned travellers is less likely to have an infective cause than acute diarrhoea and requires investigation.

Rabies

Post-exposure rabies treatment is effective and should be considered for all travellers with potential exposure.

Severe acute respiratory syndrome (SARS)

SARS, a respiratory disease caused by a coronavirus, is transmitted by contaminated aerosol droplets. Victims may have mild disease but 20% of hospitalized patients require ventilatory support.

A case is defined by:

- high fever (≥38°C)
- **and** one or more respiratory symptoms
- **and** radiographic evidence of lung infiltrates consistent with pneumonia or respiratory distress syndrome
- **and** travel within 10 days of onset of illness to a SARS endemic area **or** a location containing SARS virus isolates or diagnostic specimens.

Confirmatory investigations:

- RT-PCR test for SARSCoV (nasopharyngeal aspirate or faeces)
- seroconversion by ELISA or IFA.

Suspected cases must wear a face-mask and be isolated in a negative pressure environment. Attending staff must wear personal protective equipment (PPE) and perform impeccable hand hygiene and barrier nursing. Seek specialist advice immediately.

Treatment is largely supportive.

Avian influenza

Avian influenza A virus normally infects birds but several subtypes can infect humans, particularly the H5N1 strain, which causes severe disease with an incubation period of around 3 days.

A case is defined by:

- fever (≥38°C) **or** history of fever
- **and** respiratory symptoms requiring hospitalization **or** death from an unexplained respiratory illness
- **and** travel within 10 days of onset of illness to an area affected by avian influenza
- **and** potential viral exposure, defined by close contact (within 1 month) with:
  live or dead domestic fowl, wild birds or swine
  other cases(s) of severe respiratory illness or unexplained death within an infected area
  healthcare workers in a cluster of severe unexplained respiratory illness
  a laboratory worker with potential exposure to avian influenza.

Other symptoms include sore throat, rhinorrhoea, myalgia, conjunctivitis and diarrhoea. Severe complications include respiratory distress syndrome, multiple organ failure and sepsis. The case fatality rate is high (55–60%).

Suspected cases must wear a face-mask and be isolated in a negative pressure environment. Attending staff must wear personal protective

equipment (PPE) and perform impeccable hand hygiene and barrier nursing. Request specialist help immediately.

Investigations:

- FBC (lymphopenia) and LFTs
- Chest x-ray
- nasopharyngeal aspirate and throat swab for RT-PCR and viral culture
- rapid tests for normal human influenza should be performed as this is the most likely cause of symptoms.

Treatment is largely supportive but consider neuraminidase inhibitors (e.g. oseltamivir). Healthcare workers attending patients with suspected H5N1 should consider taking prophylactic oseltamivir. Seek specialist advice.

Pandemic influenza

Pandemic influenza will be caused by a new viral strain capable of spreading efficiently between humans. It may occur at any time of year and will affect people of all ages.

What can you do to prepare for pandemic flu?

- Be 'fit tested' for your mask.
- Ensure you are trained in the use of PPE, which must be donned and removed without contaminating yourself or others.
- Read the information on the following websites:
  www.dh.gov.uk/PolicyAndGuidance/ EmergencyPlanning/PandemicFlu
  http://www.who.int/csr/disease/avian_ influenza/guidelines/draftprotocol/ en/index.html

---

Key points

- Fever in a returning traveller requires prompt investigation to prevent significant morbidity and mortality from malaria.

- Diarrhoea is the most common health problem in returning travellers.

- All travellers bitten by an animal require evaluation for rabies prophylaxis.

- Some important chronic infections may present months or years later (e.g. schistosomiasis).

Allergy and anaphylaxis

Allergy is a state of hypersensitivity induced by exposure to a particular antigen (allergen) that leads to an exaggerated and inappropriate response of the immune system. These hypersensitivity reactions are classified into four types (Table 1). There are no differences in prevalence between races or gender. The numbers of patients suffering allergic reactions is increasing in the UK.

Anaphylaxis is a generalized, multisystem type I hypersensitivity reaction following previous exposure to the same antigen. Immediate reactions can also occur via non-IgE-mediated (IgG and IgM) mechanisms. Activated complement components C5a and C3a can directly stimulate mast cells and so release histamine.

Type I hypersensitivity reactions with degranulation of mast cells result in secretion of vasoactive and bronchoactive mediators such as histamine, prostaglandins and leukotrienes. These mediators cause vasodilatation and smooth-muscle contraction. Anaphylaxis can be rapid, slow or biphasic (rare).

Clinical features

Allergic reactions range from mild local symptoms, such as skin itching, to systemic reactions leading to anaphylactic shock. Symptoms and signs include rhinitis, conjunctivitis, cutaneous manifestations (angio-oedema, urticaria, rashes or erythema; Fig. 1), bronchospasm, gastrointestinal upset (abdominal pain/vomiting/diarrhoea), hypotension and full-blown anaphylactic shock with cardiorespiratory arrest.

Causes

The commonest allergens are drugs (antibiotics, NSAIDs, aspirin), foodstuffs (peanuts, egg, seafood) and insect stings.

Management

The management will depend on the severity of the allergic reaction. Mild and localized reactions like urticaria and nasal allergies such as hay fever can be treated with antihistamines; H1 blockers like chlorphenamine or newer and less sedating drugs like loratadine.

Allergic contact dermatitis (type IV hypersensitivity reaction) can be treated by avoidance of the causative allergen, protective clothes/gloves, regular use of emollients and, if necessary, topical steroid cream.

Treatment for allergic conjunctivitis includes the use of systemic and topical antihistamines and sodium cromoglicate eye drops.

Nasal steroids might be used in addition for allergic rhinitis, e.g. beclometasone. If bronchospasm is present, beta-2 agonists such as salbutamol are used.

Emergency management

The management of anaphylaxis should include high flow oxygen, the careful removal of any insect sting from the skin or discontinuation of the drug, and the use of intramuscular adrenaline (epinephrine) with intravenous fluids (Fig. 2). Low dose intravenous adrenaline may be used by experienced clinicians in a fully monitored setting.

Antihistamines, inhaled beta-2 agonists and corticosteroids, may be needed depending on the severity of the symptoms. The airway of the patient is at risk and special attention must be paid to its patency at all time. Early intubation before angio-oedema of the pharynx and larynx makes this intervention impossible might be necessary. If this is not possible then a surgical airway will be required.

Patients with beta-adrenoceptor blocking drug treatment are at risk of more severe and prolonged anaphylactic reactions. Patients with a history of asthma might have more severe and treatment-resistant symptoms of bronchospasm.

Glucagon might be effective, especially in patients on beta-adrenoceptor blocking drug treatment, if there is no improvement with adrenaline.

Increased airway pressure due to severe bronchospasm can be a sign of anaphylaxis in the intubated patient and might make ventilation of the patient difficult.

Differential diagnosis

Anxiety or panic attack, asthma, hereditary angio-oedema (C1 esterase inhibitor deficiency) and vasovagal syncope can all be mistaken for an allergic reaction. One feature that may

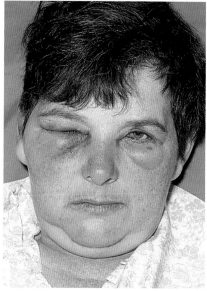

Fig. 1 **Angio-oedema involving the face.**

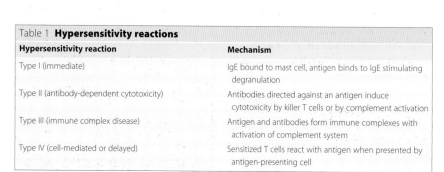

Table 1 **Hypersensitivity reactions**

Hypersensitivity reaction	Mechanism
Type I (immediate)	IgE bound to mast cell, antigen binds to IgE stimulating degranulation
Type II (antibody-dependent cytotoxicity)	Antibodies directed against an antigen induce cytotoxicity by killer T cells or by complement activation
Type III (immune complex disease)	Antigen and antibodies form immune complexes with activation of complement system
Type IV (cell-mediated or delayed)	Sensitized T cells react with antigen when presented by antigen-presenting cell

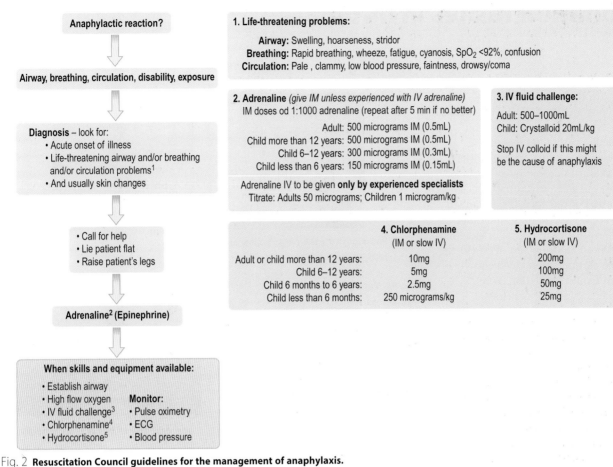

Fig. 2 **Resuscitation Council guidelines for the management of anaphylaxis.**

help to distinguish an allergic reaction is the presence of a cutaneous feature of some description (rash, urticaria and erythema).

Prevention

Allergic reaction can often be avoided by taking a clear medical history of previous drug reactions, avoidance of food in known food allergies (e.g. peanuts) and change of products used, e.g. use of non-latex gloves in known latex allergy. Skin prick testing and RAST (radio-allergosorbent) tests for IgE can help to find the causative allergen and be used to help avoid further exposure. Seasonal allergic reaction can be treated by use of oral antihistamines, nasal steroid sprays and eye drops. Some allergies might respond to hyposensitization treatment in specialist allergy centres.

Patients should discontinue the use of beta-adrenoceptor blocking drug treatment if they have had an anaphylactic reaction. For patients with a history of severe life-threatening anaphylactic reaction an EpiPen or EpiPen Jr should be prescribed for pre-hospital emergency self administration of adrenaline. The use of the Epipen should be demonstrated so it can be used for emergency treatment by the patient or his relatives.

A Medic Alert Bracelet should be worn by all patients with severe allergic reactions.

Other emergency department considerations

All patients presenting to the emergency department with anaphylaxis require follow-up in a specialist allergy clinic. Measuring a mast cell tryptase may help with confirming the diagnosis of anaphylaxis. In the UK any adverse drug reaction requires reporting to the Medicine and Healthcare products Regulatory Agency (MHRA) using the yellow card system.

Web resources

http://www.resus.org.uk
http://www.mhra.gov.uk

Paediatric considerations

The child might be too young to give a medical history. Accompanying parents or relatives might be able to give a history regarding the events leading up to developing symptoms or if the child has any known allergies.

The drug dosage and fluid boluses used will depend on the weight of the patient.

Securing the airway in a child with anaphylaxis can be challenging for any doctor and the help of an experienced paediatric anaesthetist will be invaluable.

Key points

■ A cutaneous manifestation is almost always present with allergic reactions.

■ Anaphylaxis kills if not identified and treated promptly.

■ Adrenaline and fluid are the immediate treatments for anaphylaxis.

■ The commonest allergens precipitating anaphylaxis are drugs, foodstuffs and stings.

Common rashes in adults

The skin has several important functions including thermoregulation, barrier, ultraviolet protection and protection from fluid loss. It also represents us to the outside world. The skin is inhabited by a number of microorganisms which form part of the normal skin flora. If the skin is injured, these and other organisms can cause local or systemic infection. The complaint of developing a 'rash' is a common emergency department presentation. True dermatological emergencies are uncommon but are important to recognize and treat appropriately as soon as possible. Skin changes can be important signs of serious systemic disease, such as the non-blanching, purpuric rash in meningococcal sepsis.

Minor skin problems, or exacerbations of chronic skin conditions such as eczema and psoriasis, may present to the emergency department. The long-term treatment can be continued by the patient's general practitioner after reassurance and commencement of initial treatment. Moisturizing creams or lotions, moist dressings, low dose topical steroid preparations, or antibiotics for superimposed infection may be indicated. Discussion with a dermatologist may be indicated if there has been a rapid or significant change in the skin condition, whereas the use of a pictorial library may be useful for the diagnosis of unusual rashes and skin conditions.

Knowledge of the commonly used language to describe skin changes is essential and helps in the documentation and communication with other health professionals (Table 1).

Common emergency presentations include bacterial, viral and fungal skin infections.

Bacterial infections

Impetigo

This skin infection is most commonly due to *Staphylococcus aureus* but can be caused by streptococci or may be a mixed infection. Thin-walled blisters rupture and leave yellow honey-crusted

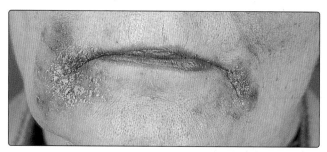

Fig. 1 **Impetigo; note the crusty yellow appearance.**

Table 1	**Types of skin lesion**
Macule	Change in colour or consistency without any elevation above the surrounding skin
Papule	Raised lesion less than 1 cm
Nodule	Raised skin lesion over 1 cm
Vesicle	Raised lesion containing fluids up to 1 cm
Bulla	Vesicle larger than 1 cm

itchy lesions, often on the face (Fig. 1). More common in children, the lesions are contagious. Treatment for localized lesions is with a topical antibacterial preparation (e.g. fusidic acid). Widespread infections are treated with oral flucloxacillin, or erythromycin in penicillin allergy.

Cellulitis

This is a deep-seated infection of the skin and subcutaneous tissue commonly caused by streptococci or *Staphylococcus aureus*. It usually affects the legs or arms. There may be an entry wound, e.g. an insect bite, small wound, skin crack, leg ulcer or injection site in an intravenous drug user. The patient will present with localized pain, swelling and erythema. On examination there will be tenderness and increased warmth. The area often has a well-demarcated edge and there may be lymphangitis or blisters over the affected skin area (Fig. 2). Systemic features such as fever or general malaise may be present. Treatment is with systemic antibiotics, either orally or intravenously depending upon severity.

Necrotizing fasciitis

This is a serious and potentially life-threatening soft tissue infection. The infection spreads along the superficial and deep fascial planes, involving muscles and causing widespread necrosis.

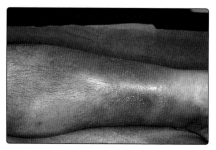

Fig. 2 **Cellulitis affecting the lower leg.**

Streptococcus pyogenes is often involved but other organisms, such as methicillin resistant *Staphylococcus aureus* (MRSA), can be the culprit. If not identified and treated aggressively, the patient has a high risk of progressing to septic shock, organ failure and death. Initially the patient may complain of flu-like symptoms with the involved skin area being swollen, with erythema and tenderness on palpation. The pain is severe, with the severity of the pain being out of proportion to the initial signs. Crepitus may be palpable and x-rays of the affected area may show gas in the soft tissues. Treatment involves intravenous antibiotics, fluids and radical debridement of the necrotic area, or amputation.

Fungal infections

Common fungal infections seen include tinea corporis (trunk and limbs), tinea capitis (scalp), tinea manuum (hand), tinea pedis (athlete's foot) and tinea unguium (nails).

Tinea corporis (ringworm)

The lesions in tinea corporis (from the Latin word for worm) can be single or multiple. The patient will present with itching, scaling and erythematous lesions which are slowly increasing in size. With central clearing the lesion can become anular in shape leaving the ring pattern which gives the infection its name (ringworm). Mild localized fungal infections of the skin are treated with topical therapy with imidazole antifungals such as clotrimazole.

Viral infections

Chickenpox (varicella zoster)

Infection by the varicella zoster virus is more common in childhood. The infection causes an itchy vesicular rash that appears in crops and mucous membranes are involved. The patient is infectious until the last vesicle has crusted over. The rash can be accompanied by fever. Treatment is symptomatic with paracetamol and calamine lotion. Oral or intravenous antivirals (aciclovir) are reserved for severe infection.

Herpes zoster (shingles)

This involves reactivation of dormant varicella zoster infection from the dorsal root or cranial nerve ganglia in a patient with previous history of chickenpox infection. The incidence increases with age and in immunocompromised patients. Precise triggers are not known. The rash is vesicular and typically affects one dermatome, most commonly in the thoracic region. Pain can precede the rash by 2 to 3 days. The pain can be severe and exacerbated by touch. Treatment is with aciclovir or famciclovir, and is most effective if started within 72 hours of the onset of the rash.

Other rashes

Erythema multiforme

This is a hypersensitivity syndrome caused by the formation and deposition of immune complexes in blood vessels of the skin and mucous membranes resulting in the classical target lesions. Mononuclear cells, deposits of IgM, fibrin and

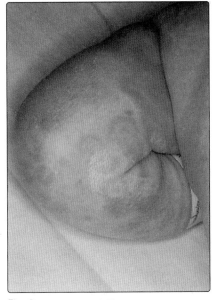

Fig. 3 **Erythema multiforme.**

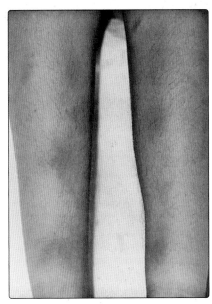

Fig. 4 **Erythema nodosum.**

complement are found around the affected blood vessels and there is epidermal necrosis and inflammatory infiltrates. The disease can be precipitated by viral, fungal or bacterial infections (especially *Mycoplasma*). Other causes include drugs, pregnancy and malignancy. No cause is found in half of patients. Stevens–Johnson syndrome and toxic epidermal necrolysis are considered to be caused by the same disease process but with a more severe presentation. Initially there may be a period of flu-like symptoms. This is followed by maculopapular lesions which appear on the hands, feet and extensor areas of the limbs. These lesions evolve into target lesions consisting of a pink-red ring and a pale centre or with vesicles and bullae (Fig. 3). The genitalia and mucous membranes may be involved. If possible, the cause should be identified and treated. Causative drugs are discontinued. Treatment is generally supportive and hospital admission may be required in more severe cases for supportive care and symptom control.

Erythema nodosum

This is an acute nodular rash that normally affects the extensor surface of the lower legs (Fig. 4). It is most often seen in young adults and is more common in females. The rash may be preceded by a flu-like illness and accompanied by arthralgia. The skin lesions have poorly defined margins and are tender to touch. Common causes include bacterial infections (especially streptococcal infections), drugs, pregnancy and sarcoidosis. Identify and treat any underlying cause, but an underlying cause is not apparent in up to half of all patients with erythema nodosum. Erythema nodosum is self-limiting and specific treatment is symptomatic, NSAIDs are particularly effective in treating any associated discomfort.

Web resource

www.dermatlas.org

Key points

- True dermatological emergencies are rare.
- Systemic disease may present initially with skin changes.
- Expert opinion and use of pictorial libraries can be useful in diagnosis.

Diabetic emergencies

Diabetes mellitus is the most common endocrine disease and results from either reduced or ineffective endogenous insulin. Untreated, diabetes will present with excessive polyuria, thirst and increased fluid intake (polydipsia), weight loss and often blurred vision as a result of hyperglycaemia.

The central nervous system (CNS) cannot synthesize glucose, and only stores a negligible amount. Glucose is its principal fuel, and even short periods of hypoglycaemia (<2.5 mmol/L or 45 mg/dL) can result in significant CNS dysfunction. Glucose regulatory mechanisms are well developed to avoid and recover from hypoglycaemia and maintain normal plasma glucose between 3.6 and 5.8 mmol/L (65–105 mg/dL).

Hypoglycaemia

Hypoglycaemia will result from an imbalance of glucose availability and insulin activity – in essence 'too much' insulin, or reduced glucose availability (Table 1).

This is most commonly seen in the diabetic patient who is on insulin therapy (Fig. 1) and misses a meal for some reason. It is not isolated to the diabetic population. Hypoglycaemia can be caused by an excess of insulin or a sulphonylurea, but not by metformin alone.

Check the blood glucose in a patient with **any** neurological symptom.

Presentation

Symptoms include behavioural changes, confusion, drowsiness, slurred speech and seizures. Focal neurological features and overt coma result from neuroglycopenia (usually glucose <2.5 mmol/L). Counter-regulatory sympathetic activity (with glucose <3.6 mmol/L) will cause tachycardia, sweating, anxiety and tremor. 'Hypoglycaemic unawareness' may occur after a single hypoglycaemic episode as a result of sympathetic desensitization, but also occurs with autonomic dysfunction and beta-blockers. This may result in rapid neuroglycopenic features without warning.

Management principles

Following an ABCDE assessment, check a capillary blood glucose (CBG) and confirm by laboratory assay.

If alcoholism or malnutrition (anorexia, malignancy) are suspected, administer 1–2 mg/kg thiamine to avoid Wernicke's encephalopathy. Give glucose either orally, buccally or intravenously. The preferred solution is 250 to 500 mL (or 3 to 5 mL/kg) of 10% glucose solution. Intramuscular glucagon can be given when there is no intravenous access. Look for causes.

Patients should recover in 10–20 minutes. If this does not occur, this may be due to recurrent hypoglycaemia, complications (such as head injury following collapse, cerebral oedema or microvascular cerebral infarction) or additional/alternative pathology (i.e. true CVA, myxoedema coma).

Long-acting hypoglycaemic agents require prolonged observation and a 10% glucose infusion may be required.

If there is no history or evidence of diabetes, consider sending a serum sample for insulin and C-peptide measurement to determine if there is excess endogenous or exogenous insulin. In the non-diabetic, if excess exogenous insulin is identified, the cause will be poisoning; either self-harm, accidental or malicious.

Diabetic ketoacidosis (DKA)

This occurs almost exclusively in type 1 diabetics due to a relative insulin deficit. It is the mode of first presentation for ~25% of type 1 diabetics. Around 20% of episodes are due to non-compliance. Symptoms are due to hyperglycaemia and osmotic load/dehydration, acidaemia, as well as any underlying precipitating pathology (sepsis in 30%). The diagnosis is made by detection of hyperglycaemia, a metabolic acidosis and ketonuria (or ketonaemia).

Symptoms
Symptoms include:

- polyuria (hyperglycaemia)
- polydipsia (osmotic load)

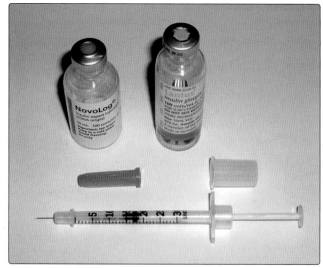

Fig. 1 **Standard insulin and syringe.**

Table 1 **Causes of hypoglycaemia**				
Poisoning/Drugs	**Reduced glucose intake**	**Reduced glucose production**	**Increased glucose utilization**	**Insulin persistence**
Insulin	Missed/delayed meal	Hepatic failure	Exertion	Insulinoma
Oral hypoglycaemics such as sulphonylureas	Vomiting	Hypopituitarism	Sepsis	Hepatic failure
Alcohol		Adrenal failure	Malaria	Renal failure
		Hypothyroidism		
		Renal failure		

Table 2 **Treatment of diabetic ketoacidosis and hyperosmolar non-ketotic state**		
Treatment	**Diabetic ketoacidosis**	**Hyperosmolar non-ketotic state**
Fluids	1000 mL 0.9% saline stat.	1000 mL 0.9% saline stat.
	2–4 × 1000 mL 0.9% saline 2-hourly with K^+	2 × 1000 mL 0.9% saline 2-hourly with K^+
	1000 mL 0.9% saline 4-hourly with K^+ until rehydrated	1000 mL 0.9% saline 6-hourly with K^+ till rehydrated over 48 h
		If Na^+ >160 mmol/L then use 0.45% saline for first 3 litres
		Convert to 5% glucose when glucose <15 mmol/L
Insulin	Initial bolus 0.1–0.15 u/kg	(Insulin infusion at 1–2 u/h until glucose <15 mmol/L, then convert to sliding scale)
	Insulin infusion at 0.1 u/kg/h – reduce by 0.05 u/kg/h if drops glucose rapidly	Sliding scale
	Sliding scale commenced when glucose <15 mmol/L (with 5% glucose infusion)	
Antibiotics	Broad-spectrum if sepsis considered	Broad-spectrum if sepsis considered
DVT prophylaxis	Consider LMWH	LMWH (i.e. enoxaparin 40 mg SC once a day)

- Kussmaul's respiration (acidaemia)
- lassitude, weakness, 'twitching' (hyponatraemia, hypokalaemia)
- weight loss (polyuria, catabolic state)
- vomiting, abdominal pain
- confusion.

Note that hyperglycaemia may be mild, even in severe DKA, if the patient continues to use insulin. Patients are fluid depleted with an average fluid loss of 3–6 litres. Thromboembolism may occur as a result of dehydration. Total body potassium is also depleted and drops further with administered insulin. Severe acidosis (pH <7.0), serum osmolality >320, anuria/oliguria and first presentation are poor prognostic factors.

Investigations

These are directed at confirming diagnosis (ketonaemia with pH ≤7.3 or HCO_3 ≤15 mmol/L), assessing severity, and searching for precipitants. Tests include:

- glucose
- arterial blood gases: pH, HCO_3, lactate
- U&Es: corrected Na = Na^+ + 1.6 × [(glucose − 5.5)/5.5]
- serum osmolality = $2(Na^+ + K^+)$ + Urea + Glucose
- septic screen: MSU, chest x-ray, blood culture
- FBC
- amylase (up to 10% have pancreatitis).

Emergency management

This involves assessment and treatment using the ABCDE approach. Invasive monitoring may be required in severe cases, patients with co-morbidity or the elderly.

Keep nil by mouth, attach a cardiac monitor and insert a urinary catheter.

Aim to replace fluid deficits over 24 hours. Start with 0.9% saline until blood glucose <12 mmol/L then convert to 5% glucose. Aim to reduce the blood glucose gently (less than 5 mmol/L/h, and keep glucose >10 mmol/L until ketoacidosis resolves). Replace K^+ early unless oliguric/hyperkalaemic. A typical regimen is shown in Table 2. Hourly assessment of acidaemia and electrolytes (potassium) is required during initial treatment. Salicylate overdose is a cause of hyperglycaemia and acidaemia, while lactic acidosis (especially in the elderly/metformin therapy) is another possibility.

Hyperosmolar non-ketotic coma (HONC)

This condition, also known as hyperosmolar non-ketotic state, usually presents in elderly patients (often first presentation of type 2 diabetes) with a long history of deterioration. The hyperglycaemia is more profound than in DKA, with associated significant dehydration and hyperosmolarity, resulting in marked thrombotic risk and a high mortality.

Symptoms

These are due to hyperglycaemia/ hyperosmolarity/dehydration, and of complications/precipitants and include:

- polyuria
- polydipsia
- reduced consciousness (coma if osmolality >430 mosm/L)
- weakness, (postural) hypotension
- thrombotic event: MI, CVA.

The hyperglycaemia is high (>40 mmol/L) and the average fluid loss is 8–10 litres. Patients are often elderly with significant co-morbidity. Fluid overload is a major risk of treatment. Rapid changes in glucose can result in CNS injury. Thrombotic risk is high, and patients should be anticoagulated. Reduced conscious level, lactic acidosis and thrombotic complications are poor prognostic factors.

Investigations

These are directed at confirming diagnosis (hyperglycaemia with plasma osmolality >350 mosm/L), severity and searching for precipitants/ complications:

- glucose
- U&Es: Corrected Na = Na^+ + 1.6 × [(glucose − 5.5)/5.5]; raised urea:creatinine ratio
- plasma osmolality: $2(Na^+ + K^+)$ + Urea + Glucose
- arterial blood gas
- FBC (sepsis, polycythaemia due to dehydration)
- septic screen: chest x-ray, MSU, blood culture
- ECG (co-morbidity, acute MI).

Emergency management

Management is similar to though less aggressive than with DKA (Table 2). Invasive monitoring is recommended in the elderly population. Keep nil by mouth, attach a cardiac monitor and insert a urinary catheter. Anticoagulate with LMWH and aim to rehydrate over 48 hours and to reduce glucose slowly.

Key points

- Patients with diabetes are at increased risk of cardiovascular disease.
- Always check bedside blood glucose in patients with altered mental status.
- Early administration of insulin switches off ketone production in DKA.
- Patients with hyperglycaemic states are usually significantly dehydrated – treat shock aggressively and then replace estimated loss more gradually.
- Remember to consider anticoagulation in hyperosmolar states.

Biochemical and endocrine emergencies

Electrolyte balance

The main electrolytes of interest in emergency medicine are potassium and sodium and to a lesser extent magnesium and calcium. Blood (serum) samples may be sent to a laboratory for analysis or be analyzed in the emergency department using point of care testing. Results should be compared with the local reference range; examples of reference ranges are shown in parentheses below.

Potassium (3.5–5.0 mmol/L)

Hyperkalaemia (raised serum potassium; K^+) may be caused by metabolic acidosis, especially if the aetiology is renal failure. Widespread cellular damage and death, e.g. rhabdomyolysis/crush injury, allows potassium to leak out of cells causing hyperkalaemia. Iatrogenic causes include drugs like ACE inhibitors, suxamethonium and massive blood transfusion.

As serum K^+ exceeds 6.5 mmol/L, cardiac dysrhythmias become more likely including VT/VF. ECG changes include tall peaked T waves, widening QRS complexes, P wave depression and eventually a sine wave pattern (Fig. 1). Treatment includes myocardial protection with an intravenous bolus of 10 ml of 10% calcium gluconate, followed by K^+ lowering with 15 units of insulin (with dextrose), bicarbonate, or 20 mg of nebulized salbutamol. Dialysis may be required.

Hypokalaemia (low serum K^+) is due to increased losses, commonly into the urine secondary to diuretic use (see Table 2 in 'Acute renal failure' chapter). Other causes include increased gastrointestinal losses through vomiting and diarrhoea and gastrointestinal fistulae. Conn's syndrome, Cushing's syndrome and steroid use also cause hypokalaemia, as can alkalosis.

Serum K^+ below 2.5 mmol/L is likely to produce cardiac dysrhythmias, especially in patients taking digoxin. ECG changes include prominent U waves, small T waves, prolonged PR segment and depressed ST segment. Treatment involves intravenous K^+ replacement at a rate not greater than 20 mmol per hour. Lesser degrees of hypokalaemia can be treated by oral supplements. Hypokalaemic patients are often deficient in magnesium and this should also be replaced.

Sodium (135–145 mmol/L)

Hyponatraemia (low serum sodium; Na^+) has a variety of causes (Table 1). Identifying the aetiology requires careful assessment of fluid balance. There may be excess sodium loss via the kidneys, skin or GI tract. Alternatively there may be an excess of water. Endocrine problems such as Addison's disease should be considered. Severe hyponatraemia <125 mmol/L is an emergency. Symptoms include weakness, nausea, headache and seizures.

Treatment depends upon the underlying cause. Chronic hyponatraemia must be corrected cautiously to avoid central pontine myelinolysis (maximum rise of 15 mmol/L daily). Acute hyponatraemia can be treated with intravenous 0.9% NaCl and even hypertonic saline in the case of ongoing seizures. The syndrome of inappropriate antidiuretic hormone secretion (SIADH) requires fluid restriction, treatment of the underlying cause and occasionally demeclocycline.

Hypernatraemia (Na^+ >155 mmol/L) usually reflects H_2O loss in excess of Na^+ loss. Serious hypernatraemia can cause seizures. Patients are usually dehydrated; causes include:

- osmotic diuresis (e.g. hyperosmolar states)
- diarrhoea and vomiting
- diabetes insipidus (low urinary osmolarity)
- excessive saline administration
- hyperaldosteronism, e.g. Conn's syndrome.

Management involves identifying and treating the underlying cause. Fluid administration is often required, including the use of half normal saline (0.45%) or even normal saline (0.9%), which in hypernatraemia is often hypo-osmolar in comparison to the patient's serum.

Calcium

The total serum calcium has a range of 2.2–2.6 mmol/L, and the ionized calcium is 1.1–1.4 mmol/L. The total calcium varies with the serum albumin such that a low total calcium may reflect hypoalbuminaemia rather than true hypocalcaemia. Clinical decisions should be based upon either a corrected total value or the ionized calcium.

Hypercalcaemia is commonly caused by malignant disease or primary hyperparathyroidism. Other causes include sarcoidosis, medications and endocrine problems (thyrotoxicosis). Most patients are asymptomatic, but may present with 'stones, bones, groans and psychic moans' (renal stones, pain, weakness, constipation and depression). Patients have an increased risk of cardiac arrest (there may be a shortened QT interval on the ECG). Initial treatment consists of rehydration with intravenous fluids, followed by a bisphosphonate or loop diuretic.

Hypocalcaemia may be caused by vitamin D deficiency, hypoparathyroidism, thyroid surgery,

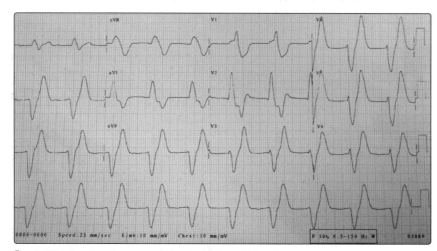

Fig. 1 **ECG showing changes associated with hyperkalaemia.**

Table 1 **Classification of hyponatraemia**			
Oedematous patient	**Euvolaemic patient**	**Dehydrated patient, urinary Na over 20 mmol/L, i.e. renal loss of Na**	**Dehydrated patient with low urinary Na, i.e. Na loss from other site**
Cardiac failure	SIADH (low urine osmolarity)	Osmotic diuresis, i.e. ↑ urea or glucose	Diarrhoea and vomiting
Renal failure	Hypothyroidism	Diuretics, e.g. thiazides	Bowel obstruction
Hepatic cirrhosis	Psychogenic polydipsia	Diuretic phase of renal failure	GI fistulae
Nephrotic syndrome		Addison's disease	Heat stroke
			Burns

pancreatitis or renal failure. Patients may complain of perioral paraesthesia (tingling) and may have signs of neuromuscular excitability and tetany. Treatment involves calcium replacement by intravenous injection of one or two ampoules of 10% calcium gluconate or chloride. Vitamin D supplementation should be considered.

Magnesium (0.70–1 mmol/L)
Hypomagnesaemia may result from an inadequate intake of magnesium, chronic diarrhoea, malabsorption, alcoholism or diuretic use. It is common in hospitalized patients, especially in intensive care units. Important problems include weakness, muscle cramps, cardiac arrhythmias and occasionally seizures. Treatment consists of intravenous or oral replacement. Always consider giving magnesium in any patient with malnutrition or alcoholism who presents with a tachyarrhythmia.

Endocrine emergencies

Thyroid
Thyroid emergencies include myxoedema coma (severe hypothyroidism) and thyrotoxic storm (severe hyperthyroidism). Both are life-threatening emergencies which require prompt recognition and expert management. Thyroid function test results are rarely immediately available.

Severe **hypothyroidism** should be suspected in any patient who presents with hypothermia, diminished reflexes or bradycardia. Cardiac failure and seizure activity may also be present. Most patients are over 65 years of age and mortality is high. Precipitants include infection (pneumonia), stroke, MI, GI bleed, heart failure, trauma or sedative drugs. The diagnosis is clinical, with confirmation by a raised thyroid-stimulating hormone (TSH) and a low serum tri-iodothyronine (T3) or thyroxine (T4). Emergency management includes airway and ventilator support, intravenous normal

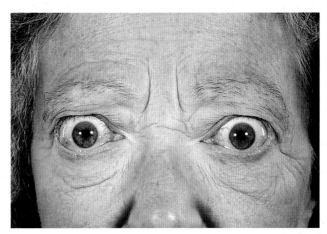

Fig. 2 **Exophthalmos as seen in Graves' disease.**

saline, but with a restricted daily amount, since patients are often water intoxicated. Gradually rewarm the patient and identify any associated adrenal or pituitary failure. Treat infection if suspected. Specifically, give intravenous hydrocortisone and T4 (or T3 (Tertroxin) by nasogastric tube).

The patient presenting with severe **hyperthyroidism** may be agitated, tachycardic, and may have a thyroid bruit. Other problems include tremor, diarrhoea, tachyarrhythmias, weight loss and anxiety. Associated problems include periodic paralysis (look for hypokalaemia) and exophthalmos seen in Graves' disease (Fig. 2). Diagnosis in the emergency department is clinical, confirmed by a low serum TSH. Emergency treatment includes supportive treatment, as well as administration of a thyrostatic drug (carbimazole or propylthiouracil) and a beta-adrenergic antagonist (propranolol or metoprolol).

Adrenal
Hypoadrenalism should be suspected in any patient with known Addison's disease, or any patient taking oral steroid therapy who presents with hypotension or shock with hyponatraemia. Emergency management of such a suspected Addisonian crisis should follow standard ABC assessment and

resuscitation including administration of intravenous fluids. A blood sample should be taken for adrenocorticotrophic hormone (ACTH) and cortisol levels, followed by administration of intravenous corticosteroids. Check for hypoglycaemia and treat with intravenous glucose if necessary.

Rarely, patients may present with a hypertensive crisis caused by a **phaeochromocytoma** (an adrenal medullary tumour). Diagnosis is by measurement of raised urine or plasma concentrations of catecholamines. Management of severe hypertension is covered in the 'Aortic, vascular and hypertensive emergencies' chapter.

Key points
- With all acute electrolyte abnormalities initiate immediate treatment, but always consider the underlying cause.
- Hyperkalaemia is a medical emergency – protect the heart with early administration of calcium (chloride or gluconate).
- Do not correct hyponatraemia too rapidly unless patient is obtunded or seizing, in which case rapid correction is necessary.
- Diagnosis of endocrine emergencies requires a high index of suspicion and careful clinical assessment.

Anaemia and bleeding disorders

Anaemia, a deficiency of haemoglobin, is the most common disorder of the blood. An initial indication of the underlying aetiology may be evident from emergency blood tests: haematocrit, red blood cell size and haemoglobin concentration, the platelet and differential white cell count and the serum bilirubin should also be noted. The three main classes of anaemia include blood loss such as acute haemorrhage (normocytic normochromic) or chronic loss (microcytic hypochromic); blood cell destruction (haemolysis – raised bilirubin); or ineffective production (often with a macrocytic picture). Asymptomatic anaemia detected in the emergency department should be noted and communicated to the patient and their primary care provider or admitting team. Symptomatic anaemia should be investigated and treated more urgently.

Sickle cell disease

Sickle cell anaemia is a haemoglobinopathy affecting people of African origin. Sickle cell syndromes are a number of related conditions resulting from the inherited presence of abnormal haemoglobin, haemoglobin S (HbS). Patients may present to the emergency department in crisis, of which there are three types:

1. vaso-occlusive crisis
2. sequestration crisis
3. haemolytic anaemia.

If deoxygenated, the HbS will develop a characteristic sickle shape. This deoxygenated HbS then polymerizes to form plugs that occlude the microcirculation. This process is responsible for the vaso-occlusive crisis which manifests with musculoskeletal pain of varying severity. Patients are generally aware of their sickle status and will have experienced similar previous episodes. Commonly affected areas are the hips, shoulders and back. Vaso-occlusive episodes are triggered by minor illness or cold, and are self-limiting. Treatment involves adequate analgesia (often intravenous opiates are required), oxygen and rehydration (intravenous if necessary).

Sequestration crisis results from sequestration of the sickle HbS within a specific organ, either the spleen (splenic sequestration) or the lungs (acute chest syndrome). These generally occur in children and severe sequestration can lead to hypovolaemic shock. Children may present in crisis as the first presentation of the disease. Acute chest syndrome is most commonly seen in children under the age of 2 years. The child presents with fever and respiratory symptoms.

With haemolytic anaemia the patient presents with jaundice and signs of severe anaemia (pallor, shortness of breath). This can be precipitated by drugs (aspirin), infections (parvovirus) and foods (fava beans). Treatment for both haemolytic anaemia and sequestration involves analgesia, oxygen, rehydration and transfusion; either straight or exchange transfusion.

Other important emergency conditions seen in sickle cell disease include priapism (see 'Male genital problems' chapter) and osteomyelitis (see 'Non-traumatic musculoskeletal emergencies' chapter).

Bleeding disorders

Haemophilia

Haemophilia A is deficiency of factor VIII and haemophilia B is deficiency of factor IX. The presentation of emergency complications is identical. Patients with haemophilia are generally aware of their condition. When a haemophiliac presents to the emergency department always consider consultation with the on-call haematologist no matter how seemingly trivial the presentation may appear as the patient may require factor VIII replacement (or IX if haemophilia B). Bleeding is the most common complication, often occurring spontaneously into a joint.

Von Willebrand's disease

This is the commonest inherited bleeding disorder and many people are unaware of their status. Approximately 1% of the population will have deficiency of their Von Willebrand factor (VWF), which has two functions: to promote platelet adhesion and to transport factor VIII. Von Willebrand's disease represents a range of conditions with a range of severity of bleeding. In its most severe form, there is spontaneous bleeding and bruising. Common sites for bleeding include the gums and nose. In a patient presenting with apparently excessive bleeding, take a careful history for previous episodes of excessive bleeding after a laceration or dental extraction. Ask about spontaneous bruising and repeated epistaxis. The full blood count will be normal as will the prothrombin time (extrinsic pathway). The activated partial thromboplastin time (APTT) will be prolonged (intrinsic pathway) and in anyone with a slightly prolonged APTT consideration needs to be given to the possibility of a milder form of Von Willebrand's disease. Such patients will require further testing and referral to a haematologist. In mild cases bleeding can easily be controlled and is self-limiting. Tranexamic acid, an anti-fibrinolytic, can be helpful. In bleeding with more severe disease, desmopressin, a synthetic drug that mimics antidiuretic hormone, is also used. Desmopressin mobilizes factor VIII and is administered either intranasally or intravenously.

Thrombocytopenia

This is a blood platelet count of less than 150×10^9/L. There are several causes (Table 1), and patients present with bleeding, purpura and petechiae. In children, alternative diagnoses must be considered (Table 2). Spontaneous bleeding occurs only with a very low platelet count (less than 20×10^9/L). Common sites are the gums and conjunctiva, and there may be epistaxis and menorrhagia. Purpura are red or purple areas of skin discoloration caused by bleeding. Small spots are called petechiae and larger ones ecchymoses (Fig. 1).

Table 1 **Causes of thrombocytopenia**	
Reason for thrombocytopenia	**Most common causes**
Production of platelet failure	Leukaemia, drugs (heparin)
Shortened lifespan of platelets	Idiopathic thrombocytopenia (ITP)
Sequestration of platelets	Hypersplenism
Dilutional effect	Massive transfusion

Table 2 Important causes of unexplained bruising or petechiae to consider in a child

- Non-accidental injury
- Leukaemia
- Idiopathic thrombocytopenia
- Henoch–Schönlein purpura
- Meningococcal disease

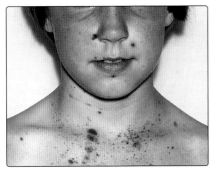

Fig. 1 **Child with idiopathic thrombocytopenia.** Note both the purpura and the petechiae.

Massive transfusion

Massive transfusion is defined as the replacement of one blood volume (equivalent to 10 units of blood) in any 24-hour period, or half of the blood volume (five units of blood) in any 4-hour period. The principal problems with a massive transfusion are:

- Depletion of coagulation factors. In stored blood the clotting factors are of a poorer quality and quantity. Anticipate the need for early administration of fresh frozen plasma (FFP contains all clotting factors) and cryoprecipitate (contains fibrinogen).
- Platelet depletion. Again stored blood is inevitably depleted of platelets.
- Citrate toxicity. Citrate is used as a preservative for stored blood. Citrate toxicity leads to hypocalcaemia. Ionized calcium levels should be monitored and replaced with calcium chloride when necessary.
- Hypothermia. Where possible use a blood warmer to administer blood products.

Coagulopathy, the dreaded complication of massive transfusion, results from haemodilution, hypothermia, use of unfractionated blood products and disseminated intravascular coagulopathy (DIC):

- Haemodilution, from excessive crystalloid or colloid use.
- Hypothermia (<35°C) slows the activity of the coagulation cascade, reduces the synthesis of coagulation factors, increases fibrinolysis, and affects platelet function.
- Blood components: stored blood is inevitably deficient in clotting factors and platelets.
- DIC: An acquired syndrome secondary to systemic and excessive activation of coagulation.

In trauma patients, tissue trauma, brain injury, shock, tissue anoxia and hypothermia all contribute to DIC. The diagnosis is based on the clinical picture together with an elevated D-dimer, prolonged prothrombin time, thrombocytopenia and reduced fibrinogen.

Recombinant coagulation factor VIIa (rFVIIa) (Novoseven®), is a vitamin K-dependent glycoprotein licensed for treatment of bleeding in haemophilia A and B. It is being increasingly utilized as an adjuvant therapy in managing massive haemorrhage due to trauma.

Anticoagulation problems
Elevated international normalized ratio (INR)

The degree of anticoagulation with warfarin is monitored using the INR. Anticoagulated patients may present with bleeding, or be found to have an elevated INR on testing. Consideration should first be given to the degree of bleeding (if any) and secondarily to the indication for anticoagulation. If bleeding is ongoing, the first priorities are haemorrhage control and resuscitation. In life-threatening haemorrhage the effect of warfarin will need to be reversed; this is achieved using either a prothrombin complex concentrate (Beriplex®) or FFP. The main advantage of a prothrombin complex concentrate is its rapid availability and action. Vitamin K is also administered but this takes several hours to take effect. If there is no active bleeding and the INR is very prolonged then either omitting a dose of warfarin or administration of vitamin K is indicated.

Heparin induced thrombocytopenia (HIT)

This can occur in anyone taking heparin. Increasingly patients are being treated with heparin on an outpatient basis. Patients present with features of thrombocytopenia. It is a well-recognized complication of heparin therapy and treatment involves cessation of heparin.

Intravenous drug users

Deep vein thrombosis is a common complication of intravenous drug use. Problems with venous access and an erratic lifestyle make monitoring of INR difficult. It is often preferable to treat with self-administration of low molecular weight heparin rather than warfarin.

Key points

- The three main classes of anaemia are blood loss, blood cell destruction and ineffective production.
- Treatment of vaso-occlusive sickle cell disease crisis involves analgesia, oxygen and rehydration.
- Massive blood transfusion (greater than one blood volume – 10 units – in an adult) is associated with numerous problems. Ensure administered blood is warmed and give FFP, cryoprecipitate and platelets.

Oncology emergencies

Oncology emergencies normally occur in patients with known malignant disease since often they are associated with either advanced disease or as a complication of treatment. When a patient with known malignancy presents to the emergency department it is important to consider that the presentation may be related to the known malignant disease. Thromboembolic disease is much more common in patients with malignant disease and is often overlooked; consider the possibility of a pulmonary embolus in any patient with malignant disease presenting with shortness of breath (see 'Thromboembolic disease' chapter).

Febrile neutropenia

Neutropenia can result from cytotoxic chemotherapy but may also occur in patients presenting with an acute haematological malignancy. Sepsis in a neutropenic patient is a true time urgent emergency and if the patient fulfils the criteria for neutropenic sepsis (Table 1) then broad-spectrum antibiotics must be administered within 30 minutes of the diagnosis. Choice of antibiotics depends upon local protocol and the patient's renal function, but they must be administered urgently.

Raised intracranial pressure

This can occur in patients with intracerebral malignant disease, either a primary brain malignancy or secondary deposits. Early on, the principal symptoms are headache and vomiting, but as the intracranial pressure increases the consciousness level may become depressed. Fundoscopy is important; the principal findings of raised intracranial pressure are loss of venous pulsations and papilloedema (Fig. 1). A CT scan of the head is usually indicated, to delineate the exact cause of the raised intracranial pressure. The raised pressure may be due to tumour and associated oedema, obstructive hydrocephalus or to another cause such as an intracranial abscess. It may be necessary to get a neurosurgical opinion since either resection or insertion of a shunt (if there is hydrocephalus) may be indicated. Other options include corticosteroids (such as dexamethasone), which may help to reduce oedema, mannitol (an osmotic diuretic) and radiotherapy. Symptom control with adequate analgesia and anti-emetics is essential.

Upper airway obstruction

Patients with a known upper airway malignancy occasionally present with upper airway obstruction, in respiratory distress with stridor. Nebulized adrenaline, intravenous corticosteroids and heliox gas are the main immediate treatment options. Summon expert help immediately, ideally the most experienced anaesthetist and ENT surgeon available. Heliox is a mixed gas containing 21% oxygen and 79% helium. Helium is much less dense than nitrogen so the airway resistance and consequently the work of breathing is reduced. The lighter heliox promotes laminar flow rather than the more turbulent flow of oxygen and nitrogen. It is slightly counter-intuitive giving someone who is hypoxic and struggling to breathe a lower inspired oxygen concentration (commonly the normal response to patients with upper airway obstruction is to give higher and higher inspired oxygen concentrations) but in selected patients with upper airway obstruction from malignant disease the use of heliox can dramatically reduce their work of breathing and make them less hypoxic.

Superior vena cava syndrome

This can be a difficult diagnosis since it tends to occur insidiously. The superior vena cava (SVC) is gradually compressed by an enlarging tumour mass. Patients present with increasing shortness of breath together with facial swelling. On examination there may be a plethoric facial appearance, distended superficial and deep veins in the distribution of the SVC together with swelling of the face, trunk and upper limbs. A chest x-ray and chest CT help to confirm the diagnosis. Treatment involves radiotherapy or insertion of an endovascular stent.

Spinal cord compression (SCC)

Consider this in any patient with malignant disease who presents with back pain. Tumour can spread to the vertebrae by the haematogenous route, direct tumour extension or by direct metastasis of tumour cells via the CSF. The haematogenous route is by far the commonest. Patients at highest risk are those with a malignancy that commonly metastasizes to bone (breast, lung, renal, thyroid and prostate). Pain is the most important symptom. Typically the pain is localized, persistent, severe at night and not relieved by rest. Weakness of the lower limbs may be present. As the compression continues, autonomic symptoms such as constipation, retention of urine or incontinence may develop. Typically these are late symptoms and are normally associated with pain and weakness. Plain x-rays can be helpful but lack sensitivity; up to 15% of bony tumours may be

Table 1 **Definition of neutropenic sepsis**
The patient must be neutropenic (neutrophil count <0.5×10⁹/L) and:
■ The body temperature greater than 38°C on two occasions at least one hour apart in any 12-hour period or greater than 38.5°C on a single occasion
■ Not febrile by the above definition but sepsis is suspected and the patient is either hypotensive (systolic BP <90 mmHg) or there is acute respiratory distress

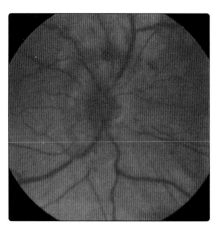

Fig. 1 **Papilloedema on fundoscopy, reddening of the disc and blurring of the disc margins.**

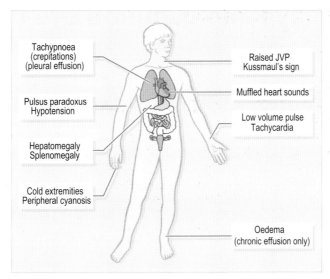

Fig. 2 **Physical signs in cardiac tamponade.**

missed. CT and bone scan can be helpful but the gold standard is MRI since this will also demonstrate direct compression of the cord. Treatment includes adequate analgesia and corticosteroids (dexamethasone). More advanced treatment options include surgical decompression, radiotherapy and chemotherapy in certain chemo-sensitive malignancies.

Hypercalcaemia

This may be the initial presentation of a patient with underlying malignant disease. The diagnosis of hypercalcaemia can be tricky since the symptoms are vague and non-specific. Nausea, vomiting, constipation, lethargy, polyuria and weakness may all occur. In extreme cases of hypercalcaemia there may be alteration of the conscious level with a reduced GCS score. There may be ECG changes

with shortening of the QT interval. Confirmation is by measurement of corrected serum calcium levels. Initial treatment involves rehydration with intravenous normal saline, use of loop diuretics and, if required, bisphosphonates.

Pericardial effusions

The patient may present with chest pain or if tamponade is present with

hypotension. Signs include pulsus paradoxus (elevation of the JVP on inspiration) and quiet heart sounds (Fig. 2). The ECG may show small voltage complexes and electrical alternans (complexes of varying size). The best initial investigation is bedside ultrasound to demonstrate the pericardial effusion. Treatment options include aspiration but a surgical pericardial window is more effective.

Key points

- Ensure adequate analgesia in patients with malignancy.

- All febrile patients undergoing chemotherapy should be considered to be neutropenic until proven otherwise and should receive early appropriate broad-spectrum antibiotics.

- Spinal metastasis and cord compression may be the first symptom of a malignancy.

- Consider cardiac tamponade in cancer patients who present with unexplained cardiopulmonary symptoms.

- Corticosteroids can provide temporary symptomatic relief from tumour-associated oedema.

The acute red eye and common eye trauma

The acute red eye

Most acutely red eyes are caused by pathology in the anterior part of the eye. Some can threaten vision and require prompt diagnosis. Many causes of red eye are easily treated in an emergency department (ED); conjunctivitis is the commonest diagnosis.

Key diagnostic points

A focused but thorough history and examination using a slit-lamp and ophthalmoscope will determine the diagnosis in most cases (Fig. 1). The initial assessment of all patients presenting with an eye problem must include measurement of visual acuity. Anterior eye symptoms include pain (often an indicator of serious pathology), photophobia, watering/tears and discharge. Table 1 lists 'red flag' signs and symptoms. Risk factors for anterior eye pathology include:

Table 1 Red flag symptoms and signs in the red eye

- Pain
- Decreased visual acuity (compared to normal)
- Fixed pupil
- Visible anterior chamber inflammation
- Corneal infiltration or oedema
- Inflammation of the limbus
- Visible ulcer on fluorescein staining

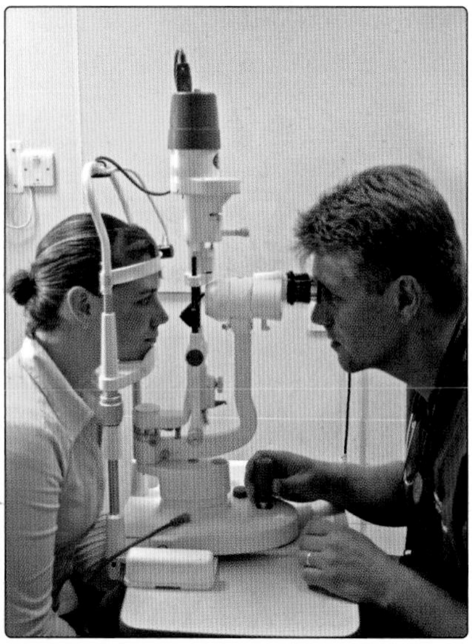

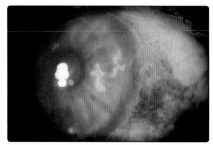

Fig. 1 **Slit lamp examination of the eye.**

- Contact lens wear. Soft contact lens wearers are at high risk for keratitis and ulcers, including acanthamoeba keratitis.
- Past medical conditions associated with eye disease, including inflammatory bowel disease, ankylosing spondylitis, and Reiter's syndrome.

Vision. Measure visual acuity both uncorrected and corrected (if patient normally wears glasses; use a pinhole if prescription glasses are unavailable). Many patients have not had their visual acuity checked for many years; a surprising number of people function very well with less than 6/6 vision.

Lids. Look for swelling, discharge or blepharospasm. Examination of the eye may be aided by resolving the blepharospasm. If topical anaesthesia with an ophthalmic preparation of local anaesthetic is not successful, mydriatics such as cyclopentolate often provide relief.

Conjunctiva/Sclera. Look for redness and inflammation of the limbus.

Cornea. Identify any clouding (oedema). Instil fluorescein stain and check for uptake patterns using cobalt blue light (on slit lamp). Small dot-like uptake of fluorescein indicates keratitis.

Also examine for reactivity and equality of **pupils** and look for cells and flare in the **anterior chamber**.

Serious causes of an acute red eye

Acute iritis

This causes pain, photophobia and blurred vision sometimes with previous similar episodes. Signs on examination are inflammation of the limbus, keratic precipitates (KPs), cells and flare in the anterior chamber. The pupil is often fixed and small due to adhesions between iris and lens (posterior synechiae). ED management involves analgesia, administration of a mydriatic, such as cyclopentolate, and referral to the ophthalmology team.

Corneal ulcers

These are common in contact lens wearers. Symptoms include pain and watering. Examination may reveal white localized inflammatory infiltrates of the cornea. If seen before fluorescein staining, this indicates a bacterial or acanthamoebic ulcer rather than simple corneal abrasion. Herpetic ulcers show a classical branching (dendritic) pattern with fluorescein staining (Fig. 2). All non-traumatic corneal ulcers will require ophthalmology review; antibacterial or antiviral agents may be indicated.

Acute glaucoma

The main symptoms are ocular pain or headache. Other symptoms include vomiting, nausea and decreased vision. The eye is red or pink with an oedematous cornea, decreased visual acuity, and a fixed/mid-dilated pupil (Fig. 3). Acute glaucoma is caused by closure of the angle of drainage of the anterior chamber and can be a complication of other pathologies, especially anterior uveitis. All patients with suspected raised intraocular pressure require applanation tonometry (normal intraocular pressure is 12–20 mmHg). ED management includes analgesia, administration of a miotic agent (such as pilocarpine), intravenous acetazolamide and urgent referral to ophthalmology.

Scleritis

History is of a severe, 'boring' pain often with a background of rheumatoid arthritis. Examination shows inflammation of the sclera that is a deeper red than in episcleritis. Patients with suspected scleritis will require ophthalmology review to decide on use of topical steroids.

Fig. 2 **Dendritic ulcer.**

Common conditions

Conjunctivitis

Symptoms include watering, sticky discharge, and a gritty sensation. Bacterial infection is usually marked by discharge or pus, redness and an inflamed conjunctiva. ED management involves administration of simple broad-spectrum antibacterial ointment or drops. Viral conjunctivitis may be similar to bacterial, but usually with less discharge and a poor or no response to antibiotics. Allergic conjunctivitis may follow exposure to known allergens. Examination will show white discharge, with a typical cobblestone appearance of the subtarsal conjunctiva or oedema of scleral conjunctiva (chemosis), which may be alarming. Allergic conjunctivitis should be treated with cromoglicate.

Episcleritis

History is of mild discomfort. Examination typically reveals a patch of pink inflammation, minimal watering or discharge. This tends to occur more frequently in women and may be associated with connective tissue or autoimmune diseases. Ophthalmology review is indicated to assess need for steroids.

> ### Paediatric considerations
>
> Infants presenting with conjunctivitis under the age of 6 weeks are likely to have chlamydial or gonococcal infection. The eye should be swabbed and the mother advised to attend a local genitourinary medicine service.

Common eye trauma

One of the commonest presentations to the ED is corneal abrasion or a suspected foreign body. The history is often of having felt something 'go into' the eye with subsequent pain, lacrimation and frequently decreased visual acuity. Determine if there is a history of high velocity impact with potential for penetration of the cornea or sclera. In such cases, orbital x-rays or CT may be required. Always document the visual acuity and seek advice if concerned.

Subconjunctival haemorrhage

The spread of blood under the conjunctiva can look serious; however, this condition is usually insignificant. Check the blood pressure, as this can be a manifestation of hypertension. Patients are often alarmed and require reassurance.

Corneal abrasion

Examine for an abrasion by using fluorescein drops and cobalt blue light. Multiple punctate abrasions can be caused by exposure to UV light. This occurs in welders where adequate eye protection was not worn and is known as 'arc eye'. Treatment is with analgesia and antibiotic drops or ointment for 5 to 7 days.

Corneal foreign bodies

Small foreign bodies may lodge on the cornea (Fig. 4). Occasionally the foreign body can hide under the tarsal plate. Always evert the upper lid and examine carefully. Most can be removed carefully using the tip of a hypodermic needle under magnification with a slit lamp. Always keep the bevel parallel to the surface to avoid puncture. Treatment is otherwise the same as for an abrasion.

Chemical burns

The eyes can be irritated by many chemicals. Serious injury can be caused by acids and alkalis, with alkalis being more dangerous as they can penetrate further. Immediate and continued irrigation with copious amounts of water is the initial treatment.

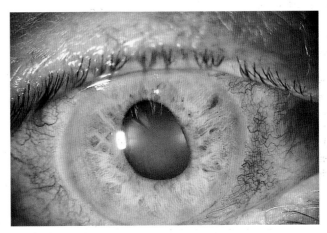

Fig. 3 **Acute angle closure glaucoma.**

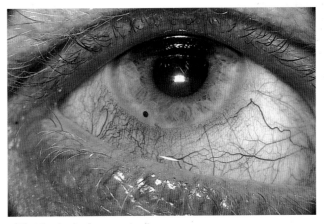

Fig. 4 **Corneal foreign body.**

> ### Key points
>
> - Look for red flag signs and symptoms.
> - Always check visual acuity.
> - Always use fluorescein stain when examining the cornea.
> - Always consider the more serious causes of the acute red eye.
> - If in any doubt, consult with an ophthalmologist.

Acute loss of vision

Sudden loss of vision is an uncommon but alarming event. The important management principles are to recognize the underlying pathology and save any residual eyesight in the affected or unaffected eye.

Traumatic loss of vision

Although rare, complete loss of vision can be caused by traumatic retinal detachment or penetrating eye injuries. Both of these are emergencies and require urgent referral to an ophthalmologist. Examination of the eye is essential in all cases of facial injury, especially if there is significant periorbital bruising. Penetrating injuries causing damage to the uvea may result in a sympathetic ophthalmitis in the other eye. This may require steroids or even surgical removal of the damaged globe. Emergency department treatment for a penetrating eye injury includes analgesia, an anti-emetic and a hard cover to prevent further herniation of eye contents.

Retinal detachment may cause visual loss of all or any part of the visual field (Fig. 1). Complete visual loss occurs when the macula is involved and implies a poor prognosis. When there is partial visual loss, it is essential to diagnose and treat the detachment early to prevent loss of central vision.

Atraumatic loss of vision

Most causes of visual loss are painless and non-traumatic. A few key questions can help narrow the differential diagnosis:

Sudden versus gradual

Sudden loss of vision is usually due to vascular or neurological pathologies, developing over seconds to minutes. Gradual visual loss in one eye is usually due to choroiditis or a progressive retinal detachment. The patient may not be aware of minor visual loss until central vision is affected and then present with 'acute' loss of vision. Gradual, bilateral vision loss is likely to be due to cataracts, senile macular degeneration, glaucoma or diabetic retinopathy.

Complete versus incomplete

Acute loss may involve the whole vision, often as a sudden blackness or greying of the vision, or involve only a portion, half or quadrant, of the vision. The pattern of loss often helps determine the cause.

Generally, where loss of vision is sudden and complete, the cause is more likely to be a vascular problem in the eye (occlusion of vessels or haemorrhage) as opposed to neurological causes (Table 1).

Table 1 **Vascular and neurological causes of sudden visual loss**	
Vascular	**Neurological**
Vitreous bleed	TIA/amaurosis fugax
Branch/central retinal artery occlusion	Cerebrovascular accident
Branch/central retinal vein occlusion	Optic neuritis
Giant cell arteritis	

Exceptions to this are optic neuritis and amaurosis fugax. Amaurosis fugax is a transient loss of vision with full recovery and should be treated as a transient ischaemic attack (TIA).

For partial loss of vision it is important to demarcate the exact portion of the visual field affected. Where the retinal vessels are involved, there tends to be horizontal demarcation. This reflects the branches supplying the retina. Remembering that the image is inverted as it passes the lens, a thromboembolism of the artery to the top half of the retina, for example, causes loss of the lower half of the visual field.

Neurological problems, arising in the visual tract will cause vertical demarcation of visual loss. The exact location of a lesion in the tract will determine the exact pattern of loss (Fig. 2). A patient may complain of only unilateral loss of vision, but when visual fields are examined there may be a hemianopia affecting both eyes.

Neurological problems

A problem in the optic nerve will cause loss of vision in one eye and loss of ipsilateral direct and contralateral consensual pupillary constriction. This can cause a relative afferent pupillary defect (RAPD); i.e. shine light in the 'good' eye and both pupils constrict, shine light in the 'bad' eye and that pupil either dilates or fails to constrict. The third nerve carries efferent fibres (sympathetic and parasympathetic) to the eye; pathology in these nerves will cause ipsilateral loss of direct and consensual reflex.

Fibres in the optic nerve carrying impulses from the nasal side of the eye (temporal vision) cross the midline just above the pituitary gland (optic chiasm). Swelling of the optic chiasm causes loss of the temporal vision in both eyes, 'bitemporal hemianopia'. The optic pathway then passes to the optic cortex of the occipital lobe. Interruptions to these neurons will cause hemianopia of either left or right side of vision (Fig. 2).

The nerves of the optic tract may be affected by various pathologies. The commonest is acute vascular occlusion

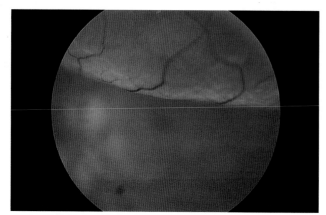

Fig. 1 **Retinal detachment.**

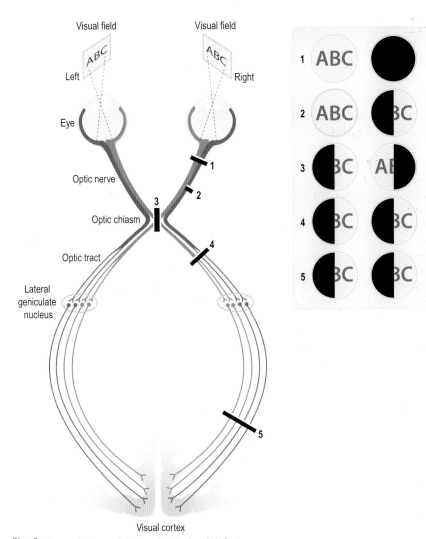

Fig. 2 **The optic tract with associated visual defects.**

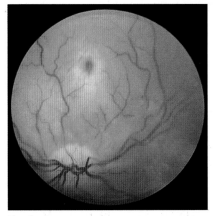

Fig. 3 **Cherry red spot in central retinal artery occlusion.**

It usually leads to a pale area of retina on fundoscopy with a 'cherry red' spot at the macula (Fig. 3). Sometimes an embolus may be visible as a gap in a branch of the retinal artery.

Occlusion of the retinal vein presents in a similar way but is more common than arterial occlusion. Examination often reveals large flame haemorrhages and yellow exudates over the affected retina ('blood and thunder' or sunset-like). There is no definitive treatment and long-term outcomes are variable.

Vitreous haemorrhages are associated with diabetic retinopathy, hypertension or bleeding disorders and if large enough can cause vision loss with an absent red reflex. The episode of vision loss may be preceded by an increase in vitreous floaters. Most vitreous haemorrhages, even if large, resolve spontaneously and treatment is directed at the underlying cause.

due to thrombus or embolus; this is more common with underlying hypertension, cardiac emboli, carotid artery dissection or vasculitis (including giant cell arteritis).

Optic neuritis is associated with demyelinating disorders and leads to degrees of visual loss ranging from mild blurring and loss of red vision to complete visual loss. Signs include swelling of the optic nerve head (although this may be absent in retrobulbar neuritis), painful eye movements, or a relative afferent pupillary defect. In young people recovery is usual, although it may be the first presentation of multiple sclerosis.

Vascular problems

Most vascular conditions causing sudden loss of vision are associated with degenerative diseases such as vasculopathy, diabetes or arteritis.

Retinal artery occlusion can present with loss of entire vision if the central retinal artery is occluded (CRAO) or a partial visual loss if a branch is occluded (BRAO).

Key points

■ Some cases of gradual vision loss may present suddenly when central vision becomes affected.

■ The pattern of partial vision loss on examination may indicate the likely diagnosis.

■ Prompt diagnosis can save further visual loss.

Obstetrics and gynaecology

Gynaecological emergencies

Always perform a urine or serum βHCG, as pregnancy will alter the differential diagnosis.

Lower abdominal pain

Pointers towards a possible gynaecological cause include: sudden onset of severe colicky pain with vomiting (ovarian torsion); vaginal discharge, a cyclical pattern to symptoms, vaginal bleeding or a missed menstrual period. Gynaecological conditions causing lower abdominal pain include ectopic pregnancy, torsion of the ovary, dysmenorrhoea, endometriosis, rupture of a corpus luteal cyst, mittelschmerz pain and pelvic inflammatory disease (PID) (see 'Acute abdominal pain' chapter).

Vaginal bleeding

A small number of women with vaginal bleeding will present in a hypotensive state either due to extensive blood loss (hypovolaemic shock) or very occasionally due to clots or products of conception in the cervical os (cervical vasovagal shock). Resuscitation and prompt removal of clots from the cervical os are required.

Pregnancy (intrauterine or ectopic) should always be excluded, even if there has been no apparent missed period. Always check the βHCG. Serum βHCG levels rise rapidly, giving a positive test within days. Be aware of false negatives with urine βHCG and perform a serum assay if clinical suspicion of pregnancy is high.

In pregnancy, causes of vaginal bleeding include miscarriage and ectopic pregnancy. In the non-pregnant patient, vaginal bleeding may be due to uterine leiomyomas (fibroids), endometriosis, PID, trauma, breakthrough bleeding on the oral contraceptive pill (OCP) or vaginal/cervical lesions such as polyps, erosions or carcinoma.

Miscarriage

This is fetal loss before viability (24 weeks gestation in the UK; Fig. 1). Bleeding is usual together with crampy, bilateral abdominal pain similar to that of a period. During the examination, assess the uterine size and the state of the cervical os. Abdominal tenderness is unusual and

if present raises suspicion of an ectopic pregnancy. Management is expectant, with early follow-up and ultrasound scanning. Check the rhesus status of all women with bleeding in early pregnancy and administer anti-D immunoglobulin if appropriate.

Ectopic pregnancy

Ectopic pregnancies are life-threatening emergencies since they invariably rupture and bleed, often catastrophically (Fig. 2). The classical presentation is of abdominal pain, vaginal bleeding and shock. Risk factors include IVF, previous ectopic pregnancy, tubal surgery, PID and unilateral pain. The diagnosis is often made by noting the **absence** of an intrauterine fetal pole on ultrasound in a patient with a positive pregnancy test. Management involves appropriate resuscitation, cross-match and immediate referral to the gynaecology team.

Emergency contraception

To decrease the chance of conception after unprotected intercourse, levonorgestrel may be given within the first 72 hours. It is important to refer to the family planning clinic for further follow-up and discuss the possibilities of sexually transmitted infection (STI).

Trauma to the genital tract

Patients may present after accidental or non-accidental injury (see 'Violence' chapter) to the genital area. Haematomas and small lacerations can often be treated conservatively. Penetrating injury should prompt assessment of the abdomen for signs of peritonism.

Obstetric emergencies

Always remember that there are two patients, the mother and the fetus. If circulatory compromise is present, tilt the mother to the left or manually displace the uterus to prevent aorto-caval compression syndrome (compression of the aorta and inferior vena cava (IVC) by the gravid uterus when supine causing a reduction in IVC filling and subsequently hypotension).

Placental abruption

Abruption of the placenta occurs when it separates from its bed in the uterine

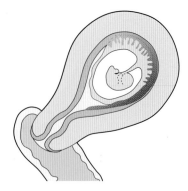
Threatened miscarriage

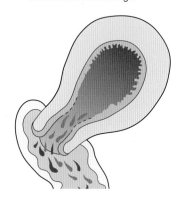
Incomplete miscarriage

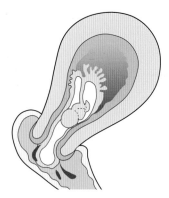
Inevitable miscarriage

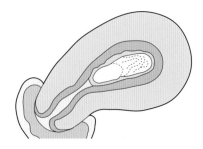
Missed miscarriage

Fig. 1 **Different types of miscarriage.**

cavity. This can be caused by bleeding from a malformed vessel or as a result of blunt abdominal trauma. Abruption, a clinical diagnosis, can cause death of

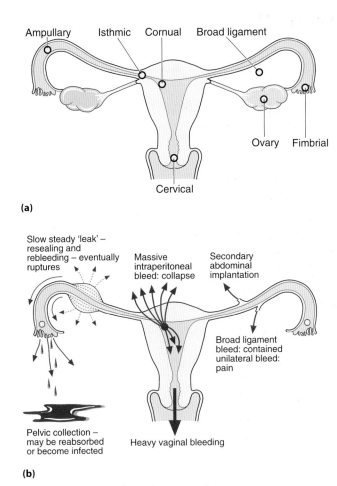

(a)

(b)

Fig. 2 **Sites (a) and sequelae (b) of ectopic pregnancies.**

the fetus and is life-threatening to the mother. Symptoms include abdominal pain, vaginal bleeding, and symptoms of shock more severe than the visualized blood loss. On examination the mother may be shocked, have a tender hard abdomen and uterus, fetal parts may be difficult to feel and the fetal heartbeat may be absent or abnormal. If suspected, resuscitate, urgently involve the obstetric team, cross-match blood and administer analgesia.

Placenta praeviae

Occasionally the placenta may lie in the lower part of the uterus. The stretching and thinning of the lower segment may result in shearing of some placental attachments resulting in painless, often recurrent, fresh red vaginal bleeding. On examination the uterus is generally soft and non-tender. It is easy to feel the fetus as the head is high, breech or transverse. If suspected do **not** perform a digital vaginal examination. Management involves resuscitation, admission and vaginal ultrasound.

Postpartum haemorrhage

Primary postpartum haemorrhage is defined as a blood loss of >500 mL measured clinically in the first 24

hours of delivery. Following delivery, up to 300 mL of blood is commonly lost. Resuscitate and manually stimulate the uterus by rubbing up a contraction; this may help since uterine atony is common. Further oxytocics may be required. If the placenta is incomplete, remaining lobules in the uterine cavity may prevent it from contracting down. Examine for trauma to the lower uterus, cervix, or upper vagina.

Secondary postpartum haemorrhage is defined as bleeding after the first 24 hours post delivery. It is often associated with infection, and in the first instance is treated with antibiotics.

Amniotic fluid embolism

This occurs late in the third trimester or during labour. Patients present with shock in the absence of blood loss, collapse while having strong contractions, sudden dyspnoea, and produce frothy sputum. Treatment is supportive with resuscitation, corticosteroids and urgent delivery.

Cord prolapse

This is more likely with twins, polyhydramnios or malpresentation. Displace the presenting part upwards (manually with a hand or retrograde

filling of the bladder). Do not handle the cord itself due to risk of spasm. Call for senior obstetric support and aim for urgent delivery.

Pre-eclampsia and eclampsia

This is a multisystem disorder which is characterized by hypertension, proteinuria and fluid retention. There is intravascular coagulopathy which may lead to diffuse intravascular coagulation, glomerular damage (proteinuria), liver dysfunction (HELLP syndrome – Haemolysis, Elevated Liver function tests, Low Platelets), cardiac failure, pulmonary oedema and seizures. It has a broad range of severity and is unpredictable resulting in rapid deterioration in some patients. The definitive treatment is delivery of the baby but it may occur postpartum.

The management of eclampsia involves resuscitation and administration of intravenous magnesium.

The management of pre-eclampsia involves obtaining intravenous access, checking LFTs, U&Es, FBC and coagulation screen. Monitor blood pressure and aim to reduce it slowly (hydralazine, labetolol or nifedipine); monitor the fetus and involve obstetric team immediately.

Trauma

The management of trauma in pregnancy follows the same principles as that of non-pregnant patients. Avoid aorto-caval compression, institute fetal monitoring and check if anti-D immunoglobulin is indicated. Abruption may be very covert and any pregnant woman in the second or third trimester who sustains blunt abdominal trauma requires obstetric team review and probable admission for observation of both mother and fetus.

Cardiac arrest in pregnancy

The principles of resuscitation in pregnancy are similar to those in a non-pregnant individual. Important additional considerations include early obstetric, neonatal and anaesthetic involvement and optimizing venous return by avoiding aorto-caval compression. Peri-mortem caesarean delivery must be considered, ideally within 4 minutes of maternal cardiac arrest.

Key points

- Always perform a urine or serum βHCG.
- Liaise with the on-call obstetric and gynaecology team, early pregnancy assessment unit (EPAU) and delivery suite as soon as possible.
- Remember both your patients!

Dental emergencies

The commonest dental emergencies presenting to the emergency department are dental pain, dental injury or bleeding. Patients with bleeding have normally recently had a dental extraction.

Although the tooth is often the source of pain it is important to consider non-dental causes for apparent dental pain such as maxillary sinusitis, temporomandibular joint pathology and trigeminal neuralgia.

Dental anatomy

Human teeth are made up of three layers: the hard outer enamel, the core structure composed of dentine, and at the centre the pulp chamber, which contains the neurovascular bundle (Fig. 1).

Dental pain (toothache)

The main causes of toothache are (Fig. 2):

- pulpitis
- apical periodontitis
- pericoronitis.

Pulpitis

Dental caries result in demineralization of the enamel and dentine. Pulpitis develops when the caries begin to impinge on the pulp and neurovascular bundle. Pulpitis may be either reversible or irreversible. Reversible pulpitis is triggered by hot, cold or sweet stimuli and resolves quickly once the stimulus has been removed. Patients usually present to the emergency department when this early stage is ignored and the caries develop further, encroaching on the pulp and progressing to irreversible pulpitis. Irreversible pulpitis causes a throbbing aching pain that may begin spontaneously or persist long after the stimulus has been removed. Definitive treatment is either root canal treatment (removal of the pulp and filling) or dental extraction. The emergency treatment involves analgesia and advice to seek dental treatment within the next few days. Warn the patient that if they fail to seek early dental treatment the pulp may necrose and apical periodontitis ensue.

Apical periodontitis

Apical periodontitis is severe inflammation at the apex of the tooth, presenting with persistent, spontaneous severe pain localized to the tooth. Definitive management is root canal treatment or extraction. Antibiotics are not always necessary unless the patient has features of spreading cellulitis. An apical abscess may develop with a fluctuant buccal or palatal swelling. Regional lymphadenopathy is often present. Once the pus drains, the pain will improve. If a tense localized fluctuant swelling is present, incise and drain the abscess, prescribe antibiotics (amoxicillin or metronidazole) and analgesics, and advise the patient to seek dental treatment within a couple of days. If localized cellulitis is present, as indicated by diffuse tense painful swelling in the surrounding soft tissues, it is important to prescribe antibiotics. If the cellulitis is localized, oral antibiotics are acceptable as long as the patient is systemically well. Occasionally infection may be more severe and, although rare, it may spread into the fascial spaces of the head and neck, with the risk of airway compromise. Infection in the maxillary region may spread to the periorbital region, leading to vision loss and cavernous sinus thrombosis. If a more

Fig. 1 **The structure of a normal tooth.**

Enamel

Dentine

Pulp

Neurovascular bundle

Tooth apices

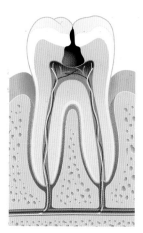 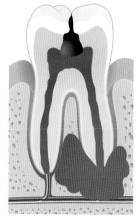 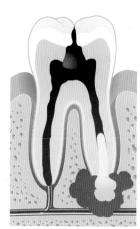

Irreversible pulpitis   Apical periodontitis   Periapical abscess

Fig. 2 **Stages of tooth decay and causes of toothache.**

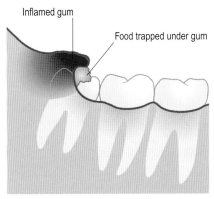

Fig. 3 **Pericoronitis.**

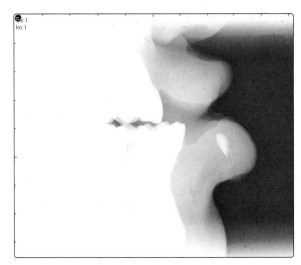

Fig. 4 **Avulsed tooth fragment seen on soft tissue x-ray of lips.**

serious infection is suspected inpatient treatment is needed with intravenous antibiotics and a CT scan to look for any abscesses suitable for surgical drainage. Refer to a maxillofacial surgeon.

Pericoronitis

Pericoronitis is due to inflammation around the crown of a partially erupted tooth, commonly wisdom teeth (Fig. 3). Food debris and bacteria accumulates beneath a gum flap leading to inflammation, pain and tenderness. Patients often complain of pain and have an unpleasant taste in their mouth from pus formed under the flap. Treatment is directed at removing all food debris by brushing regularly and using an antibacterial mouthwash. Symptoms often resolve once the tooth has fully erupted. In recurrent severe cases, a dentist can excise the gum flap or remove the tooth. Once again antibiotics are only indicated in cases with evidence of cellulitis.

Dental trauma

Dental trauma is common; a tooth may fracture, loosen, or be avulsed.

Tooth fractures and loosening

Tooth fractures may involve the enamel, dentine or pulp. Fractures involving the enamel and small amounts of dentine that are not sensitive do not require immediate treatment but should be checked by a dentist. If the fracture involves the dentine, same-day or next-morning dental input is necessary. Ideally fractures of the root require same-day

dental attention. Any tooth fragments should be kept hydrated as they could possibly be reattached. Patients with loosened teeth should be advised to visit a dentist. If a portion of tooth is missing it is important to consider the possibility that it has been inhaled or buried in a lip. Consider the need for a chest or soft tissue x-ray (Fig. 4).

Avulsed teeth

A tooth avulsion is a true dental emergency; a permanent tooth re-implanted within 15 minutes stands over a 90% chance of surviving. Never re-implant deciduous (primary) teeth. If visibly contaminated, rinse the tooth under cold running tap water. Do not rub or touch the root as this compromises the chance of the tooth taking hold. Irrigate the socket to remove the haematoma and place the tooth firmly into the socket. The tooth then needs to be stabilized; arrange urgent dental review. If it is not possible to re-implant the tooth, transport it in a moist environment. The best place is in the patient's own mouth; the buccal sulcus. Alternatively transport it in an isotonic fluid such as milk, saline or contact lens fluid. Prolonged contact with water damages the tooth. If not re-implanted immediately, prescribe antibiotics, check tetanus status and refer as an emergency to a dental surgeon for re-implantation and splinting. Do not

discard the tooth even if it has been transported suboptimally; it may still be used.

Dental bleeding

This normally follows from a recent dental extraction and on occasions can be quite profuse. Stop the bleeding by applying firm pressure, roll up some gauze and place over the socket, asking the patient to bite down onto it. Soaking the gauze in a solution of lidocaine (1%) and adrenaline (epinephrine) (1 in 100 000) may assist haemostasis by vasoconstriction. If bleeding is profuse and prolonged, resuscitate as for any trauma haemorrhagic shock patient and assess ABCs (see 'Initial approach to the trauma patient' chapter). Occasionally the socket will require a suture to achieve haemostasis.

> **Key points**
>
> - In patients with dental pain always consider the need for analgesia and oral antibiotics.
> - Patients with dental infection and systemic features may need to be admitted under the maxillofacial surgeons
> - An avulsed permanent tooth is a true emergency.

Ear, nose and throat, and facial emergencies (1)

Epistaxis

Nose bleeds can be divided into bleeding from the anterior aspect of the nose (Little's area) or posterior aspect of the nose. Important points in the history include details about previous episodes, the quantity of blood lost, duration of bleeding and history of bleeding disorders. A comprehensive medication history is essential, particularly regarding anticoagulant or antiplatelet drugs. Enquire about possible cocaine use.

Anterior bleeds account for 80% of nose bleeds. Pinch the soft part of the nose, sit the patient forward and apply cold to the bridge continuously for 15 minutes (Fig. 1). Spray a combination of local anaesthetic and vasoconstrictor, such as lidocaine and phenylephrine, into the nose. This can reduce the bleeding sufficiently to identify the site of bleeding. If a discrete bleeding point is seen, cauterize it using a silver nitrate stick. Do not cauterize the nose blindly, only cauterize if a discrete bleeding point is identified. If unsuccessful and the bleeding persists pack the anterior nasal cavity. Most commonly this is achieved using a nasal tampon; ribbon gauze is an alternative method. If bleeding continues pack the other nostril to evenly spread the pressure across the septum. This will control most, but not all, nose bleeds. If bilateral anterior packing fails, the bleed is most likely to be posterior. In order to pack the posterior aspect of the nose a special nasal catheter is inserted into the nostril, inflated and pulled gently back to have a tamponade effect. If a specialized catheter is not available, use a urinary catheter. The anterior aspect of the nose can then be packed. It is sensible to involve an ENT surgeon in the management of any patient requiring insertion of a nasal pack. While dealing with the nose bleed, resuscitate the patient by placing a wide-bore intravenous cannula; at the same time take blood for a full blood count, group and save, and check the coagulation profile.

Foreign bodies

The first attempt to remove a foreign body from the nose or ear of a child has the highest chance of success. If you hurt or scare the child they will likely require a general anaesthetic for removal. Customize your extraction method to the personality of the child, parent and foreign body concerned. If it is an insect in the ear it can be killed by drowning it; pour some lidocaine into the ear.

Techniques of removal:

- Irrigation – useful for foreign bodies in the ear.
- Positive pressure techniques – for nasal foreign bodies, ask the patient to blow their nose. If that fails, try a 'magic kiss': ask the parent to block the child's contralateral nostril and blow gently into the mouth.
- Negative pressure techniques – suction is best suited to small round objects.
- Glue – cyanoacrylate, tissue adhesive is good for smooth dry round objects. Place a little on a stick and glue it to the object.
- Surgical instruments – crocodile forceps are perfect for arms of toy soldiers but not good for marbles. Hooks can be pushed past round objects and then withdrawn.

Foreign bodies, commonly coins, may also be swallowed. It is essential to identify the size and shape of the object, and to ensure that it has passed through the lower oesophageal sphincter into the stomach. This can be confirmed on chest x-ray (Fig. 2) for radio-opaque objects. Objects lodged in the oropharynx, upper oesophagus or upper airway require urgent ENT referral.

Sore throats

In the history note the duration of sore throat, previous treatments and whether the pain is unilateral or bilateral. Can the patient swallow food, liquid or saliva?

Examine for peritonsilar redness or swelling and for pus or exudates on the tonsils (tonsillitis or glandular fever). If swelling is present, is it bilateral or unilateral? Is the pharynx red (pharyngitis), are there any white spots (candida) or ulcerated areas? Presence of trismus (spasm of the pterygoid muscles) suggests a possible quinsy. Do a thorough general examination and look for systemic signs of sepsis, such as fever and tachycardia.

The vast majority of sore throats (over 90%) are viral in nature and require only symptomatic treatment. Mild cases of bacterial tonsillitis will also respond to conservative treatment. If the patient is significantly unwell and there are no signs of a viral upper respiratory tract infection consider prescribing antibiotics (Fig. 3).

Patients that have difficulty swallowing may benefit from corticosteroids. Patients with complete dysphagia, including an inability to swallow saliva, will require admission for intravenous fluids and antibiotics.

Quinsy is a localized collection of pus above the tonsil. This may require drainage (by either aspiration or incision), intravenous antibiotics, and fluids.

Consider non-infective causes of sore throat such as gastro-oesophageal

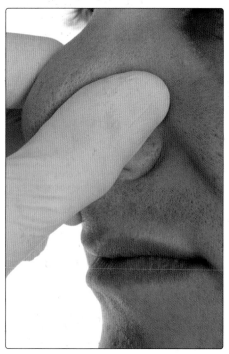

Fig. 1 **Pinch the soft part of the nose continuously for 15 minutes,** apply cold to the bridge of the nose.

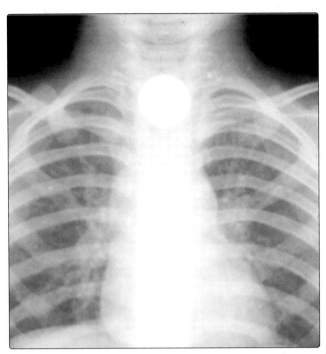

Fig. 2 **Chest x-ray showing a coin lodged in the upper oesophagus.**

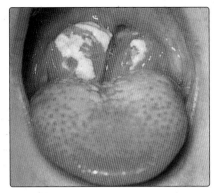

Fig. 3 **Acute tonsillitis.**

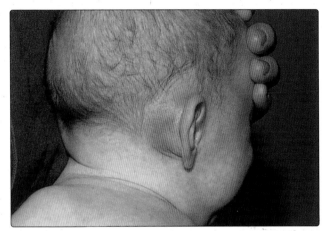

Fig. 4 **Child with acute otitis media progressed to mastoiditis.**

reflux disease and occupational irritants; heavy smokers may develop a chronic pharyngitis.

Ear pain

In taking the history ask about previous surgery, recent ear syringing, cotton bud use, recent swimming, diving, or flying, associated hearing loss and whether there is any discharge.

Examine for scars and the appearance of the external auditory canal and tympanic membrane, and palpate the neck for lymph nodes. Note if tugging on the pinna or pressure on the tragus causes discomfort (suggestive of otitis externa). Look behind the ear at the mastoid process for swelling or redness and palpate for tenderness (mastoiditis; Fig. 4).

Otitis externa is inflammation, usually infective, of the external auditory canal. It is common in patients with eczematous ear canal skin and patients who use cotton buds. Treat with topical antibiotic and corticosteroid drops.

Furunculosis is an infection of hair follicles and can cause a severe throbbing pain. A red lump, with or without pus, may be visible in the ear canal. Initial treatment is with analgesics; the abscess usually discharges spontaneously.

Otitis media

Acute otitis media is inflammation of the middle ear, most commonly seen in children. There is ear ache, irritability and ear tugging. Examination reveals a bulging tympanic membrane with loss of landmarks and changes in membrane colour; there may be a perforated tympanic membrane with discharge of pus. Otitis media is mostly viral in origin. Acute otitis media is usually a self-limiting illness, resolving in over 80% of patients within 3 days without antibiotic treatment. The mainstay of treatment is analgesia, reassurance and education on the pros and cons of antibiotic treatment. Antibiotics have been shown to reduce the duration of the illness but do not reduce the incidence of complications. Consider antibiotic use in: child under 2 years, patients with systemic symptoms (high temperature, vomiting) and those with local signs of tympanic perforation and discharge of pus.

Mastoiditis is rare and may complicate acute otitis media (Fig. 4). Patients present with severe pain over the mastoid process and are systemically unwell. Early signs include oedema and redness over the mastoid, and oedema of the posterior ear canal wall. Urgent ENT referral is required.

A perforated tympanic membrane may be traumatic or associated with otitis media. Perforations associated with acute otitis media are treated with antibiotics. In traumatic perforations, advise the patient not to put anything in the ear and not to submerge the ear under water. All perforations require review by the patient's GP to ensure that they have healed.

Ramsey Hunt syndrome

Herpes zoster infection of the facial (VII) nerve produces a facial nerve palsy associated with a shingles rash in the ear and often on the soft palate together with loss of taste on the anterior two-thirds of the tongue. Treatment is with antiviral medication such as aciclovir.

Facial pain

Common causes of facial pain include: sinusitis and dental abscesses (see 'Dental emergencies' chapter). Sinusitis presents with facial pain, blocked nose, nasal discharge and anosmia (loss of smell). Referred pain may be present to

Ear, nose and throat, and facial emergencies (2)

the teeth and ears. Sinusitis may be viral or bacterial in origin. Treatment consists of simple analgesia/NSAID and antibiotics.

Trigeminal neuralgia presents with paroxysms of severe unilateral pain in the trigeminal nerve distribution lasting only seconds separated by pain-free periods. Spasm of the facial and masticatory muscles may occur during an episode.

Facial weakness

Bell's palsy is a lower motor neuron paralysis of the facial (VII) nerve. It is commonest between the ages of 10 and 40 years. The cause is unknown but may be associated with herpes infections. Pain behind or in front of the ear may precede the weakness by 1 to 2 days. Patients may have loss of taste to the anterior two-thirds of the tongue (sensory component VII nerve) and sensitivity to sound, hyperacusis (VII nerve – motor to stapedius). The paralysis is lower motor neuron and so will involve upper and lower facial weakness.

If associated with a blistering rash typical of herpes zoster, Ramsey Hunt syndrome should be suspected (Fig. 5). Most cases resolve spontaneously within 3 weeks. If a patient with a Bell's palsy presents early in the course of the disease, prednisolone and aciclovir are of benefit.

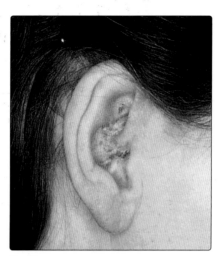

Fig. 5 **Florid case of herpes zoster.**

Difficult noisy breathing/stridor

Epiglottitis

This is a life threatening condition caused by *Haemophilus influenzae* infection of the epiglottis. It is usually seen in 3–7 year olds, but may occur in adults. With Hib vaccination the incidence is decreasing. The onset of symptoms is rapid with high fever and sore throat being the earliest features. The patient may develop stridor and their voice may become muffled or absent. Tachycardia, tachypnoea, swallowing difficulties, and drooling may then ensue. Patients are toxic, apprehensive, and pale; they sit upright, leaning forward with neck extended, mouth open and jaw thrust forward in an attempt to maximize the diameter of the airway. There is usually no cough. Cyanosis, shock, loss of consciousness, and complete airway obstruction may ensue unless intervention by a senior doctor with airway expertise. Do not attempt to examine the throat. Refer immediately to an ENT surgeon. Give oxygen but do not cause distress to the child and allow the patient to maintain their upright posture.

See 'Cough and breathlessness in children' chapter for management of croup; and 'Oncology emergencies' chapter for compressive airway obstruction.

Vertigo

(See 'Vertigo and giddiness' chapter.)

> ### Key points
> - Most ENT emergencies can be dealt with in the emergency department with resuscitation and first aid measures.
> - If no obvious local cause is found for pain consider referred pain.

Emergency paediatric presentations

It is not the strongest of the species that survive, nor the most intelligent, but the ones most responsive to change

Charles Darwin

Fever and sepsis in children

Fever in infants is a rectal temperature of 38°C or higher. In older children, a rectal temperature of 38.4°C or an oral temperature of 37.8°C is generally considered abnormal. Fever is the most common reason for parents to seek medical attention for their child and there are many serious causes (Table 1). In the vast majority of cases the fever will be due to a benign viral infection. Children older than 3 years often have more specific symptoms and a clear focus may be apparent, but up to 20% of febrile children will lack a clear focus for their temperature. Where there is no focus, approximately 3–5% of children will have an occult bacteraemia. The vast majority of these children will recover spontaneously, but a small number (2–3%) will develop a serious bacterial infection. Other non-infective causes may also induce fever including inflammatory conditions, autoimmune disease, malignancy, drugs and heat stroke.

The key to safe assessment of a febrile child is careful history taking, thorough clinical examination and accurate risk stratification. Generally, the younger the child, the higher the risk of occult bacterial infection.

Important points
The higher the temperature, the more likely there is a serious bacterial infection. The response to antipyretics does not differentiate between viral and bacterial aetiology.

In young children the signs of serious infection may be subtle or atypical. An infant may present with a serious infection without having significant pyrexia. Recent or current antibiotic therapy may obscure clinical signs of sepsis.

A small number of children who are febrile (but otherwise well) may later develop more serious illness. A thorough examination, including all skin areas, tympanic membranes and oropharynx (Fig. 1) is essential for every febrile child.

Antipyretics
Antipyretics may be used to treat obvious discomfort or pain associated with high fever; however, routine use is not recommended. Treating fever does not prevent febrile convulsions. Parents should be advised not to exceed the recommended doses, and not to continue antipyretics for more than 2–3 days without medical review.

If antipyretics are deemed necessary the drugs of choice are paracetamol or ibuprofen. Tepid sponging does not reduce temperature more effectively than antipyretics and is associated with more discomfort and is not recommended.

The management of children with fever should be directed by the level of risk. The traffic light system published by NICE aids risk assessment (see www.nice.org.uk/CG47).

Children with fever without an apparent source with one or more high risk features (Table 2) should have the following investigations performed: a full blood count, blood cultures, CRP and urinalysis.

The following investigations should also be considered in children with 'red' high risk features, as guided by the clinical assessment:

- chest x-ray
- serum electrolytes and blood gases
- lumbar puncture in children of all ages (if not contraindicated).

Table 1 **Specific serious diseases causing fever**

Diagnosis to be considered	Symptoms and signs *along with fever*
Meningococcal disease	Non-blanching rash, particularly with one or more of the following: ill-looking child lesions larger than 2 mm in diameter (purpura) a capillary refill time of ≥3 seconds neck stiffness
Meningitis	Neck stiffness Bulging fontanelle Decreased level of consciousness Convulsive status epilepticus
Herpes simplex encephalitis	Focal neurological signs Focal seizures Decreased level of consciousness
Pneumonia	Tachypnoea Crackles Nasal flaring Chest indrawing Cyanosis Oxygen saturation ≤95%
Urinary tract infection	Vomiting Poor feeding Lethargy Irritability Abdominal pain or tenderness Urinary frequency or dysuria Offensive urine or haematuria
Septic arthritis	Swelling of a limb or joint Not using an extremity Non-weight bearing
Kawasaki disease	Fever for more than 5 days and at least four of the following: bilateral conjunctival injection change in mucous membranes change in the extremities polymorphous rash cervical lymphadenopathy

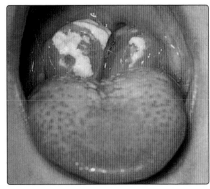

Fig. 1 **Acute bacterial tonsillitis.** Bacterial and viral pharyngeal infections are a common cause of fever in children.

Table 2 'Red flag' features for identifying high likelihood of a serious cause in fever

- Pale/mottled/ashen/blue skin colour
- Reduced skin turgor
- Prolonged capillary refill time
- No response to social cues
- Appears ill to a healthcare professional
- Unable to rouse or if roused does not stay awake
- Weak, high-pitched or continuous cry
- Grunting
- Tachypnoea: respiratory rate >60 breaths/minute
- Moderate or severe chest indrawing
- Age 0–3 months, temperature ≥38°C
- Age 3–6 months, temperature ≥39°C
- Non-blanching rash
- Bulging fontanelle
- Neck stiffness
- Status epilepticus
- Focal neurological signs
- Focal seizures
- Bile-stained vomiting

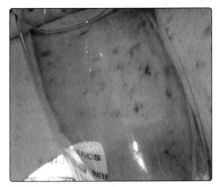

Fig. 2 **Non-blanching rash in meningococcal disease.**

Meningococcal disease

Meningococcal disease in children may present with predominant septicaemia (with shock), meningitis (with raised intracranial pressure) or both. A purpuric or petechial, non-blanching rash is typical (Fig. 2), but the rash may be atypical or absent.

Any child with meningococcal disease, including one who appears non-toxic, may deteriorate rapidly.

Initial management

Always summon senior help. Assess ABCs, look for features of shock or raised intracranial pressure. Give intravenous antibiotics (ceftriaxone) as soon as possible. Intravenous fluid boluses should be initiated (20 mL/kg crystalloid). Even if responding well to fluid boluses and appearing stable, close observation is required since deterioration may be delayed by 4 to 6 hours after presentation. Antibiotic prophylaxis of household and close contacts may be required (rifampicin or ciprofloxacin); seek advice from the Public Health team.

Urinary tract infection

Urinary tract infection (UTI) in the first years of life is common but potentially serious. The diagnosis of UTI should be considered in all febrile infants and young children as well as in all babies who are non-specifically unwell.

A proven UTI is a pure growth of >10⁵ organisms per mL of urine. Common organisms include *E. coli* (80% of UTIs), *Proteus*, staphylococci and *Klebsiella* species.

Diagnosis of urinary tract infection

A reliable urine sample is required to establish the diagnosis. Urine bag samples are unreliable (high false positive rate) and are not recommended. Clean catch samples are more reliable and the preferred method. If samples are required urgently, bladder catheterization or supra-pubic aspiration (SPA) may be considered (the yield from SPA is markedly improved by using pre-procedure ultrasound to confirm a full bladder).

Antibiotic treatment

Antibiotic treatment should start promptly. Awaiting urine culture results in the presence of other positive indicators for UTI should not delay treatment.

Further management

Confirmed UTIs should be followed up for further investigation including renal ultrasound and other renal tract imaging.

Kawasaki disease

Kawasaki disease is a systemic vasculitis which predominantly affects children under 5 years of age, with a peak incidence at 9–11 months. It is characterized by persistent fever (of at least 5 days' duration), swelling of the mouth and lips, bilateral non-purulent conjunctivitis, and acute cervical lymphadenopathy. There is no diagnostic laboratory test. The most serious complication is the formation of coronary artery aneurysms, potentially leading to thrombosis, myocardial infarction and sudden death. (See also 'Rashes in children' chapter.)

Key points

- Febrile infants under 1 month old should be admitted to hospital and treated with antibiotics.

- All febrile children under 3 years old who have toxic manifestations should be admitted to hospital, be fully investigated for sepsis and meningitis, and receive antibiotic treatment.

- The risk of bacterial infection is very low in children over 3 years old who seem well, and follow-up without laboratory tests or treatment is generally adequate.

- Give antibiotics early if meningitis is suspected.

Coma and seizures in children

Coma

Coma is a state of profound unconsciousness from which the child cannot be roused.

The main causes of coma in children include:

- hypoxic brain injury – following respiratory or circulatory failure
- infection (meningitis, encephalitis)
- seizures
- trauma
- poisoning such as carbon monoxide or an ingested substance
- raised intracranial pressure – shunt blockage, intracranial bleeding, brain tumours
- metabolic causes such as hypoglycaemia, renal or hepatic failure, Reye's syndrome.

Emergency assessment

The emergency assessment of the child with altered consciousness involves a primary survey using the ABCDE approach, alongside a focused history and an early bedside blood glucose reading (DEFG – Don't Ever Forget Glucose).

Primary survey

- ABC: Assess and support airway, breathing and circulation.
- D: Assess level of consciousness using the AVPU (Table 1) or Paediatric Glasgow Coma Scale (Table 2). Check eye movements, pupil size and reaction to light; unilateral or bilateral dilation suggests raised intracranial pressure (ICP; Fig. 1). Look for retinal haemorrhages (strongly suspicious of non-accidental injury). The three absolute signs of raised ICP, papilloedema, bulging fontanelle and absence of various pulsation in retinal vessels, are often absent in acutely raised ICP. Look for abnormal posturing and for neck stiffness in a child and full fontanelle in an infant. A noticeable odour may indicate metabolic disorders and poisoning.
- E: Expose and examine head to toe looking for rashes; if purpuric, consider meningitis or non-accidental injury. Fever suggests an infective cause, although its absence does not rule this out.

Key points in the focused history will include enquiry about health and activity over the past 24 hours, infectious contacts, any recent trauma or potential poisoning. A family and travel history may be useful. If there is a vague or inconsistent history, remember to consider non-accidental injury. It is often not possible to ascertain the diagnosis in the first hour of managing a child in a coma.

Initial investigations

Perform blood glucose, U&Es, blood cultures, FBC, renal and liver function tests and arterial blood gases. Consider plasma ammonia if a metabolic cause is suspected.

Emergency management

Ensure the airway is patent. If the child has an AVPU score of P or U, their airway is not protected. Give high-flow oxygen via face-mask with a reservoir if the airway is patent. If not, consider supporting respiration with a bag-valve-mask device or intubation and ventilation. Establish IV access quickly. Give 20 mL/kg rapid bolus of crystalloid if signs of shock are present. If hypoglycaemia is present give an IV bolus of 5 mL/kg of 10% dextrose.

Broad-spectrum antibiotics (ceftriaxone) should be given along with aciclovir if encephalitis suspected. If meningitis cannot be excluded it ought to be treated, as the consequence of missing this diagnosis is disastrous.

If the ICP is suspected of being raised, discuss management with a senior doctor and a neurosurgeon as appropriate.

Options include:

- intubation and ventilatory support (aim for PCO_2 4.0–4.5 kPa)
- nursing the child in 20–30° head-up position (to help cerebral venous drainage)
- mannitol
- if not controlled, dexamethasone may be required.

Seizures

Introduction

Around 3% of all children will have a seizure before the age of 15 years.

Table 1	**AVPU assessment tool**
A (alert)	Patient is alert and conscious
V (verbal)	Patient responds to verbal stimulus
P (pain)	Patient responds to painful stimulus
U (unresponsive)	Patient is unresponsive to any form of stimulus

Table 2	**The Paediatric Glasgow Coma Scale (PGCS)**		
	Infant <1 year	Child 1–4 years	Age 4 to adult
Eyes			
4	Open	Open	Open
3	To voice	To voice	To voice
2	To pain	To pain	To pain
1	No response	No response	No response
Verbal			
5	Coos, babbles	Oriented, speaks, interacts, social	Oriented and alert
4	Irritable cry, consolable	Confused speech, disoriented, consolable	Disoriented
3	Cries persistently to pain	Inappropriate words, inconsolable	Nonsense words
2	Moans to pain	Incomprehensible, agitated	Moans, unintelligible
1	No response	No response	No response
Motor			
6	Normal, spontaneous speech	Normal spontaneous speech	Follows commands
5	Withdraws to touch	Localizes pain	Localizes pain
4	Withdraws to pain	Withdraws to pain	Withdraws to pain
3	Decorticate flexion	Decorticate flexion	Decorticate flexion
2	Decerebrate extension	Decerebrate extension	Decerebrate extension
1	No response	No response	No response

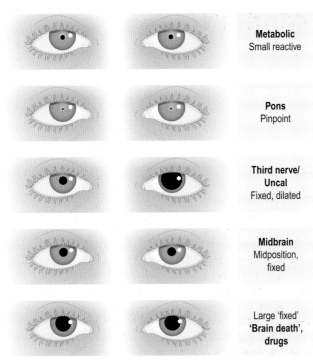

Metabolic
Small reactive

Pons
Pinpoint

**Third nerve/
Uncal**
Fixed, dilated

Midbrain
Midposition,
fixed

Large 'fixed'
'Brain death',
drugs

Fig. 1 **Pupillary changes in coma.**

Diagnosis requires a detailed history, with an eyewitness account if possible. It can be difficult to differentiate seizure activity from other causes of collapse and loss of consciousness.

- A seizure is an involuntary alteration in motor activity, behaviour, sensation or autonomic function. It may be convulsive or non-convulsive.
- A convulsion is involuntary contraction of body muscles.
- Epilepsy is defined as two or more unprovoked, recurrent seizures. Seventy-five per cent of epilepsy is primary (idiopathic); 25% is secondary to another CNS disorder.
- A simple seizure is one with no alteration of consciousness.
- In a complex seizure there is alteration of consciousness.
- Status epilepticus is defined as an epileptic seizure that lasts more than 30 minutes or seizures that occur so frequently that consciousness is not restored between seizures.

Seizures are generally divided into partial (focal) seizures involving a limited brain region, and generalized seizures involving the entire brain and therefore associated with loss of consciousness.

Non-epileptic seizures
These are seizures that are secondary to an underlying cause such as CNS infection (meningitis, encephalitis, cerebral abscess); trauma (head injury, non-accidental injury, post-traumatic intracerebral haemorrhage); metabolic abnormalities (diabetic ketoacidosis, electrolyte disturbances, Reye's syndrome); vascular pathology (non-traumatic intracerebral haemorrhage and stroke, hypertension) and febrile seizures.

Febrile seizures
Around half of all seizures in children are febrile in nature. Simple febrile seizures are benign and are defined as: a single seizure occurring between the ages of 6 months and 6 years in children, with no history of chronic neurological disease, with evidence of fever (temperature >38°C); they are generalized, usually tonic-clonic; are self-limiting, lasting less than 15 minutes, with a full recovery.

Some children may have complex febrile seizures. Complex features include a duration of more than 20 minutes, focality when the seizure occurs on one side of the body and multiplicity, when more than one seizure occurs during a 24-hour period. The significance of the complex features is that of a higher risk for future epilepsy.

Treatment for simple febrile seizures is usually unnecessary. For complex febrile seizures or if in doubt, further investigation should be considered to rule out possible more serious causes such as meningitis.

Assessment
The initial assessment is similar to that of the unconscious child: an ABCDE approach and early bedside assessment of the blood glucose. The primary survey should also note pupil size and response to light, as well as muscle tone. A careful examination for signs of sepsis such as a purpuric rash or fever should be completed.

Management
Treat any underlying cause (such as hypoglycaemia) while supporting ventilation and circulation and terminating any ongoing seizure activity. Benzodiazepines (such as midazolam) are the first line drugs. A repeat dose is administered before proceeding to secondary drugs such as rectal paraldehyde or IV phenytoin. Rapid sequence induction of anaesthesia with thiopental may be required (see Appendix 1, p. 176).

> **Key points**
> - Use the ABCDE approach.
> - Don't Ever Forget Glucose.
> - Diagnosis of the cause of coma is often not possible in the first hour.
> - The absolute signs of raised ICP are often absent in acutely raised ICP.
> - Always consider non-accidental injury as a possible cause.

Cough and breathlessness in children

Introduction

Children presenting to the emergency department (ED) with coughing or breathlessness may have one or more problems involving their upper or lower respiratory tract. These include such varied causes as acute infection, asthma or an inhaled foreign body. The principles of assessment include reassurance alongside an ABC approach.

Cough

An acute episode of cough is defined as a clinical event lasting less than 3 weeks. Chronic cough is described as a cough lasting more than 8 weeks. Young children experience up to 7 to 12 viral upper respiratory tract infections a year, many associated with cough. In 50% of cases, the cough resolves within 10 days, in 90% by 25 days. Causes may be respiratory or non-respiratory (Table 1).

History

A clear history of the quality of the cough is vital in eliciting the cause. Ideally, a cough should be heard rather than purely described. *Bronchiolitis* (wet, fruity cough), *croup* (harsh, barking cough), *Pertussis* or *'whooping cough'* (paroxysmal whoop), *psychogenic cough* (bizarre or honking) can sometimes be diagnosed before even seeing the patient, due to the pathognomonic quality of the coughs.

The patient's age and the duration of the cough are important. A cough that presents soon after birth or within the first few months of life is suggestive of

a congenital anomaly such as a *tracheo-oesophageal fistula*. *Pertussis, bronchiolitis, Chlamydia* and *Mycoplasma* classically present in infants and young children. *Bacterial tracheitis* tends to occur in children aged between 1 and 5 years and *croup* in children aged between 6 months and 3 years. *Foreign body inhalation* should be ruled out in any child from the age of 6 months to 5 years with a sudden history of a cough. Nocturnal coughs can be indicative of *asthma, gastro-oesophageal reflux* and *croup*. Other features may be associated with a specific underlying diagnosis: shortness of breath with asthma; stridor with laryngomalacia, croup, epiglottitis and bacterial tracheitis; wheeze with foreign body inhalation and mediastinal masses; chronic sputum production and chest infections with cystic fibrosis and recurrent aspiration; apnoea with bronchiolitis and whooping cough; cyanosis with foreign body aspiration; and haemoptysis with TB.

Examination

Recognition of potential respiratory failure is vital. Examination of the child should be age-appropriate and non-threatening. Injudicious examinations of the upper airway can precipitate the sudden need for urgent intubation or needle cricothyrotomy. Assess airway patency and stability, breathing rate, effort and associated sounds, skin colour, chest movement, mental status and tone. Asking the patient to cough or 'huff' can be very helpful in precipitating the cough. Unilateral wheeze and difficulty ventilating implies a foreign body.

Investigations

Consider chest x-ray to rule out collapse/consolidation or a pneumothorax.

Emergency management

The classic management approach of ABC (airway, breathing and circulation) should be used. Consider high flow oxygen via a facemask with a reservoir bag.

Further treatment depends on the underlying diagnosis: oral/nebulized

steroids for croup; broad-spectrum intravenous antibiotics for pneumonia or bacterial tracheitis; nebulized/ intramuscular adrenaline, nebulized salbutamol and intravenous corticosteroids for anaphylaxis; and inhaled/nebulized beta agonists, such as salbutamol, oral/IV corticosteroids for asthma. Encourage a calm environment and involve parents in the management (Fig. 1).

If in doubt, admit for observation.

Breathlessness

Breathlessness or dyspnoea is defined as perceived difficulty in breathing. It is often associated with lung or heart disease, is a very common symptom encountered in the emergency medical setting, and can be fatal if not adequately managed. There is a large differential diagnosis for the breathless child (Table 2).

History

A complete history should reveal any pre-existing cardiac or pulmonary symptoms. Onset, duration and occurrence at rest or on exertion should be determined. Associated features such as cough may imply *pneumonia* or *asthma*. Fever usually suggests an infectious cause, such as *pneumonia, croup* or *bronchiolitis*. Pleuritic chest pain may be due to

Table 1 **Important causes of acute cough in children**	
Respiratory	**Non-respiratory**
Laryngotracheobronchitis (croup)	Impaired gag reflex/ Unsafe swallow
Bacterial tracheitis	Congestive cardiac failure
Epiglottitis	Pulmonary hypertension
Pertussis	
Inhaled foreign body	
Aspiration	
Pneumonia	
Bronchiolitis	
Post-infectious	
Asthma	
Anaphylaxis	

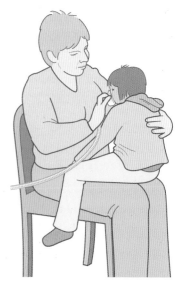

Fig. 1 **A mother holding a child with croup, while helping to administer a nebulizer.**

Table 2 **Causes of breathlessness in children**
Respiratory
Croup/epiglottitis/bacterial tracheitis
Asthma
Bronchiolitis
Congenital malformations
Cystic adenoid malformation
Congenital emphysema
Pneumonia
Pleural effusion
Gastro oesophageal reflux disease with aspiration
Foreign body
Trauma
Accidental
Pneumothorax
Haemothorax
Traumatic diaphragmatic rupture
Non-accidental
Cardiac
Congenital heart defects
Dysrhythmias
Cardiomyopathy
Myocarditis
Neurological
Seizure
Neuromuscular disorders
CNS infection
Brain tumour
Hydrocephalus
Drug ingestion
Aspirin
Sepsis
Psychogenic
Panic attacks
Hyperventilation
Pain
Anxiety
Endocrine
Metabolic acidosis
Medications

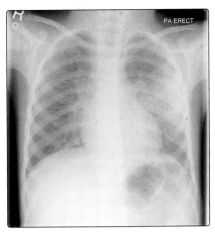

Fig. 2 **Chest x-ray showing consolidation in a child with left lower lobe pneumonia.**

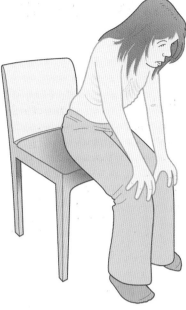

Fig. 3 **Tripod position adopted by a child with respiratory distress.** Note the intercostal recession.

pericarditis, pneumonia, pulmonary embolism, pneumothorax or *pleuritis. Pulmonary embolisms* are rare in children. A sudden onset of breathlessness is more likely to be because of a *spontaneous pneumothorax*, especially if accompanied by chest pain. Dyspnoea and a severe sore throat suggests *epiglottitis*. Previous Hib immunization does not preclude it, as the child may have been a non-responder.

Examination

The patient's general appearance, vital signs, pulse oximetry and cardiac rhythm should be noted. Airway patency, effort, efficacy and effect of breathing, mental status and ability to speak should be assessed. Peak flow measurement can be helpful.

Wheezing, pulsus paradoxus and accessory muscle use is suggestive of an *acute exacerbation of asthma.* A *pneumothorax* is implied by absent breath sounds and hyper-resonance. Stridor, wheeze, persistent pneumonia with difficulty breathing could be due to foreign body inhalation. Nasal flaring, recurrent apnoeas, and wheeze may indicate *bronchiolitis*.

Congestive cardiac failure presents with oedema, bibasal crepitations, wheeze, hepatomegaly, hepatojugular reflux, murmurs, hypertension, third or fourth heart sounds and a raised jugular venous pressure. This last sign can only be found in children over 4 years.

Investigations

A raised white cell count occurs in infectious processes and foreign body aspirations. The chest x-ray may show hyperinflation in asthma. A pneumonic process causes infiltrates, collapse/consolidation and effusions on the chest radiograph (Fig. 2). Bronchiolitis can be indicated by hyperinflation and atelectasis on the chest x-ray. Pulmonary oedema, effusions and cardiomegaly can be seen in congestive cardiac failure. Lateral neck X-rays can be helpful in the diagnosis of croup (subglottic oedema, enlarged epiglottis).

Emergency management

Continuous monitoring is vital, as children can rapidly deteriorate. Consider airway opening manoeuvres, suction, high concentration oxygen, airway adjuncts and assisted ventilation. Emergency intubation/needle cricothyrotomy are rarely required. There are no absolute criteria for mechanical ventilation as the decision to intubate is based on the clinical condition of the patient and the patient's response to treatment already received.

Consider intubation if there are signs of respiratory failure, recurrent apnoeas, oxygen saturations are decreasing or the $PaCO_2$ is increasing. If in doubt, admit for clinical observation.

Key points

Cough

- Beware of the six 'd's: **d**yspnoea, **d**rooling, **d**ysphonia, **d**usky colour, **d**ysphagia and **d**eath.

Look for signs of respiratory failure

- Increasing effort of breathing: nasal flaring, accessory muscles, tracheal tug, chest recession inspiratory and expiratory stridor at rest adoption of the tripod position (Fig. 3).

- Decreasing efficacy/effect of breathing: hypoxia, mottled, blue, pale skin, poor tone.

- Any signs of exhaustion: agitation, sleepiness, unresponsiveness.

- Beware the silent chest: breathing effort without air movement or exhaustion.

Vomiting and diarrhoea in children

Vomiting with or without diarrhoea may be the presenting symptoms of a variety of illnesses especially in the very young, for example gastroenteritis, urinary tract infection, meningitis, appendicitis and intussusception. Be very cautious about diagnosing gastroenteritis in a child with vomiting but who has no diarrhoea. Persistent or projectile vomiting in the first two months of life, with failure to thrive, may be due to gastric outlet obstruction, such as pyloric stenosis. Always consider intussusception, particularly in children aged 6–18 months.

Acute infectious gastroenteritis is one of the major causes of morbidity and mortality during childhood in developing countries. The number of children worldwide who die each year from gastroenteritis is estimated to be between one and three million.

In the UK, acute gastroenteritis accounts for over 20% of GP consultations for children aged 5 years and under and for almost 2% of all paediatric hospital admissions.

Diarrhoea

Diarrhoea is, for clinical purposes, a change in bowel habit for the child that results in substantially more frequent and looser stools. It is the consistency of the stools rather than the number that is more important. Passing formed stools frequently is not diarrhoea. Babies fed exclusively on breast milk tend to have loose, pasty stools, and this also is not considered diarrhoea.

Diarrhoeal episodes can be divided into:

- acute, if it has persisted for less than 10–14 days
- chronic or persistent, if it has persisted for more than 2–4 weeks (definitions vary with respect to duration).

Vomiting and diarrhoea may be as a result of an infection or alternatively be non-infectious in nature. Non-infectious causes of acute diarrhoea are uncommon in children. Using routine laboratory tests, pathogens are found in about 25% of cases (Table 1). Viral infections are commonly the cause of diarrhoea in children. Dysentery is

Table 1 **Laboratory reports of common intestinal infections, England and Wales, January to June 2006. Data from Health Protection Agency**	
Infecting organism	**Isolates**
Campylobacter	17 791
Cryptosporidium	976
Escherichia coli O157:H7	296
Giardia	1 068
Norovirus	2 990
Rotavirus	11 887
Non-typhoidal salmonellosis	3 644
Shigella sonnei	253

diarrhoea associated with intestinal inflammation resulting in the presence of mucus and/or blood in the stool and is a notifiable disease. Examples of organisms that can cause bloody diarrhoea include: *Shigella*, *Campylobacter*, enterohaemorrhagic *Escherichia coli* O157:H7, enteroinvasive *Escherichia coli*, *Salmonella* (non-typhoidal) serotypes, *Balantidium coli* (balantidiasis) and *Entamoeba histolytica* (amoebiasis).

Diarrhoea is a common consequence of treatment with antibiotics. The frequency of diarrhoea associated with a number of commonly used antibiotics has been reported to range from 2 to 25%.

Non-gastrointestinal infections, for example urinary tract infection, pneumonia, otitis media and other systemic infection, can present with vomiting and diarrhoea. In these conditions vomiting is usually more prominent than diarrhoea. Also consider other gastrointestinal conditions such as ulcerative colitis/Crohn's disease, Hirschsprung's enterocolitis, irritable bowel syndrome, short bowel syndrome, food-sensitive enteropathy (e.g. lactose intolerance), and coeliac disease. Younger children can present with 'toddler's diarrhoea', or constipation with overflow.

Haemolytic uraemic syndrome (HUS) is rare, but is one of the most feared complications of acute infectious gastroenteritis. HUS is characterized by acute renal failure, haemolytic anaemia and thrombocytopenia. It occurs mostly in young children, and is the most common cause of renal failure in children in the UK.

Assessment

When assessing a child with vomiting and diarrhoea it is important to differentiate causes other than infective. The next step is to consider the hydration and electrolyte state. Dehydration and electrolyte disturbance can progress to acidosis and circulatory failure, with hypoperfusion of vital organs, renal failure and eventual death if not promptly treated. WHO classifies dehydration as:

- no dehydration
- mild to moderate
- severe dehydration.

Prolonged skinfold recoil, dry mucous membranes, sunken eyes and altered mental status are reliably associated with dehydration. A prolonged capillary refill time (>2 seconds) and raised respiratory rate may also be useful (Table 2).

Always perform a bedside glucose test. Collect stool samples for microbiology (very important if diarrhoea and vomiting is associated with abdominal pain or blood/mucus in stools) and obtain a urinary specimen.

Initial management

In severely dehydrated or shocked children, intravenous access and administration of one or more 20 mL/kg boluses of normal saline is indicated. In mild to moderate dehydration, give oral fluids 50–75 mL/kg over 4 hours – divide this volume into small volumes given every 10 minutes (Table 3).

There is no evidence that milk or other fluids should be diluted or excluded to improve tolerance. A light diet, however, may be sensible. Avoid fizzy and natural fruit juice drinks. Mothers should be advised to continue breastfeeding and to supplement with bottle feeds if necessary. Oral rehydration fluid may be useful and can be given by nasogastric tube if the child has a poor oral intake.

Many children with gastroenteritis can be managed at home after observation and rehydration in the emergency department. Ice lollies can help rehydrating children (Fig. 1).

Table 2 Clinical assessment of dehydration

Signs and symptoms	No dehydration (<3% loss total body water)	Mild to moderate dehydration (3–9% loss total body water)	Severe dehydration (>9% loss total body water)
Mental status	Alert and well	Normal, fatigued or restless, irritable	Apathetic, lethargic, comatose
Thirst	Drinks normally, might refuse liquids	Thirsty	Drinks poorly, unable to drink
Cardiovascular status	Normal heart rate and pulse, CRT <2 seconds	Normal to increased, pulse quality normal to decreased, CRT >2 seconds	Tachycardia, bradycardia in extremis, weak, thready or impalpable pulse, CRT ≫2 seconds
Extremities	Warm	Cool	Cold, mottled
Respiratory status	Normal	Normal to tachypnoeic	Deep and rapid breathing
Eyes	Normal	Slightly sunken	Deeply sunken
Tears	Present	Decreased	Absent
Mucous membranes	Moist	Dry	Parched
Urine output	Normal to decreased	Decreased	Absent
Pinched skin fold	Immediate recoil	Recoil in <2 seconds	Recoil in >2 seconds

CRT, capillary refill time.

Table 3 Initial management of child with vomiting and diarrhoea in the emergency department

Mild dehydration	Oral intake – small amounts frequently, ice lolly
Moderate dehydration and still drinking	Use oral rehydration solutions
Moderate/severe dehydration/not drinking	Consider nasogastric tube or intravenous rehydration
Shocked child	Immediate intravenous access and fluid bolus

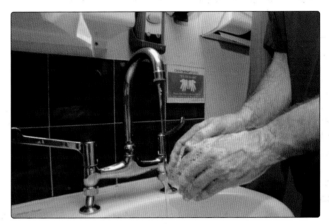

Fig. 2 **Hand washing.**

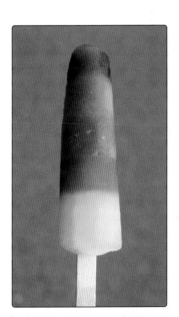

Fig. 1 **Ice lollies help replace fluid and may lower a fever.**

There is some evidence that probiotic treatment may reduce the frequency and duration of diarrhoea.

Parents can help to protect young children against diarrhoea by ensuring that hands are washed carefully after toileting and before handling food and before feeding. Good hand washing requires the use of soap and water (Fig. 2).

Inpatient management
This is indicated if:

■ there is suspicion of serious bacterial infection (e.g. suspected meningitis or urinary tract infection)

■ there are any signs of toxicity
■ there is any vomiting of blood or bile
■ there is severe abdominal pain or abdominal signs.

Other reasons for admission include moderate or severe dehydration and poor oral intake, concerns regarding parental care or access to emergency services or telephone. Be especially wary of children with chronic illnesses, poor growth and the very young.

Key points

■ Few children with vomiting and diarrhoea need a cannula; try oral rehydration first.

■ Small volumes of fluid given frequently are tolerated better.

■ Frequently reassess children during rehydration therapy.

■ Early resumption of a normal diet should be encouraged.

■ Breastfeeding should not be stopped.

■ Always look for underlying sepsis; avoid diagnosing gastroenteritis in children who present with vomiting without diarrhoea.

Rashes in children

Most rashes in children are caused by viruses, are benign and resolve over time without any treatment. However, some childhood rashes have serious or even life-threatening causes and many different conditions result in rashes that look the same. Often, the symptoms and signs other than the rash help make the diagnosis.

Viral rashes

Most viral rashes are associated with a period of infectivity and such children should avoid contact with those at risk (immunosuppression, pregnancy etc.). Advise to avoid school attendance while infective.

Chickenpox (varicella zoster)

This contagious viral illness is generally not a serious disease in healthy children. The vesicular itchy rash first appears on the scalp, armpits or groin area and progresses, to spread over the entire body (Fig. 1).

An area of redness with a small, superficial blister in the centre eventually ruptures, forming a crust. Other symptoms include low-grade fever, malaise, sore throat and red eyes. Incubation period is about 1 week and symptoms last 2 weeks. Treatment is symptomatic.

Measles

Caused by a paramyxovirus. Despite an effective vaccine, outbreaks continue to occur in under-immunized populations.

The measles vaccine is part of the MMR (measles-mumps-rubella) vaccine given at age 12–15 months and repeated at age 4–6 years.

The disease usually begins with coryzal symptoms and fever. After 3 or 4 days, a facial macular erythematous rash develops (Fig. 2) which spreads down the body and lasts more than 3 days. Koplik's spots (red spots with a minute bluish white speck seen on the buccal mucosa and lingual mucosa) are diagnostic. Complications include diarrhoea, pneumonia and encephalitis.

Rubella

A much milder disease caused by Rubivirus. Begins with a pink rash to the face, then spreads to the body and gets better in less than 3 days. The major danger is of congenital abnormalities to the unborn child of an infected mother.

Erythema infectiosum (fifth disease or slapped cheek syndrome)

This is caused by parvovirus B19. Initial presentation is with bright red cheeks followed by a lacy rash over the body (Fig. 3). The rash fades when the skin is cool, but becomes more pronounced with warmth. Once the rash appears, the child is no longer contagious.

Roseola infantum

A common early childhood virus caused by the human herpesvirus 6. Classically a high, spiking fever for 2–4 days is followed by the onset of a small, pink, flat or slightly raised rash on the trunk that spreads to the extremities.

Hand, foot and mouth disease

This is caused by a coxsackie virus. A prodrome of fever and non-specific symptoms such as lethargy and anorexia is followed by the development of small vesicles in the mouth and on the hands and less commonly on the feet. The distribution of the vesicles is characteristic and aids the diagnosis.

Bacterial rashes

Scarlet fever

This is the association of a streptococcal throat infection with a macular rash, usually with a fever. The main concern is of associated immune reactions such as rheumatic fever. Proven streptococcal infections should receive a full course of penicillin.

Impetigo

A superficial skin infection due to streptococci or staphylococci. It is commonly found around the nose and mouth but can occur anywhere. The rash begins as small blisters that rupture leaving red, open patches of skin, often with a yellow crust. The rash is highly contagious. Treatment is with topical or oral antibiotics (such as mupirocin, fucidin topically or oral flucloxacillin).

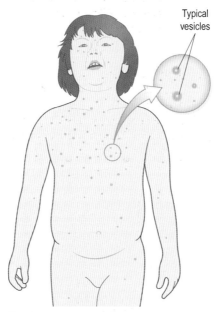

Typical vesicles

Fig. 1 **Chicken pox.**

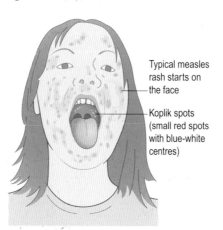

Typical measles rash starts on the face

Koplik spots (small red spots with blue-white centres)

Fig. 2 **Measles.**

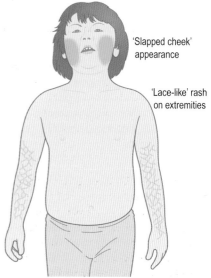

'Slapped cheek' appearance

'Lace-like' rash on extremities

Fig. 3 **Erythema infectiosum.**

Lyme disease

Caused by the spirochete bacteria *Borrelia*, typically from the bite of an infected tick. Presentation includes a rash and flu-like symptoms, followed by the possibility of musculoskeletal, arthritic, neurological, psychiatric and cardiac manifestations. The classical reddish 'bull's-eye' rash known as erythema chronicum migrans appears anywhere from one day to a month after a tick bite. Antibiotics such as doxycycline (not for children under 8 years), amoxicillin and ceftriaxone are the primary treatment for Lyme disease.

Toxic shock syndrome

A life-threatening disease caused by a toxin produced by *Staphylococcus aureus* or a streptococcal bacteria. A high fever, sore throat, arthralgia and gastrointestinal upset may occur. The source may be relatively inconspicuous such as a burn or abrasion or classically a retained tampon in an adolescent girl. The rash resembles sunburn but may involve any area of the body. Treatment involves circulatory support and treatment of the underlying infection.

Life-threatening rashes

Often the clue to a life-threatening cause for a rash is the systemic condition of the child. Occasionally a rash may precede the systemic symptoms and offer an opportunity for early treatment.

Fever and petechiae

These may be present with many rashes and are often signs of a more serious condition.

Petechiae may occur from a number of causes:

- forceful coughing or vomiting causes petechiae on the face and chest
- Henoch–Schönlein purpura
- thrombocytopenia (including idiopathic thrombocytopenia purpura, ITP)
- leukaemia.

Petechiae with fever is concerning. Although most of these children will have a viral illness, a small number will have diseases that need immediate treatment. The main concern is meningococcal sepsis with *Neisseria meningitides* (see 'Fever and sepsis in children' chapter).

Other infective rashes

Parasites and fungal infections may cause skin rashes. Common causes are ringworm (tinea corporis: body; and tinea capitis: scalp) and athlete's foot. Lesions start as itchy red, slightly scaly, areas that get bigger over time. Topical antifungals are normally sufficient to treat these infections.

Scabies is an itchy rash caused by a mite (*Sarcoptes scabiei*) that burrows beneath the top layer of skin. It is spread by close bodily contact. The rash tends to be found between the fingers, in the armpits, or on the inner wrists and arms (Fig. 4). Treatment is by application of topical lotions or creams such as malathion. Good hygiene is essential to prevent recurrence.

Non-infective rashes

Many systemic conditions are associated with a rash. Examples include systemic lupus erythematosus (SLE), Kawasaki disease, coeliac disease and allergies (see 'Allergy and anaphylaxis' chapter).

Kawasaki disease (mucocutaneous lymph node syndrome)

Of unknown aetiology, this condition usually affects children younger than 9 years.

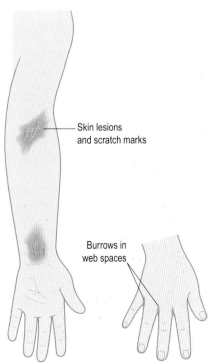

Fig. 4 **Scabies.**

Skin lesions and scratch marks

Burrows in web spaces

The disease is defined by a fever for 5 days associated with four of the following five diagnostic criteria:

- conjunctivitis
- lymphadenopathy
- red mucous membranes/strawberry tongue
- palmar or plantar erythema/swelling/desquamation
- a macular erythematous rash.

Complications include coronary artery aneurysms and thrombocytosis. Treatment is with intravenous gamma globulin and high-dose aspirin.

Neonatal rashes

Common neonatal rashes include:

- milia (small yellow to white dots on the face and the gums occur in healthy newborns)
- seborrhoeic dermatitis (cradle cap; a greasy, scaly, red, bumpy rash on the scalp)
- infantile acne
- erythema toxicum (small blisters on a red base) seen in about half of all newborns
- miliaria (prickly heat; small, clear blisters usually on the nose)
- candidal rashes (fungal infection of the skin by *Candida albicans*, involving the creases in the nappy area and often associated with oral thrush)
- nappy rash (the effects of urine and faeces on the sensitive skin of the neonate sparing creases and folds).

> **Key points**
>
> - Always consider the general state of the child as well as the rash.
> - Always use caution when assessing a child with a non-blanching (petechial or purpuric) rash.
> - Meningococcal sepsis may take several hours to develop.
> - Contact, family and travel histories are important.
> - A blanching erythematous rash in a **well** child is usually benign.

Limb injuries and the limping child

The unique feature of paediatric injuries is the excellent healing potential and the presence of the growth plate (physis). The presence of the physis is a double-edged sword: remaining growth around the physis will often allow some deformity to remodel; however, if the physis is damaged, growth disturbance may occur. Always consider non-accidental injury in all children presenting to the emergency department with an injury (see 'Child protection' chapter).

Upper limb

Most fractures of the distal radius in children are unicortical (affect a single cortex of the bone), buckle or greenstick fractures. These are stable injuries and require symptomatic treatment only. Two other common patterns of distal radial fractures are Salter Harris type II fractures (Figs 1 and 2) through the distal physis, and complete metaphyseal fractures. Treatment depends on the age of the patient, the degree of fracture displacement and the potential for remodelling. Displaced fractures of both forearm bones may require manipulation under anaesthetic (MUA).

The injured paediatric elbow can be very challenging; the majority of the joint is cartilage, it has multiple growth centres and interpreting radiographs can be difficult. The most commonly used mnemonic for the sequence of ossification around the elbow is CRITOL (Capitelum, Radial head, Internal (medial) epicondyle, Trochlea, Olecranon, Lateral epicondyle). These ossification centres generally appear at 2-yearly intervals starting at approximately 2 years of age.

The commonest elbow injury seen in children under 5 years is the pulled elbow. This is generally caused by a longitudinal force on an extended limb. The child holds the arm at their side and is not keen to flex the affected arm at the elbow. Radiographs are normal. It is thought to be caused by the radial head slipping out from the annular ligament. Reduce by applying an axial force at the wrist, flexing and supinating the elbow.

Supracondylar distal humeral fractures are the most common elbow fracture. If displaced, they require reduction under anaesthetic and if unstable, K-wire fixation. It is important to examine the neurovascular status of the arm carefully.

Humeral shaft fractures are relatively rare. The humerus either fractures at the elbow or through the proximal humeral physis. It has an excellent remodelling potential and is often treated conservatively. Fractures of the clavicle are common and normally caused by a fall. Generally they are treated with analgesia and a broad arm sling.

Lower limb injuries

Injuries resulting in long bone fractures of the lower limb are generally high energy injuries. Initial treatment for femoral shaft fractures involves adequate analgesia (intravenous opiates, Entonox and femoral nerve block); splint the leg in a Thomas splint. Specific treatment is very dependent on the age of the child.

Injuries around the knee may be bony or soft tissue. The cruciate ligaments may rupture mid substance, but often the bone fails first, leading to an avulsion fracture of the tibial eminence. Physeal fractures around the knee are caused by considerable energy transfer. Be vigilant for neurovascular injury in proximal tibial physeal fractures. If the tibial shaft is fractured, administer analgesia and splint the limb above the knee.

Most ankle injuries in children are simple ligamentous injuries. Occasionally it can be difficult to differentiate an undisplaced Salter Harris type I fracture of the distal fibular physis from a ligament injury. If suspected treat symptomatically, splinting the ankle, and arrange follow-up in clinic a few days later. Examination a few days after injury is easier as the area of tenderness becomes more localized; anterolateral for ligament injuries, and more posterior for bony injuries.

The limping child

The limping child is a common presentation, often benign and self-limiting, but always consider and exclude serious pathology. The differential diagnosis is extremely wide (Table 1).

History

The age is very important. Very young children find it difficult to localize pain and may merely present with a refusal to use the affected limb. Certain

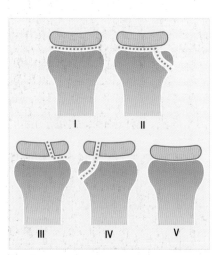

Fig. 1 **Salter Harris classification of growth plate (physeal) injuries.** I, Through the physis but not through the epiphysis or metaphysis. II, Through the physis and the metaphysis (commonest). III, Through the physis and the epiphysis. IV, Oblique fracture across the metaphysis, physis and epiphysis. V, Vertical compression to the physis.

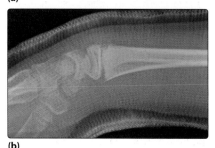

HBL

(a)

(b)

Fig. 2 **Lateral radiograph of a wrist; (a)** showing dorsally displaced physeal fracture of the distal radius; **(b)** Post-reduction radiograph showing fracture reduced.

Table 1 Common causes of a painful limp in children		
All ages		
Trauma		
Infection (septic arthritis, osteomyelitis, discitis)		
Secondary to various viral illnesses		
Tumour		
Sickle cell disease		
Toddler (1–3 years)	**Child (4–10 years)**	**Adolescent (11–16 years)**
Transient synovitis	Transient synovitis	Slipped upper femoral epiphysis
Toddler's fracture	Perthes disease	Overuse syndromes
Child abuse	Juvenile arthritis	Osteochondritis dissecans
Juvenile arthritis	Rheumatic fever	
Haemophilia	Haemophilia	
Henoch–Schönlein purpura	Henoch–Schönlein purpura	

conditions affect the hips at different ages: Perthes disease in younger children, slipped upper femoral epiphysis (SUFE) in adolescents and infective causes in all ages. Ask about any recent infections, particularly upper respiratory tract infection, and diarrhoea and vomiting. Is the limp or pain getting better, worse or no different? Is it intermittent? Is the limp worse in the mornings? Consider the possibility of referred pain; hip pain may be felt as knee pain and vice versa. Abdominal pathology may present with hip pain, for example psoas abscess, retrocaecal appendix and discitis.

Examination

Examine the whole lower limb systematically, beginning at the feet and working your way up the leg. Look for any obvious swelling or bruising, and note the resting position of the limb. Palpate, looking for areas of tenderness, and move all the joints through a full range of motion. Do a thorough general examination, including the abdomen and testes in a boy. Check for any systemic features of infection, e.g. tachycardia or temperature.

Special investigations

Further investigations are based on the findings of the history and physical examination. If a clear history of trauma is offered obtain plain radiographs. A prepubertal limping adolescent with hip or knee pain needs an anteroposterior and 'frog-leg' lateral radiograph of the hip to exclude a SUFE (Fig. 3).

A child of any age with temperature or systemic toxicity needs exclusion of infection; do FBC, ESR, CRP and blood

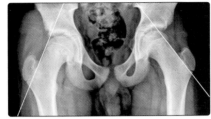
(a)

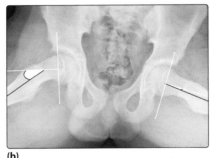
(b)

Fig. 3 **(a) AP radiograph demonstrating early SUFE.** Note how Klein's line – a line drawn up the lateral aspect of the femoral neck – cuts through the normal head on left hip. **(b) Frog-leg lateral radiograph of same patient.** Note how it is easier to see the slip on the lateral view. Note the increased shaft epiphyseal angle of Southwick on the right.

cultures. An ultrasound of deep joints such as the hips with ultrasound-guided aspiration may be indicated. A bone scan may be hot, normal or cold in the presence of septic arthritis or osteomyelitis depending on the phase of the disease. An MRI of the affected area is the best investigation but this may be difficult to obtain out of hours and in young children who may require sedation.

Transient synovitis

Most common diagnosis but a diagnosis of exclusion, once sinister pathology has been ruled out. Treatment is symptomatic, rest and NSAIDs, symptoms improving within 48 hours and resolving totally over 2 weeks.

Infection

Septic arthritis and osteomyelitis may present at any age in any bone or joint. Haematogenous osteomyelitis in children occurs in the metaphysis of the long bones and as such pain may be felt in the adjacent joint. The cardinal signs are pain, fever, pseudoparalysis in the neonate or infant; antalgic limp in the older child (See chapter on 'Non-traumatic musculoskeletal emergencies').

Slipped upper femoral epiphysis

This occurs in prepubertal patients, and is more common in boys than girls. The patient has no systemic symptoms, is apyrexial and has normal inflammatory markers. It is important to get a 'frog-leg' lateral view of both hips as it may be missed on a single AP radiograph (Fig. 3). The patient may only complain of knee pain; always consider hip pathology in a patient presenting with knee pain.

Perthes disease

This is avascular necrosis of the femoral head, and occurs in children aged 4 to 10 years. Radiographs may initially be normal. If symptoms persist or recur after an initial episode, orthopaedic follow-up is required (Fig. 4).

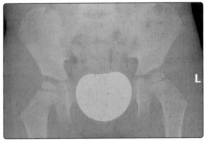
(a)

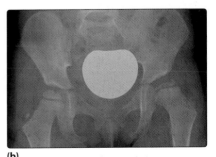
(b)

Fig. 4 **(a) Perthes disease; initial radiograph normal. (b) Follow-up radiograph of same patient 6 months later;** note sclerosis and collapse of left femoral epiphysis.

Neonatal emergencies

The neonatal period is characterized by transition from the intrauterine to the extrauterine environment. Problems related to this transitional process are unique to the neonatal period. Some phenomena encountered in this period are common and often resolve with no or little intervention, such as physiological jaundice. There are other conditions which are acutely life-threatening if not recognized and treated appropriately. Cardiac problems, sepsis and metabolic disease may all manifest themselves as an extremely unwell, shocked neonate and differentiation may be difficult at first.

Neonatal resuscitation at birth

Neonatal (or newborn) resuscitation differs from that in older children and adults in that there is a greater emphasis on temperature homeostasis and lung aeration. Only a few newborns need support at birth and the majority of these respond to lung inflation and oxygenation with spontaneous establishment of cardiac output. Even fewer need further intervention like cardiac compressions or drug therapy. Newborn resuscitation is approached in a stepwise manner (Fig. 1).

Cardiac problems in the neonatal period

Cardiac problems that may manifest within the first 2 weeks of life include:

- hypoplastic left heart
- transposition of the great arteries
- coarctation of the aorta
- multiple other structural cardiac abnormalities (Fig. 2).

Cyanosis may not be a regular feature. A history of slow feeding, exhaustion and sweating brought on by feeding may suggest cardiac disease.

Symptoms and signs of cardiac failure in neonates other than poor feeding include sweating, tachycardia, tachypnoea, liver enlargement, fine crackles on lung auscultation and oedema. Palpation of the peripheral pulses and a four limb blood pressure are essential in order not to miss critical aortic coarctation.

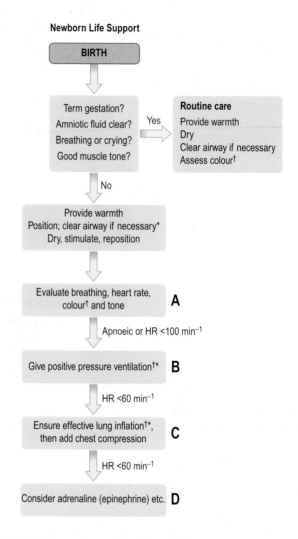

Fig. 1 **Newborn life support algorithm.**

Echocardiography will lead to the definitive diagnosis. Chest x-ray may show a characteristic heart silhouette suggesting a particular cardiac defect; for example a 'boot shaped' heart in tetralogy of Fallot.

In many cases an acute deterioration is brought on by the closure of the ductus arteriosus. Pending definitive paediatric cardiology evaluation, prostaglandin E1 infusion will maintain ductus arteriosus patency. Newborns in shock will require input from the paediatric intensive care unit and early involvement of a paediatric cardiologist.

Neonatal sepsis

Prematurity, prolonged rupture of membranes and positive maternal group B streptococcal status all place the neonate at increased risk of sepsis. The septic neonate may present with poor feeding, lethargy, tachycardia, tachypnoea and poor perfusion.

The most common pathogens for early onset neonatal sepsis are:

- group B *Streptococcus*
- *Escherichia coli*
- *Listeria monocytogenes*.

In addition, late onset sepsis can be due to staphylococci, streptococci and a variety of other organisms. This is reflected in the first line antibiotic treatment; either a third generation cephalosporin or a combination of a penicillin with an aminoglycoside. A full septic screen is desirable provided the neonate is stable enough. This includes blood cultures, urine for

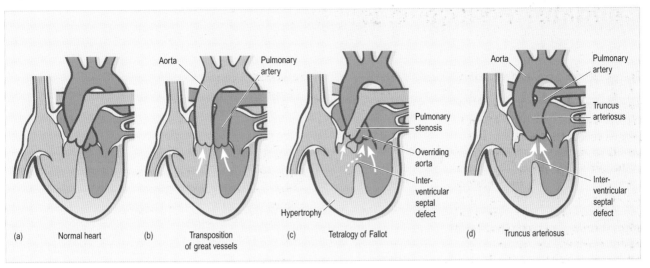

Fig. 2 **Congenital cardiac abnormalities.**

culture and microscopy (obtained by catheter or suprapubic aspiration), chest x-ray and cerebrospinal fluid obtained by lumbar puncture.

Metabolic problems

Inborn errors of metabolism are rare. Affected babies can be clinically indistinguishable from the sick neonate with sepsis or cardiac failure. Features in the history that should alert to the possibility of an inborn error of metabolism include consanguinity, previous neonatal deaths and onset of symptoms when first exposed to feeds. In this case feeds should be stopped and the neonate started on intravenous dextrose solution (10%) with regular monitoring of blood glucose levels. The baseline investigations for suspected metabolic conditions are urea and electrolytes, liver function tests, ammonia level, urine and blood for amino and organic acids as well as a blood spot on filter paper for an acyl-carnitine profile, and, if possible, saved serum for later analysis. The timing of these specimens is crucial: The sooner obtained, if a neonate presents in crisis, the more likely are the tests to pick up a metabolic abnormality.

A much more commonly encountered problem in neonates is hypoglycaemia (blood glucose level <2.6 mmol/L). In the vast majority of newborns presenting to the emergency department this will be due to insufficient calorie intake. Because of its detrimental effect on brain development, hypoglycaemia needs to

be identified and treated promptly in every unwell neonate.

Jaundice

Jaundice in the well neonate is due to physiological hyperbilirubinaemia in the majority of cases, and this needs only minimal investigation. The onset of physiological jaundice is from 24 hours of age. It can last for up to 2 weeks and sometimes longer in breastfed and premature neonates. Hyperbilirubinaemia can be either conjugated or unconjugated. In the unwell jaundiced neonate, in severe

jaundice, or when presenting with jaundice outside the usual time frame, more uncommon causes for hyperbilirubinaemia need to be considered (Table 1). Investigations depend on the age at presentation, the severity of jaundice and whether the neonate is sick or well. Initially a full blood count and a split bilirubin level should be performed. If there is predominantly conjugated hyperbilirubinaemia (over 25% of total bilirubin or more than 25 μmol/L), early involvement of a specialist in paediatric liver disease is required.

Table 1 **Neonatal jaundice**

Causes for unconjugated hyperbilirubinaemia:

- Breastfeeding jaundice (physiological)
- Breakdown of haem (following a cephalohaematoma)
- Haemolysis (rhesus, ABO and other blood group incompatibilities, spherocytosis)
- Sepsis (urinary tract infection)
- Metabolic and endocrine causes (hypothyroidism, can be mixed, conjugated/unconjugated)
- Gilbert's, Crigler–Najjar syndrome (usually presenting as prolonged jaundice)
- Gastrointestinal obstruction

Causes for conjugated hyperbilirubinaemia (>25% of total bilirubin level):

- Biliary atresia (pale stools)
- Choledochal cyst
- Neonatal hepatitis syndrome (idiopathic, alpha-1-antitrypsin deficiency, congenital infection)
- Galactosaemia

Key points

- Ventilation is key in newborn resuscitation.
- In neonates, poor feeding may be a manifestation of sepsis, cardiac disease or a metabolic disorder.
- Distinction between sepsis, cardiac disease and metabolic disease can be challenging.
- Check blood glucose in an unwell neonate.
- Attend to ABC, keep warm and dry, correct hypoglycaemia.
- Involve senior help early.

Child protection

Background

The emergency department may be the first and the only place where an abused child presents. All health professionals who see children have a responsibility to consider the possibility of non-accidental injury or child abuse and to ensure that an appropriate assessment takes place when there is a suspicion that a child may have been subjected to abuse.

Child abuse is categorized as physical abuse, emotional abuse, sexual abuse or neglect.

Physical abuse can take the form of hitting, shaking, thermal injury, drowning, suffocating or otherwise causing physical harm to the child. A particular form of physical abuse is when a carer fabricates symptoms or induces symptoms of illness in a child.

Emotional abuse can take many forms: conveying that the child is worthless and unloved, age-inappropriate expectations, but also witnessing the ill-treatment of others in the context of domestic violence.

Sexual abuse involves children in sexual activities whether the child is aware of it or not. It does not necessarily require physical contact.

Neglect is probably the most common form of abuse. It is defined as a persistent failure to meet a child's basic physical or psychological needs. This includes lack of supervision.

Child abuse may be suggested by the child, a parent, a fellow professional or be picked up incidentally. There is no need to make a firm diagnosis of child abuse in the setting of the emergency department but it is the duty of every professional to safeguard a child even in the case of a mere suspicion of abuse. The interest of the child is paramount and overrules all other concerns. Early consultation with paediatric colleagues and involvement of the relevant statutory agencies like social services or the police are essential: it must not be assumed that someone else will raise the alarm. Clear, comprehensive and contemporaneous documentation is important.

History

The following features should raise suspicion when taking a history:

- inconsistent, unwitnessed and discrepant history of the event
- history is not consistent with the injury/presenting problem or the developmental stage of the child
- inappropriate and unexplained late presentation to medical services
- history of inappropriate child response to injury
- previous concerns relating to this or other children (child protection register) and involvement of social services
- multiple previous attendances to the emergency department
- adverse carer's attributes: substance abuse, mental illness, domestic violence, young and unsupported parents
- adverse child's attributes: prematurity, feeding difficulties, disability, chronic illness and children who are in care.

Talk and listen to the child but don't probe if information is not volunteered. The carers should not be confronted or accused of having harmed the child. Instead they require a calm and clear explanation of the concerns and the consequent steps that will need to be taken in order to investigate these concerns further. When dealing with children at risk of significant harm, siblings or other children looked after by the same carers need to be considered.

Examination

When examining children the following features (not exhaustive) should raise concerns with regard to the possibility of child abuse:

- presence of other, unexplained injuries
- injuries not in keeping with the history given
- injuries or bruising in a non-mobile child or infant
- patterned bruises or those showing an imprint suggestive of finger marks or an object
- bruises on unusual parts of the body (neck, face, abdomen, chest and buttocks)
- bite marks
- contact burns (cigarette) and immersion scalds
- abnormal child/parent interaction (emotional abuse)
- unkempt and dirty appearance of child, failure to thrive (neglect)
- evidence of self-harm in adolescents, inappropriate, sexualized behaviour (sexual abuse).

Examination of children suspected of having been sexually abused should be left to specially trained professionals. Documentation of examination findings is paramount and handwritten entries in the notes assisted by body charts for a drawing of the injuries are essential. Photography is merely an adjunct.

Investigations

Initial investigations should aim to identify injuries that require immediate treatment (Fig. 1). Further investigations such as a radiological skeletal survey and clotting screen may be indicated as part of the assessment for non-accidental injury.

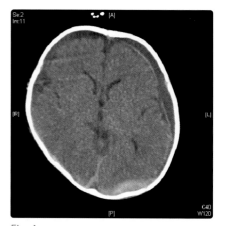

Fig. 1 **CT scan showing subdural haematomas caused by non-accidental injury.**

Key points

- Consider the possibility of child abuse/non-accidental injury.
- Discuss early with a senior/paediatrician.
- Liaise with social services and police.
- Keep the parents (and child) informed.
- Document your findings well.
- Do not discharge if you have concerns.
- Remember: the child's safety is more important than parental concerns or sensitivities.

Social issues

Mistakes are a fact of life.
It is the response to error that counts
Nikki Giovanni

Violence

Intentional injury is a common underlying cause of many emergency department attendances. Broadly, violence can be categorized into community violence (where the perpetrator is usually unknown by the victim), domestic violence (which is usually a pattern of coercive, abusive behaviours and the perpetrator is well known by the victim), sexual assault, non-accidental injury in children and elder abuse. The emergency physician's primary role is to provide initial medical care. The secondary role is to provide forensic recording of the injuries; this may require additional training. Good quality documentation, ideally with photographs, can increase the chances of successful prosecution if the victim decides to press charges. The police are unaware of the majority of assault victims who require emergency department treatment. Emergency physicians should encourage victims to report assaults to the police, as this is the most effective form of injury control. Psychological disturbances are common after an assault and the emergency physician should be prepared to support a victim.

Domestic abuse

Background
The scale of domestic abuse is staggering. One woman in 10 will be physically assaulted by a partner or family member each year. Domestic abuse refers to a wide range of abusive behaviours; physical abuse, sexual abuse, emotional abuse and financial abuse. Emergency physicians are much more likely to encounter physical assault rather than other forms of abuse. Physical assault is often only part of domestic abuse with emotional, financial and sexual abuse commonly coexisting. Domestic abuse is best viewed as a coercive pattern of behaviours where a (usually male) partner aims to dominate and control a (usually female) weaker partner.

History/risk factors
On average, 15–20 episodes of physical abuse will occur before a victim seeks help. Domestic abuse occurs in all cultures and socio-economic strata, but is more prevalent and severe involving women, poor people and where there is cultural endorsement of violence. Patients with psychiatric and substance misuse problems are particularly vulnerable. It is not feasible to ask every woman about domestic violence, but **confidential** inquiry should be considered when the patient has: multiple attendances, an inconsistent mechanism of injury, a delayed presentation, no clear diagnosis, a history of self-harm, psychiatric co-morbidity, or presents following an assault. Pregnancy and the immediate postnatal period are times of increased risk. Simple and direct questions are appropriate and acceptable:

> 'We know that violence at home is a problem for many women, is there anyone who is hurting you in any way?'

Most victims will not volunteer domestic abuse unless asked specifically.

Examination
There are no patterns of injury that can reliably identify domestic abuse. Multiple injuries and injuries to the face are more common, as are bruises around the neck from attempted throttling (Fig. 1). The majority of domestic abuse injuries will be relatively minor. If domestic abuse is disclosed, photographs (ideally by a trained medical photographer) can increase the chances of a successful prosecution.

Emergency management
Emergency department staff must treat victims in a supportive and non-judgemental manner. It should be explained to the victim that physical assault is a crime. Contact with the police should be offered from the safety of the emergency department. This is frequently declined and may frustrate emergency department staff. Information about local support agencies and shelters should be widely available in the emergency department. Information is ideally printed on credit sized cards; larger information sheets are thought to be a risk for the victim. Even if a victim does not wish to take further legal action at this stage, it is important that there is a good record of injuries, since this may be referred to in future legal proceedings. Less than 1% of domestic assaults treated at the emergency department will result in a conviction. Local law varies as to whether a clinician is required to report suspected domestic violence to the police or social services, and the evidence that this reduces violence is limited. There is good quality evidence that domestic violence advocacy workers can reduce violence. The role of advocacy workers varies, but they are usually able to get non-molestation orders (or the equivalent) quickly and navigate and support victims through the criminal justice system. If there is good reason to suspect that the victim lacks capacity, then the emergency physician can inform the police, though this is unusual. Emergency department staff may become frustrated with women who appear not to want to leave a clearly abusive partner. Experience indicates that women leave when they feel ready, not when healthcare staff believe they should.

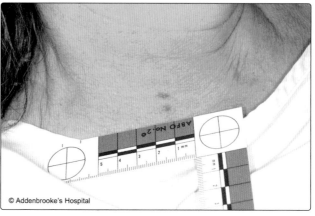

© Addenbrooke's Hospital

Fig. 1 **Point bruising to the neck,** typical of attempted strangulation.

Sexual assault

Definition

Rape is defined in English law as the non-consensual penetration of the vagina, mouth or anus by a penis. Assault by penetration is the non-consensual, intentional insertion of an object other than the penis into the vagina or anus. Victims may be any age and either sex, although females are more commonly assaulted.

Presentation

Disclosure by male victims is lower. Approximately 50% of reported cases involve violence and victims have injuries to genital or central areas.

Emergency management

If the assault occurred within 7 days of presentation, treat injuries, offer pregnancy and STI prophylaxis, refer to Genitourinary Medicine (GUM) or the Sexual Assault Referral Centre (SARC) and encourage police involvement (Table 1).

For victims presenting earlier, attend to life-threatening injuries, regardless of the need for forensic investigation, before collecting early evidence (mouth swab for DNA and urine sample for toxicology). Then involve police or SARC, provided the victim consents. Respect a victim's right to refuse treatment or forensic investigation but advise it is best performed within 72 hours of the assault. Medical care proceeds once forensic investigations

are complete or if the victim declines participation. If clothes have to be cut, cut away from holes and blood stains.

History and examination

Consider the need for privacy and that the patient may feel ashamed or be unwilling to cooperate. Document a detailed history accurately and complete a disclosure record. Include assault nature, timing, location, perpetrator details and whether the victim has changed clothes or washed since. Sensitively take a sexual (STIs, hepatitis B, contraceptive, last consensual intercourse) and gynaecological (last menstrual period, parity) history. During the examination, gain consent at each stage and offer a chaperone. Document evidence of force, resistance and injuries.

Investigations

- Urine/serum HCG in women of childbearing age.
- Colposcopy/anoscopy to photograph evidence of penetrative trauma. (In this case, it is advisable to defer speculum examination for accuracy.)
- Serology for hepatitis B status in previously vaccinated patients.
- Pre-screening and pre-treatment serology for existing syphilis, hepatitis B, hepatitis C, HIV.
- STI screening, ideally 10–14 days after assault, comprising cultures from penetration site(s) (gonorrhoea, *Chlamydia, Trichomonas*) and serology (syphilis, hepatitis B, hepatitis C, HIV) with subsequent repeat serology.
- Toxicology screen if drug-assisted assault.

Treatment

Following assault involving vaginal penetration, 1–5% of women become pregnant. Postcoital contraception is contraindicated in existing pregnancy, but should be offered to all other at-risk victims. Within 5 days, offer

levonorgestrel (efficacy decreases beyond 12 hours) or an intrauterine device (with antibiotic prophylaxis).

Assess HIV risk and consider post-exposure prophylaxis. Hepatitis B immunoglobulin can be administered within 7 days of assault. Where a patient has already been vaccinated, test serum anti-HBs. STI risk reflects local prevalence. Offer victims antibiotic prophylaxis, screening or both. A blood sample should be stored for future testing.

Finally, consider tetanus vaccination based on injuries and status. Refer to GUM for post-exposure prophylaxis follow-up (after 2–3 days), STI screening (after 10–14 days) and repeat serological testing. Advise the patient of sources of psychosocial support and involve a social worker if he/she feels unsafe at home or if the victim is a minor.

Table 1 **Aims of emergency management**

- Respectful, non-judgemental, empathic assessment in safety and privacy, considering culture and religion
- Psychosocial support
- Full, accurate documentation, avoiding discrepancy with police report
- Evidence preservation
- Involvement of police or Sexual Assault Referral Centre (SARC)
- Injury management
- Postcoital contraception
- Sexually transmitted infection (STI) prophylaxis
- Referral: GUM, Obstetrics and Gynaecology, counselling, social worker

Paediatric considerations

If domestic abuse is disclosed and there are children living with the victim or the perpetrator, then local child protection procedures must be activated, ideally with the consent of the victim.

Children are at risk in a number of ways: they can be injured as the parents fight; witnessing violence between parents has psychological effects on the children; and child abuse is much more common where there is violence between the parents.

Please also refer to the 'Child protection' chapter.

Key points

- Always consider the possibility of domestic abuse.
- Take a direct yet sympathetic and confidential approach.
- Record your findings accurately.
- Ensure the victim has a safe place to return to.

Alcohol and drug related problems

The use of alcohol and illicit drugs contributes significantly to the number of patients presenting to the emergency department. Around 3% of emergency department attendances are directly related, and 4% are indirectly related to drug use. Common presentations are acute injuries and assault, overdose, and medical complications of drug use.

Around 5% of emergency department attendances are related to alcohol. One in four male acute hospital admissions are alcohol related. Alcohol related attendances can be categorized as:

1. A direct result of alcohol poisoning.
2. A medical complication of persistent alcohol abuse, such as variceal haemorrhage or bleeding peptic ulcer.
3. A psychiatric complication resulting from persistent alcohol abuse, such as Wernicke–Korsakoff syndrome or acute alcohol withdrawal.
4. An injury resulting from intoxication.
5. An assault resulting from intoxication.

It is crucial that the emergency physician considers alcohol or drug misuse as a potential contributing factor when assessing almost all patients. Never be judgemental or make assumptions regarding alcohol or drug use; other serious medical conditions may require urgent consideration. An example of this is when managing an unconscious patient, where an assumption of intoxication, without adequate assessment and investigation, could potentially miss serious diagnoses such as an extradural haematoma or meningitis. Approximately 30% of patients with a mental illness will abuse either alcohol or drugs. More than a third of alcohol abusers and nearly two-thirds of drug abusers have one or more serious mental health disorders (see 'The patient with disturbed behaviour' chapter). Alcoholics and drug addicts are more likely to suffer injuries and illnesses than the non-addicted population. By taking an appropriate alcohol history, and providing non-judgemental and supportive advice at the time of presentation, the emergency physician can positively impact on a patient's drinking and future risk of illness and injury.

Alcohol intoxication

The effects of alcohol vary according to the level of consumption: low doses promote mild euphoria and uninhibited behaviour, while substantial consumption may trigger irrational thinking, problematic behaviour, psychomotor difficulties, and in rare cases, coma.

Treatment is supportive, with careful monitoring of airway and breathing as well as prevention of hypoglycaemia, and thiamine supplementation. If the patient is hypoglycaemic, thiamine administration should precede glucose infusion. Remember that alcohol is an analgesic and sedative and can mask potentially serious illnesses and injuries.

Alcohol withdrawal

Symptoms of alcohol withdrawal can vary but usually begin within 24 hours of the last intake of alcohol. Symptoms include restlessness, tremor, sweating, anxiety, nausea, vomiting, loss of appetite and insomnia. Generalized seizures occur rarely. In delirium tremens ('DTs'), there is confusion, agitation, tachycardia and hypertension, with fever being common. Treatment of alcohol withdrawal should include a benzodiazepine such as chlordiazepoxide, thiamine supplementation (parenterally initially), vitamin supplementation and fluid replacement. If this is inadequately treated with vitamin supplementation, Wernicke's encephalopathy or Korsakoff's psychosis can result.

Wernicke's encephalopathy

The classic triad for this disease is encephalopathy (confusion), ophthalmoplegia and ataxia. Untreated, this may progress to coma or Korsakoff's psychosis. Korsakoff's psychosis is characterized by disabling memory deficits, out of proportion to other cognitive deficits. Confabulation, where the patient invents plausible explanations to cover gaps in their memory, is common.

Treatment includes prompt intravenous thiamine supplementation and rehydration. Electrolyte depletion, particularly of magnesium and phosphate, is common and should be corrected. Assess for other CNS pathology or metabolic disturbances. If treated early, recovery may be rapid and complete.

Common drug related problems

Drug misuse should always be suspected in the patient who presents with bizarre behaviour, or if their presenting features match a known toxidrome caused by drug use (see 'The poisoned patient and toxidromes' chapter).

Emergency presentations secondary to drug misuse include coma and respiratory arrest from opiates or benzodiazepines. Pinpoint pupils (Fig. 1) will be noted in opiate overdose, and a response to intravenous naloxone is usual. Administration of naloxone should be by careful intravenous titration. Alternative routes such as nasal or IM administration may be considered if IV access is difficult.

Intoxication with stimulant drugs such as amphetamines or cocaine causes restlessness, anxiety, hyperactivity, dysphoria, hypertension and tachycardia. Overdose may lead to cardiac arrhythmias and extreme hypertension, myocardial infarction and cardiac arrest.

Other drugs that are popular at clubs include MDMA (ecstasy), GHB

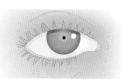
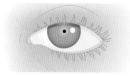
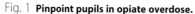

Fig. 1 **Pinpoint pupils in opiate overdose.**

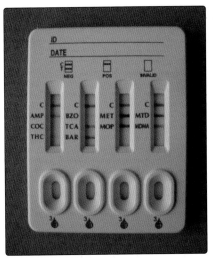

Fig. 2 Point of care urine toxicology test.
Absence of a line indicates a positive result.

Table 1 **The Fast Alcohol Screening Test (FAST)**				
For the following four questions please choose the answer which best applies (1 drink = ½ pint of beer or 1 glass of wine or 1 single spirits)				
1. MEN: How often do you have EIGHT or more drinks on one occasion? WOMEN: How often do you have SIX or more drinks on one occasion?				
0	1	2	3	4
Never	Less than monthly	Monthly	Weekly	Daily or almost daily
2. How often during the last year have you been unable to remember what happened the night before because you have been drinking?				
0	1	2	3	4
Never	Less than monthly	Monthly	Weekly	Daily or almost daily
3. How often during the last year have you failed to do what was normally expected of you because of drinking?				
0	1	2	3	4
Never	Less than monthly	Monthly	Weekly	Daily or almost daily
4. In the last year has a relative or friend, or a doctor or other health worker been concerned about your drinking or suggested you cut down?				
0	2	4		
No	Yes, once	Yes, more than once		
A total score of 3 or more indicates probable hazardous drinking				

(gammahydroxybutyrate), ketamine and LSD. They may have stimulating or hallucinogenic properties. Rehydration, cooling and supportive care are important management principles. Point of care urine toxicology tests may aid the diagnosis (Fig. 2).

Patients with opiate addiction require a specialist approach in the emergency department. They may present with symptoms or signs of withdrawal such as yawning, abdominal cramps, nausea, vomiting and diarrhoea, tremor, insomnia and restlessness, generalized aches and pains, tachycardia, hypertension, piloerection and dilated pupils. It is advisable to have protocols in place to manage such patients. Symptomatic treatment and cautious use of an opiate substitute, such as methadone, under specialist supervision is required.

Assessment for alcohol and substance use disorders in the emergency department can be effective as a first step toward recovery. A simple questionnaire such as the Paddington Alcohol Test (PAT) or FAST (Table 1) improves the identification of harmful drinkers. A large proportion of patients with drug or alcohol dependency problems can be managed in the community. Liaison with local support services and teams is very important.

Key points

- Always consider intoxication in unresponsive patients.
- Never assume intoxication in unresponsive patients.
- Prevent hypoglycaemia.
- Always give intravenous thiamine before glucose infusions in patients with a history of alcohol abuse.

Legal and ethical aspects of emergency medicine

General principles

Medico-legal problems are more frequent in emergency medicine for several reasons: the high volume of medical activity, mostly out of hours; anxious patients with high expectations; injuries from assaults and road traffic crashes that often result in requests for police statements or medico-legal reports. The emergency physician can avoid a legal quagmire (Fig. 1) by adopting best practice rules and a common-sense approach: be aware of your own limitations, follow departmental protocols, ask for help from more senior emergency department staff and hospital specialists, take care when handing over patients, make good contemporaneous notes and be familiar with common 'pitfalls'. Common errors include missed injuries (digital nerve/tendon damage, retained foreign bodies, torn quadriceps/Achilles tendon), misdiagnoses (leaking AAA with back pain, head injury in a drunk patient, testicular torsion thought to be orchitis), radiographic misinterpretations or mismanagement such as failure to admit a patient.

Dealing with the police

In the UK, the GMC good medical practice advice should be followed at all times. The confidentiality rule occasionally brings the emergency physician into conflict with police or lawyers. Clinical details and information to third parties can be released only with the written explicit consent of the patient or at the request of a court of law to satisfy a statutory requirement. Information can be

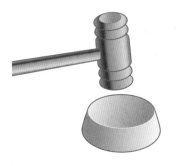

Fig. 1 **An awareness of the law** is essential in emergency medicine.

Table 1 **Situations and circumstances where breaching patient confidentiality is clinically, legally and ethically justified**	
With the patient's consent	E.g. for insurance companies or employers
For the patient's benefit	E.g. for healthcare decisions when the patient lacks capacity Consent is implied when care is shared among healthcare professionals
To prevent harm to others	Possible harm to others may override duty to the patient
When required by law	E.g. for notifiable infectious diseases, gunshot wounds, victims of abuse, and under anti-terrorism laws
For medical research, audit and registry	Ensure approval from the research/ethics committee Remove identifiable data Never publish an identifiable case without the patient's consent

shared with other clinicians or nurses to assist the care of the patient but the doctor is duty bound to ensure all abide by the rule of professional secrecy. Rarely, disclosure is required in the public interest when a serious crime (murder, rape, armed robbery, terrorist activities) is committed or its detection or prevention will be seriously compromised (Table 1). The information released should be used solely for this purpose and must be destroyed at the end of the legal process. Information is frequently asked by the traffic police for patients involved in motor vehicle accidents. It is acceptable to provide the name and age of the patient, general description of injury (e.g. head or leg injury), the severity (critical, serious, or minor) and the disposal of the patient (admitted, discharged, transferred). Gunshot injuries must be reported to the police. The emergency physician is under no obligation to perform blood tests in suspected drunk drivers; these and any other sampling for other offences, e.g. sexual assaults, are carried out by a police surgeon.

Consent and capacity

The expressed consent of all patients should be sought for examination, investigations and treatments. This can be implied, verbal or written. Written consent is commonly sought for procedures that require general anaesthesia or sedation. For consent to be valid, the patient must be competent and be informed of the true nature of the procedure and inherent risks (no requirement that every possible complication must be explained). To be competent, an adult must be able to understand what is said, retain the information, be made aware of the options and be able to make a decision. For children (age <16), parents or legal guardians should provide the consent. Minors may give their consent if they are 'Gillick' competent, i.e. they fulfil the above criteria of competence. Under the Children and Young Persons Act 1933, parents cannot refuse treatment if it is considered to be in the best interest or health of a child. Likewise, Jehovah's Witness parents cannot refuse blood transfusions or an operation that may require a transfusion for their child. In an emergency, the emergency physician is duty bound to act as the custodian or legal guardian of a child or of an adult who lacks capacity. Patients can refuse emergency treatment if they are deemed to be competent. Such refusal should be clearly documented in the patient's notes and preferably witnessed. The emergency physician should respect the wishes of patients with advanced directives or 'living wills' but must ensure that these are relevant to the emergency department attendance or presenting circumstances. The Mental Capacity Act 2005 (England) formalized common law guidance and also introduced lasting Power of Attorney nomination.

Key ethical points

- Beneficence – act in the best interest of the patient.
- Non-maleficence – 'first, do no harm'.
- Autonomy – the patient's right to refuse or choose their treatment.
- Justice – fairness and equality for all.
- Dignity.
- Truthfulness and honesty – the concept of informed consent.

Treatment of status epilepticus in children

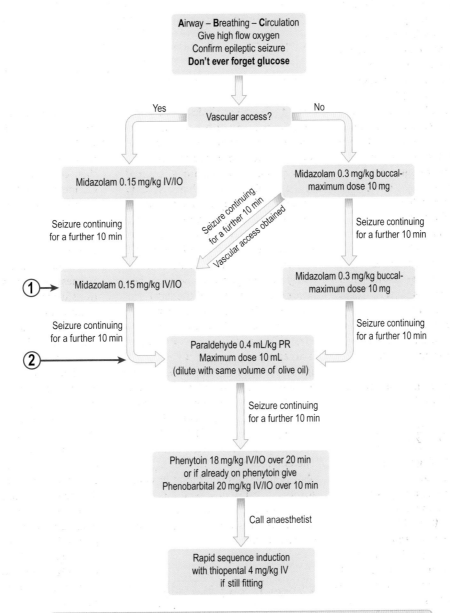

For children who have already received 1 dose of diazepam or midazolam prior to admission start at stage ① of algorithm.

For children who have already received 2 doses of diazepam or midazolam prior to admission start at stage ② of algorithm.

Airway – **B**reathing – **C**irculation
Give high flow oxygen
Confirm epileptic seizure
Don't ever forget glucose

Vascular access?

Yes → Midazolam 0.15 mg/kg IV/IO

No → Midazolam 0.3 mg/kg buccal- maximum dose 10 mg

Seizure continuing for a further 10 min

Seizure continuing for a further 10 min
Vascular access obtained

① → Midazolam 0.15 mg/kg IV/IO

Midazolam 0.3 mg/kg buccal- maximum dose 10 mg

Seizure continuing for a further 10 min

Seizure continuing for a further 10 min

② → Paraldehyde 0.4 mL/kg PR
Maximum dose 10 mL
(dilute with same volume of olive oil)

Seizure continuing for a further 10 min

Phenytoin 18 mg/kg IV/IO over 20 min
or if already on phenytoin give
Phenobarbital 20 mg/kg IV/IO over 10 min

Call anaesthetist

Rapid sequence induction
with thiopental 4 mg/kg IV
if still fitting

Seizure terminated
- Position child in Trendelenburg position, on left side
- Maintain airway (jaw thrust, chin lift, suction)
- History/examination – search for underlying cause (head injury, sepsis, meningitis, metabolic)
- Investigations – full blood count, electrolytes, calcium, magnesium, blood culture, cerebral imaging if focal seizure, blood pressure
- Treat underlying cause if identified, e.g. consider antibiotics if bacterial sepsis cannot be excluded

Index